Human Labor and Birth

HARRY OXORN B.A., M.D., C.M., F.A.C.S., F.R.C.S.(C),
Assistant Professor of Obstetrics and Gynecology, McGill
University;
Obstetrician and Gynecologist-in-Chief, Reddy Memorial
Hospital;
Associate Obstetrician and Gynecologist, Royal Victoria
Hospital; Junior Assistant Obstetrician and Gynecologist,
Montreal General Hospital, Montreal, Canada

WILLIAM R. FOOTE B.A., M.D., C.M., F.A.C.S., F.R.C.O.G.,
F.R.C.S.(C). Associate Professor of Obstetrics and Gyne-
cology, McGill University;
Obstetrician and Gynecologist, Royal Victoria Hospital;
Assistant Obstetrician and Gynecologist, Montreal General
Hospital, Montreal, Canada

Illustrations by DOROTHY IRWIN

Human Labor and Birth

SECOND EDITION

APPLETON-CENTURY-CROFTS
Division of Meredith Corporation
NEW YORK

PREFACE

In step with modern scientific advances, many textbooks of obstetrics devote more and more space to the exciting new knowledge of the physiology and biochemistry of pregnancy and placental function, and to the medical, surgical, and metabolic conditions which may complicate or be associated with the pregnant state. There being a limit to the size of a textbook, correspondingly fewer pages are given to the mundane topic of the passage of the fetus through the pelvis.

The main stimulus for the preparation of this book having come from our medical students, their needs (as well as those of the general practitioner) have been uppermost in our minds. Hence we have concentrated on the basic details of the mechanisms of normal and abnormal labor and their management, and have avoided long descriptions of complicated operations which should be performed by specially trained obstetricians..

Often forgotten or ignored is the sine qua non that the student must pass his examinations. We have tried to organize our material in such a way that students will be enabled to answer logically questions dealing with the mechanisms and forces concerned with labor. To obviate the tiresome task of turning pages to find illustrations referred to in the text, the book is arranged so that text and related drawings are on facing pages.

The use of this type of book will reduce the need for didactic lectures and frantic (often garbled) note-taking by the students. The valuable, and usually too short, classroom contact between the student and the instructor can be spent to greater advantage by discussion of problems, and practical demonstrations on the manikin and the living model.

Since most medical undergraduates are less than affluent, our publishers have done their utmost (even allowing us the use of the excellent illustrations on forceps from one of their other publications) to keep the price of the book at a level which the student can afford.

We wish to express our sincere appreciation to Mrs. Dorothy Irwin, who prepared all the new illustrations and supervised the use of the others, and

v

to Miss Helen T. MacArthur, of the Department of Illustration of the Royal Victoria Hospital, for her helpful suggestions and advice.

Our thanks go to our colleagues for their advice and encouragement; to Dr. George B. Maughan, Professor of Obstetrics and Gynecology; and to Dr. J. E. Wynands, who reviewed the manuscript of the chapter on analgesia and anesthesia.

We are grateful to Mrs. Rose Slapak, who typed most of the manuscript, and to Miss Betty Hughes, who helped.

Finally, we are most appreciative of the assistance, cooperation, and encouragement of our publisher.

Harry Oxorn
William R. Foote

CONTENTS

Human Labor and Birth

1 The Pelvis: Bones, Joints, Ligaments

THE PELVIC BONES

Definition: The pelvis is the bony basin in which the trunk terminates and through which the body weight is transmitted to the lower extremities. In the female it is adapted for childbearing. The pelvis consists of four bones—the two innominates, the sacrum, and the coccyx. These are united by four joints.

The Innominate Bones

The innominate bones are placed laterally and anteriorly. Each is made up by the fusion, around the acetabulum, of three bones.

The Ilium

The ilium is the upper bone. It has a body (which is fused with the ischial body) and an ala. Points of note concerning the ilium include:

1. The anterior superior iliac spine gives attachment to the inguinal ligament.
2. The posterior superior iliac spine marks the level of the second sacral vertebra. Its presence is indicated by a dimple in the overlying skin.
3. The iliac crest extends from the anterior superior iliac spine to the posterior superior iliac spine.

The Ischium

The ischium consists of the body, in which the superior and inferior rami merge.

1. The body forms part of the acetabulum.
2. The superior ramus is behind and below the body.
3. The inferior ramus fuses with the inferior ramus of the pubis.
4. The ischial spine separates the greater sciatic from the lesser sciatic notch. It is an important landmark. Part of the levator ani muscle is attached to it.
5. The ischial tuberosity is the lower part of the ischium and is the bone on which humans sit.

The Pubis

The pubis consists of the body and two rami.

1. The body has a rough surface on its medial aspect. This is joined to the corresponding area on the opposite pubis to form the symphysis pubis. The levator ani muscles are attached to the pelvic aspect of the pubis.
2. The pubic crest is the superior border of the body.
3. The pubic tubercle, or spine, is the lateral end of the pubic crest. Here are attached the inguinal ligament and the conjoined tendon.
4. The superior ramus meets the body of the pubis at the pubic spine and the body of the ilium at the iliopectineal line. Here it forms a part of the acetabulum.
5. The inferior ramus merges with the inferior ramus of the ischium.

Landmarks to be identified include:

1. The iliopectineal line extends from the pubic tubercle back to the sacroiliac joint. It forms the greater part of the boundary of the pelvic inlet.
2. The greater sacrosciatic notch is between the posterior inferior iliac spine above and the ischial spine below.
3. The lesser sacrosciatic notch is bounded by the ischial spine superiorly and the ischial tuberosity inferiorly.
4. The obturator foramen is delimited by the acetabulum, the ischial rami, and the pubic rami.

The Sacrum

The sacrum is a triangularly shaped bone with the base above and the apex below. It consists of five vertebrae fused together. Rarely, there are four or six. The sacrum lies between the innominate bones and is attached to them by the sacroiliac joints.

The upper surface of the first sacral vertebra articulates with the lower surface of the fifth lumbar vertebra. The anterior (pelvic) surface of the sacrum is concave, while the posterior surface is convex.

The sacral promontory is the anterior superior edge of the first sacral vertebra. It protrudes slightly into the cavity of the pelvis, and this reduces the anteroposterior diameter of the inlet.

The Coccyx

The coccyx (tail bone) is composed of four rudimentary vertebrae. The superior surface of the first coccygeal vertebra articulates with the lower surface of the fifth sacral vertebra to form the sacrococcygeal joint. Rarely there is fusion between the sacrum and coccyx, with resultant limitation of movement.

The coccygeus muscle, the levator ani muscles, and the sphincter ani externus are attached to the coccyx from above downward.

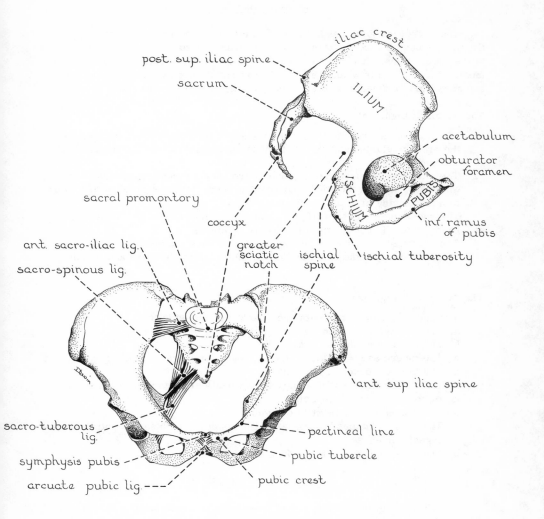

Fig. 1.   The bones and joints of the pelvis.

THE JOINTS AND LIGAMENTS OF THE PELVIS

The sacrum, the coccyx, and the two innominate bones are linked together by four joints: 1, the symphysis pubis; 2, the sacrococcygeal; and 3, the two sacroiliac synchondroses.

The Sacroiliac Joint

The sacroiliac joint lies between the articular surfaces of the sacrum and ilium. Through it the weight of the body is transmitted to the pelvis, and thence to the lower limbs. It is a synovial joint and permits a small degree of movement. The capsule is weak, and stability is maintained by four primary and two accessory ligaments, and especially by the muscles around it.

The Primary Ligaments

1. The anterior sacroiliac ligaments are short and transverse, running from the preauricular sulcus on the ilium to the anterior aspect of the ala of the sacrum.
2. The interosseus sacroiliac ligaments are short, strong transverse bands which extend from the rough part behind the auricular surface on the ilium to the adjoining area on the sacrum.
3. The short posterior sacroiliac ligaments are short, strong transverse bands which lie behind the interosseus ligaments.
4. The long posterior sacroiliac ligaments are each attached to the postero-superior spine on the ilium and to the tubercles on the third and fourth sacral vertebrae.

The Accessory Ligaments

1. The sacrotuberous ligaments are attached on one side to:
   a. The posterior superior iliac spine
   b. The posterior inferior iliac spine
   c. The tubercles on the third, fourth, and fifth sacral vertebrae
   d. The lateral border of the coccyx
   On the other side the sacrotuberous ligaments are attached to the pelvic aspect of the ischial tuberosity.
2. The sacrospinous ligament is trangular.
   a. The base is attached to the lateral parts of the fifth sacral and first coccygeal vertebrae.
   b. The apex is attached to the ischial spine.

The Sacrococcygeal Joint

The sacrococcygeal is a synovial hinge joint between the fifth sacral and the first coccygeal vertebrae. It allows both flexion and extension. Extension, by increasing the anteroposterior diameter of the outlet of the pelvis, plays an important role in parturition. Overextension during delivery may break the small cornua by which the coccyx is attached to the sacrum.

This joint has a weak capsule which is reinforced by anterior, posterior, and lateral sacrococcygeal ligaments.

The Symphysis Pubis

The symphysis pubis is a cartilaginous joint with no capsule and no synovial membrane. Normally there is little movement. The posterior and superior ligaments are weak. The strong anterior ligaments are reinforced by the tendons of the rectus abdominis and the external oblique muscles. The strong inferior ligament in the pubic arch is known as the arcuate pubic ligament. It extends between the rami and leaves a small space in the subpubic angle.

MOBILITY OF THE PELVIS

During pregnancy all the joints are relaxed, the bones are held together less tightly, and the pelvis is capable of expansion to make more room. This property is increased by exercises, certain postures, and a hormone known as relaxin which causes the ligaments to soften.

BIBLIOGRAPHY

Eastman, N. J., and Hellman, L. M. Williams Obstetrics, 13th ed. New York, Appleton-Century-Crofts, 1965.
Smout, C. F. V., and Jacoby, F. Gynaecological and Obstetrical Anatomy and Functional Histology, 3rd ed. Baltimore, The Williams & Wilkins Co., 1953.

2 The Floor of the Pelvis

The pelvic floor is a muscular diaphragm which separates the pelvic cavity above from the perineal space below. It is formed by the levator ani and coccygeus muscles, covered completely by parietal fascia.

The urogenital hiatus is an anterior gap through which the urethra and vagina pass. The rectal hiatus is posterior, and the rectum and anal canal pass through it.

FUNCTIONS OF THE PELVIC FLOOR

1. In the human it supports the pelvic viscera.
2. To build up effective intra-abdominal pressure the muscles of the diaphragm, the muscles of abdominal wall, and those of the pelvic floor must contract together.
3. The pelvic floor helps the anterior rotation of the presenting part, and directs it downward and forward along the birth passage.

MUSCLES OF THE PELVIC FLOOR

1. The levators ani, each of which is composed of two muscles:
   a. The pubococcygeus has three divisions: pubovaginalis, puborectalis, and pubococcygeus proper.
   b. The iliococcygeus
2. The coccygeus (ischiococcygeus)

The Levator Ani Muscle

The levator ani muscle has a lateral origin and a central insertion, where it joins with the corresponding muscle from the other side. The direction of the muscle from origin to insertion is downward and medial.

The origin of each levator ani is from:

1. The posterior side of the pubis
2. The arcuate tendon of the pelvic fascia (the white line of the pelvic fascia)
3. The pelvic aspect of the ischial spine

6

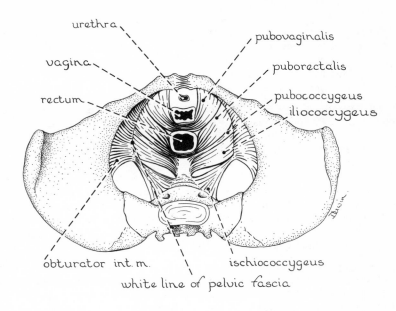

urethra

vagina

rectum

pubovaginalis

puborectalis

pubococcygeus

iliococcygeus

obturator int. m.

ischiococcygeus

white line of pelvic fascia

Fig. 1. The pelvic floor.

The insertion, from front to back, is into:

1. The vaginal walls
2. The central point of the perineum
3. The anal canal
4. The anococcygeal body
5. The lateral border of the coccyx

The Pubococcygeus

The pubococcygeus is the most important, the most dynamic, and the most specialized part of the pelvic floor. It lies in the midline, is perforated by the urethra, vagina, and rectum, and is often damaged during delivery. It originates from the posterior side of the pubis, and from the part of the white line of the pelvic fascia in front of the obturator canal. The muscle passes backward and medially in three sections, 1, the pubovaginalis; 2, the puborectalis; and 3, the pubococcygeus proper.

The Pubovaginalis Muscle: The most medial section of the pubococcygeus, this muscle is shaped like a horseshoe and is open anteriorly. The fibers make contact and blend with the muscles of the wall of the urethra. Then they form a loop around the vagina.   They insert into the sides and back of the vagina, and into the central point of the perineum.

The principal function of the pubovaginalis is to act as a sling for the vagina.   Since the vagina helps to support the uterus and appendages, the bladder and urethra, and the rectum, this muscle is the main support of the female pelvic organs.   Tearing or overstretching predisposes to prolapse, cystocele, and rectocele.   The muscle also functions as the vaginal sphincter, and when this muscle goes into spasm, the condition is called vaginismus.

The Puborectalis Muscle: The intermediate part of the pubococcygeus, this muscle forms a loop around the anal canal and rectum.   The insertion is into the lateral and posterior walls of the anal canal between the sphincter ani internus and externus, with whose fibers the puborectalis joins.   It inserts also in the anococcygeal body.

The puborectalis suspends the rectum, but since this organ does not support the other pelvic viscera, the puborectalis plays a small role in holding up the pelvic structures.   The main work of this muscle is in controlling the descent of the feces, and in so doing it acts as an auxilliary sphincter for the anal canal.   When the anococcygeal junction is pulled forward, the puborectalis increases the anorectal flexure and retards the descent of feces.

The Pubococcygeus Proper: This muscle is composed of the most lateral fibers of the pubococcygeus muscle.   It has a Y-shaped insertion into the lateral margins of the coccyx.   When it contracts it pulls the coccyx forward, increasing the anorectal juncture.   Thus, in combination with the external sphincter ani, it helps control the passage of the feces.

The Iliococcygeus

The iliococcygeus muscles arise from the white line of the pelvic fascia behind the obturator canal.   They join with the pubococcygeus muscle proper, and insert into the lateral margins of the coccyx.   These are less dynamic than the pubovaginalis, and act more like a musculofascial layer.

The Ischiococcygeus

The ischiococcygeus or coccygeus muscles originate from the ischial spines and insert into the lateral borders of the coccyx and the fifth sacral vertebra.   These muscles supplement the levators ani and occupy most of the posterior part of the pelvic floor.

THE PELVIC FLOOR DURING PARTURITION

When the presenting part has reached the proper level during the second stage, the central point of the perineum becomes thin.   The levator ani muscles and the anal sphincter relax, and the muscles of the pelvic floor are drawn over the advancing head.   Tearing and overstretching of these muscles weaken the pelvic floor and may cause extensive and irreparable damage.

3   The Perineum

The perineum is a diamond-shaped space which lies below the pelvic floor. Its boundaries are:

1. Superiorly, the pelvic floor, made up of the levator ani muscles and the coccygei
2. Laterally, the bones and ligaments which make up the pelvic outlet. Going from front to back, these are:
   a. The subpubic angle
   b. The ischiopubic rami
   c. The ischial tuberosities
   d. The sacrotuberous ligaments
   e. The coccyx
3. Inferiorly, the skin and fascia

This area is divided into two triangles: anteriorly, the urogenital triangle; posteriorly, the anal triangle. These are separated by a transverse band composed of the transverse perineal muscles and the base of the urogenital diaphragm.

THE UROGENITAL TRIANGLE

The urogenital triangle is bounded:

1. In front, by the subpubic angle
2. At the sides, by the ischiopubic rami and the ischial tuberosities
3. Behind, by the transverse perineal muscles and the base of the urogenital diaphragm

The urogenital triangle contains:

1. The opening of the vagina
2. The terminal part of the urethra
3. The crura of the clitoris with the ischiocavernosus muscles
4. The vestibular bulbs (erectile tissue) covered by the bulbocavernosus muscles
5. The Bartholin glands and their ducts
6. The urogenital diaphragm
7. The muscles which constitute the central point of the perineum (perineal body)
8. The perineal pouches, superficial and deep
9. Blood vessels, nerves, and lymphatics

The Urogenital Diaphragm

The urogenital diaphragm (triangular ligament) lies in the anterior triangle of the perineum.   It is composed of muscle tissue covered by fascia.

1. The two muscles are the deep transverse perineal and the sphincter of the membranous urethra.
2. The superior layer of fascia is thin and weak.
3. The inferior fascial layer is a strong fibrous membrane. It extends from a short distance beneath the arcuate pubic ligament to the ischial tuberosities. The fascial layers fuse superiorly and form the transverse perineal ligament. Inferiorly, they join together in the central point of the perineum.

The deep dorsal vein of the clitoris lies in a small space between the apex of the urogenital diaphragm and the arcuate pubic ligament.   Through the diaphragm pass the urethra, the vagina, blood vessels, lymphatics, and nerves.

The Superficial Perineal Pouch

The superficial perineal pouch is a space which lies between the inferior layer of the urogenital diaphragm and Colles' fascia.

The Superficial Transverse Perineal Muscles

The superficial transverse perineal muscles are the superficial parts of the deep muscles, and have the same origin and insertion.   These are outside of the urogenital diaphragm.   Sometimes they are entirely lacking.

The Ischiocavernosus Muscles

The ischiocavernosus muscles cover the clitoral crura.   The origin of each is the inferior ramus of the pubis.   The insertion is the lateral aspect of the crus.   These muscles compress the crura, and by blocking the venous return cause the clitoris to become erect.

The Bulbocavernosus Muscle

The bulbocavernosus muscle surrounds the vagina.   With the external anal sphincter it makes a figure of 8 around the vagina and rectum.   It is also called the bulbospongiosus.   It originates from the central point of the perineum, and inserts into the dorsal aspect of the body of the clitoris.   The muscle passes around the orifice of the vagina and surrounds the bulb of the vestibule.

The bulbocavernosus muscle compresses the erectile tissue around the vaginal orifice (bulb of the vestibule), and helps in the erection of the clitoris by closing its dorsal vein.   It acts as a weak vaginal sphincter.   The real sphincter of the vagina is the pubovaginalis section of the levator ani.

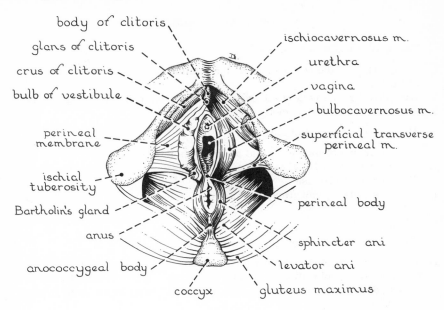

Fig. 1. The perineum.

The Deep Perineal Pouch

The deep perineal pouch lies between the two fascial layers of the urogenital diaphragm.

The Sphincter of the Membranous Urethra

The sphincter of the membranous urethra lies between the layers of the fascia of the urogenital diaphragm. It is also called the compressor of the urethra.

The voluntary fibers have their origin from the inferior rami of the ischium and pubis. They join together with the deep transverse perineal muscles. Their action is to expel the last drops of urine.

The involuntary fibers surround the urethra, and act as its sphincter.

The Deep Transverse Perineal Muscles

The deep transverse perineal muscles lie between the layers of fascia of the urogenital diaphragm. They blend with the sphincter of the membranous urethra. The origin is the ischiopubic ramus on each side. The insertion is the central point of the perineum (perineal body).

THE ANAL TRIANGLE

The anal triangle is bounded:

1. Anteriorly, by the transverse perineal muscles and the base of the urogenital diaphragm
2. Laterally, by the ischial tuberosities and the sacrotuberous ligaments
3. Posteriorly, by the coccyx

The anal triangle contains:

1. The lower end of the anal canal and its sphincters
2. The anococcygeal body
3. The ischiorectal fossa
4. Blood vessels, lymphatics, and nerves.

The Sphincter Ani Externus

The sphincter ani externus has two parts:

1. The superficial portion surrounds the anal orifice. Its fibers are voluntary and act during defecation or in an emergency. The origin is the tip of the coccyx and the anococcygeal body. The insertion is in the central point of the perineum.
2. The deep part is an involuntary muscle which surrounds the lower part of the anal canal, and acts as a sphincter for the anus. It blends with the levators ani and the internal anal sphincter. In the inactive state the deep circular fibers are in a state of tonus, occluding the orifice of the anus.

The Anococcygeal Body

The anococcygeal body is composed of muscle tissue (levators ani and external sphincter ani) and fibrous tissue. It is placed between the tip of the coccyx and the anus.

THE PERINEAL BODY

The central point of the perineum or perineal body lies between the posterior angle of the vagina in front and the anus behind. In obstetrics it is referred to as the "perineum." It is often torn at delivery. The following muscles meet to form this structure:

1. The sphincter ani externus
2. The two levator ani muscles
3. The superficial and deep transverse perineal muscles
4. The bulbocavernosus muscle

4 The Uterus and Vagina

THE UTERUS

The normal uterus is a small muscular organ in the female pelvis. It is composed of three layers:

1. An outer, covering, serous peritoneal layer, the perimetrium
2. A thick middle layer made up of muscle fibers and called the myometrium
3. An inner mucous layer of glands and supporting stroma, called the endometrium, which is attached directly to the myometrium

The myometrium is made up of three layers of muscle:

1. An outer layer of mainly longitudinal fibers
2. An inner layer whose fibers run, for the most part, in a circular direction
3. A thick middle layer, whose fibers are arranged in an interlacing pattern, and through which the blood vessels course. When these fibers contract and retract after the products of conception have been expelled, the blood vessels are kinked and constricted. In this way postpartum bleeding is controlled.

Uterine Shape

In the nonpregnant condition and at the time of implantation the uterus is pear-shaped. By the third month of gestation the uterus has become globular. From the seventh month to term the contour is again pyriform.

Uterine Size

The uterus grows from the nonpregnant dimensions of about 7.5 x 5 x 2.5 cm to 28 x 24 x 21 cm. The weight rises from between 30 and 60 g to 1,000 g at the end of pregnancy. The uterus changes from a solid organ in the nullipara to a large sac, the capacity increasing from almost nil to 4,000 cc.

Location of the Uterus

Normally the uterus is entirely in the pelvis. As it enlarges it gradually rises, and by the fourth month of gestation it has extended into the abdominal region.

Divisions of the Uterus

1. The fundus is the part above the openings of the fallopian tubes.
2. The body (corpus) is the main part, which has thick walls and lies between the tubal openings and the isthmus. This is the main contractile portion. During labor the contractions force the baby downward, distend the lower segment of the uterus, and dilate the cervix.
3. The isthmus is a small constricted region of the uterus. It is about 5 to 7 mm in length, and lies above the internal os of the cervix.
4. The cervix is composed of a canal with an internal os in its upper portion separating the cervix from the uterine cavity, and an external os below which closes the cervix from the vagina. The cervix is about 2.5 cm in length. The lower part pierces the anterior wall of the vagina, and its tissue blends with that of the vagina.

The Myometrium of the Body and the Fundus

In the myometrium of the body and the fundus most of the growth of the uterus takes place. There is both hypertrophy of the existing muscle fibers and formation of new ones. There is also an increase in the number and size of the blood vessels and lymphatics, as well as a marked overgrowth of the connective tissue. In early pregnancy the uterine walls are thicker than in the non-pregnant woman. As gestation continues the lumen becomes larger and the walls become thinner. At the end of the fifth month they are 3 to 5 mm thick and remain so until term. Thus in late pregnancy the uterus is a large muscular sac with thin, soft, easily compressible walls. This makes the corpus indentable, and enables the fetus to be palpated by the examining fingers. The walls of the uterus are so malleable that the uterus changes shape easily and markedly to accommodate itself to changes in fetal size and position.

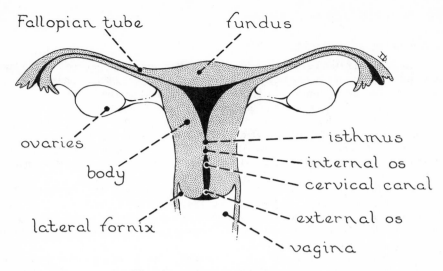

Fig. 1. Uterus, cervix, vagina.

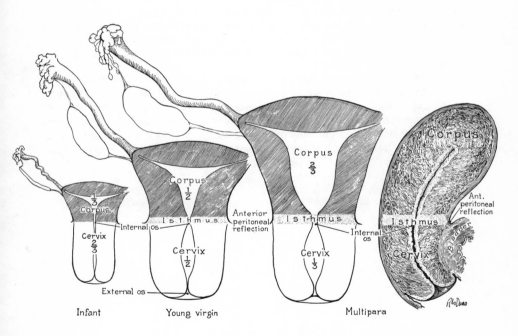

Fig. 2. Normal uterus and cervix. (From Eastman and Hellman. Williams Obstetrics, 12th ed., Appleton-Century-Crofts, 1961.)

The Isthmus

The isthmus lies between the body of the uterus and the cervix. In the human its boundaries are not well defined, and it is important as a physiologic rather than as an anatomic entity. In the nonpregnant uterus it is 5 to 7 mm long. It differs from the corpus in that it is free of mucus-secreting glands. The upper limit of the isthmus corresponds to a constriction in the lumen of the uterus which marks the lower boundary of the body of the uterus (the anatomic internal os of Aschoff). The lower limit is the site of transition from the mucosa of the isthmus to the endocervical mucous membrane (histologic internal os).

While the isthmus is of small moment in the normal state, in pregnancy it plays an important role. As the uterus grows the isthmus increases in length to about 25 mm, and becomes soft and compressible. Hegar's sign of early pregnancy depends upon the palpation of the soft isthmus between the body of the uterus above and the cervix below.

The ovum implants, in the great majority of cases, in the upper part of the uterus. At about the third month the enlarging embryo grows into the isthmus which unfolds and expands to make room for it. As this process continues, the isthmus is incorporated gradually into the general uterine cavity, and the shape of the uterus changes from pyriform to globular. The expanded isthmus forms part of the lower uterine segment of the uterus during labor. The histologic internal os becomes the internal os of pregnancy, while the anatomic internal os becomes the physiologic retraction ring of normal labor (and pathologic retraction ring of obstructed labor).

The unfolding of the isthmus continues until it has reached the firm cervix where it stops. After the seventh month most of the enlargement takes place in the body and fundus, and the uterus becomes pear-shaped once more. At the onset of labor the lower uterine segment comprises about one third of the whole uterus. While this area is not the passive part that it was once thought to be, its contractions during normal labor are extremely weak when compared with those of the body.

8 weeks

12 weeks

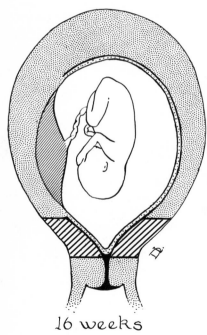

16 weeks

Fig. 3.   Isthmus of pregnant uterus.

The Cervix

The cervix is composed mostly of connective tissue interspersed with muscle fibers. It feels hard and fibrous in the nonpregnant state. During pregnancy the cervix becomes progressively softer. This is caused by increased vascularity, general edema, and hyperplasia of the glands. The compound tubular glands become overactive and produce large quantities of mucus. In the cervical canal the secretion accumulates and thickens to form the so-called mucous plug. This inspissated mucus effectively seals off the canal from the vagina, and prevents the ascent of bacteria and other substances into the uterine cavity. This plug is expelled early in labor.

At the end of gestation and during labor the internal os gradually disappears, and the cervical canal also becomes part of the lower uterine segment, leaving only the external os.

THE VAGINA

The vagina is a fibromuscular membranous tube which is surrounded by the vulva below, the uterus above, the bladder in front, and the rectum behind. Its direction is obliquely upward and backward. The cervix uteri enters the vagina through the anterior wall, and for this reason the anterior wall of the vagina (6 to 8 cm) is shorter than the posterior wall (7 to 10 cm). The protrusion of the cervix into the vagina divides the vaginal vault into four fornices: an anterior, a posterior, and two lateral fornices. The posterior fornix is much deeper than the others.

The wall of the vagina is made up of four layers:

1. The mucosa is the epithelial layer.
2. The submucosa is rich in blood vessels.
3. The muscularis
4. The outer connective tissue layer connects the vagina to the surrounding structures.

Even in the normal condition the vagina is capable of great distension, but in pregnancy this ability is increased many times. In the pregnant state there is greater vascularity, thickening and lengthening of the walls, and increased secretion, so that most women have varying quantities of vaginal discharge during the period of gestation.

5 The Obstetric Pelvis

The pelvis is made up by the two innominate bones, which occupy the front and sides, and the sacrum and coccyx behind. The bones articulate through four joints. The sacroiliac joint is the most important, linking the sacrum to the iliac part of the innominate bones. The symphysis of the pubis joins the two pubic bones. The sacrococcygeal joint attaches the sacrum to the coccyx.

The false pelvis lies above the true pelvis, superior to the linea terminalis. Its only obstetrical function is to support the enlarged uterus during pregnancy. Its boundaries are:

1. The lumbar vertebrae posteriorly
2. The iliac fossae laterally
3. The anterior abdominal wall anteriorly

The true pelvis lies below the pelvic brim, or linea terminalis, and is the bony canal through which the baby must pass. It is divided into three parts:

1. The inlet
2. The pelvic cavity
3. The pelvic outlet

1. The <u>inlet</u> (pelvic brim) is bounded:
   a. Anteriorly, by the pubic crest and spine
   b. Laterally, by the iliopectineal lines on the innominate bones
   c. Posteriorly, by the anterior borders of the ala and promontory of the sacrum

2. The <u>pelvic cavity</u> is a curved canal.
   a. The anterior wall is straight and shallow.   The pubis is 5 cm long.
   b. The posterior wall is deep and concave.   The sacrum is 10 to 15 cm in length.
   c. Laterally are the ischium and part of the body of the ilium.

3. The <u>pelvic outlet</u> is diamond-shaped.   It is bounded:
   a. Anteriorly, by the arcuate pubic ligament and the pubic arch
   b. Laterally, by the ischial tuberosity and the sacrotuberous ligament
   c. Posteriorly, by the tip of the sacrum

The <u>axis of the birth canal</u> is the course taken by the presenting part as it passes through the pelvis.   At first it moves downward and backward to the level of the ischial spines, which is the area of the bony attachment of the muscles of the pelvic floor.   Here the direction changes and it proceeds downward and forward.

The <u>pelvic inclination</u> is assessed when the woman is in the upright position.   The plane of the pelvic brim makes an angle of about 60 degrees with the horizontal.   The anterior superior iliac spine is in the same vertical plane as the pubic spine.

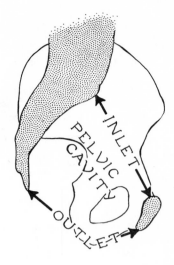

Fig. 1. True pelvis.

Fig. 2. Pelvic cavity.

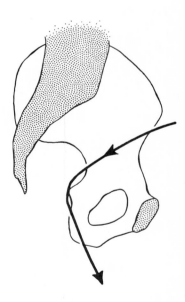

Fig. 3. Pelvic inclination.

Fig. 4. Axis of birth canal.

The pelvic planes are imaginary flat surfaces passing across the pelvis at different levels. They are used for the purposes of description. The important ones are:

1. The plane of the inlet or superior strait
2. The pelvic cavity has many planes, two of which are:
   a. The plane of greatest dimensions
   b. The plane of least dimensions
3. The plane of the outlet or inferior strait

The diameters are distances between given points. Important ones are:

1. The anteroposterior diameters
2. The transverse diameters
3. The left oblique: Oblique diameters are designated "left" or "right" according to their posterior terminal.
4. The right oblique
5. The posterior sagittal diameter: This is the back part of the anteroposterior diameter, and it extends from the intersection of the transverse and anteroposterior diameters to the posterior limit of the latter.
6. The anterior sagittal diameter: This is the front part of the anteroposterior diameter, and it extends from the intersection of the transverse and anteroposterior diameter to the anterior limit of the latter.

Fig. 5A. Sagittal section.

Fig. 5B. Coronal section.

THE INLET OF THE PELVIS

The Plane of the Obstetric Inlet

The plane of the obstetric inlet is bounded:

1. Anteriorly, by the posterior superior margin of the pubic symphysis
2. Laterally, by the iliopectineal lines
3. Posteriorly, by the promontory and ala of the sacrum

The Diameters of the Inlet

The diameters of the inlet are:

1. The anteroposterior diameters:
   a. The anatomic conjugate extends from the middle of the sacral promontory to the middle of the pubic crest (superior surface of the pubis). It measures 11.5 cm. It has no obstetrical significance.
   b. The obstetric conjugate extends from the middle of the sacral promontory to the posterior superior margin of the pubic symphysis. This point on the pubis, which protrudes back into the cavity of the pelvis, is about 1 cm below the pubic crest. The obstetric conjugate is about 11.0 cm in length. This is the important anteroposterior diameter, since it is the one through which the fetus must pass.
   c. The diagonal conjugate extends from the subpubic angle to the middle of the sacral promontory. It is 12.5 cm in length. This diameter can be measured manually in the patient. It is of clinical significance because by subtracting 1.5 cm an approximate length of the obstetric conjugate can be obtained.
2. The transverse diameter is the widest distance between the iliopectineal lines, and is 13.5 cm.
3. The left oblique diameter extends from the left sacroiliac joint to the right iliopectineal eminence. It is about 12.5 cm.
4. The right oblique extends from the right sacroiliac joint to the left iliopectineal eminence. It is about 12.5 cm.
5. The posterior sagittal extends from the intersection of the anteroposterior and transverse diameters to the middle of the sacral promontory. It is about 4.5 cm.

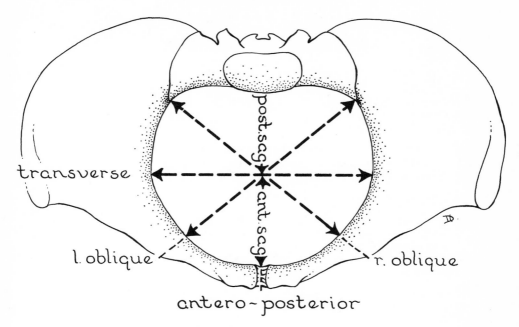

transverse

post.sag.

ant.sag.

l. oblique

r. oblique

antero-posterior

Fig. 6A. Antero-posterior view.

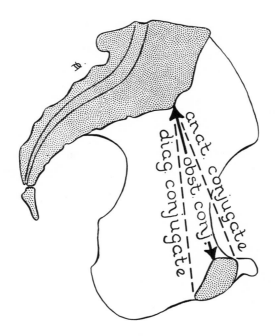

anat. conjugate

obst. conj.

diag. conjugate

Fig. 6B. Sagittal section.

THE CAVITY OF THE PELVIS

The pelvic cavity extends from the inlet to the outlet.

The Plane of Greatest Dimensions

This is the roomiest part of the pelvis and is almost circular. Its obstetric significance is small.
Its boundaries are:

1. Anteriorly, the midpoint of the posterior surface of the pubis
2. Laterally, the upper and middle thirds of the obturator foramina
3. Posteriorly, the junction of the second and third sacral vertebrae

The diameters of importance are:

1. The anteroposterior diameter extends from the midpoint of the posterior surface of the pubis to the junction of the second and third sacral vertebrae and measures 12.75 cm.
2. The transverse diameter is the widest distance between the lateral aspects of the plane and is 12.5 cm.

The Plane of Least Dimensions

This is the most important plane of the pelvis. It has the least room, and it is here that the majority of arrests of progress take place. This plane extends from the apex of the subpubic arch, through the ischial spines, to the sacrum, usually at or near the junction of the fourth and fifth sacral vertebrae.
The boundaries are, from front to back:

1. The lower border of the pubic symphysis
2. The white line on the fascia covering the obturator foramina
3. The ischial spines
4. The sacrospinous ligaments
5. The sacrum

The diameters of importance are:

1. The anteroposterior extends from the lower border of the pubic symphysis to the junction of the fourth and fifth sacral vertebrae. It measures 12.0 cm.
2. The transverse diameter lies between the ischial spines and is 10.5 cm. wide.
3. The posterior sagittal extends from the bispinous diameter to the junction of the fourth and fifth sacral vertebrae and measures 4.5 to 5.0 cm.

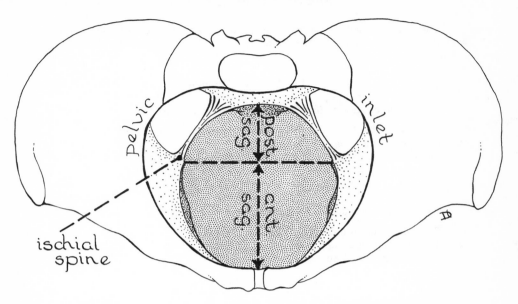

Fig. 7A. Antero-posterior view showing the antero-posterior and transverse diameters.

Fig. 7B. Sagittal section showing the antero-posterior diameter.

THE OUTLET OF THE PELVIS

The outlet is made up of two triangular planes, having as their common base and most inferior part the transverse diameter between the ischial tuberosities.

The Anterior Triangle

The anterior triangle has the following boundaries:

1. The base is the bituberous diameter (transverse diameter).
2. The apex is the subpubic angle.
3. The sides are the pubic rami and ischial tuberosities.

The Posterior Triangle

The posterior triangle has the following boundaries:

1. The base is the bituberous diameter.
2. The obstetric apex is the sacrococcygeal joint.
3. The sides are the sacrotuberous ligaments.

The Diameters of the Outlet

1. The anteroposterior diameter:
   a. The anatomic anteroposterior diameter is from the inferior margin of the pubic symphysis to the tip of the coccyx. It measures about 9.5 cm.
   b. The obstetric anteroposterior diameter is from the inferior margin of the pubic symphysis to the sacrococcygeal joint. This measures 11.5 cm. Because of the mobility at the sacrococcygeal joint, the coccyx is pushed out of the way by the advancing presenting part, and this increases the available space.
2. The transverse diameter is the distance between the inner surfaces of the ischial tuberosities and measures about 11.0 cm.
3. The posterior sagittal diameter extends from the middle of the transverse diameter to the sacrococcygeal junction and is 9.0 cm.
4. The anterior sagittal diameter extends from the middle of the transverse diameter to the subpubic angle and measures 6.0 cm.

IMPORTANT MEASUREMENTS

In assessing the obstetric capacity of the pelvis the most important measurements are:

1. The obstetric conjugate of the inlet
2. The distance between the ischial spines
3. The subpubic angle and bituberous diameter
4. The posterior sagittal diameters of the three planes
5. The curve and length of the sacrum

Fig. 8A. Inferior view.

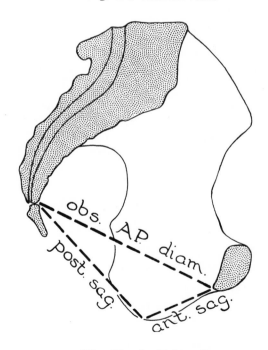

Fig. 8B. Sagittal section.

CLASSIFICATION OF THE PELVIS

Variations in the female pelvis and in the planes of any single pelvis are so great that a rigid classification is not possible. A pelvis which is of the female type in one plane may be predominantly male in another. Many pelves are mixed in that the various planes do not conform to a single parent type.

For the purpose of classification the pelvis is named on the basis of the inlet, and mention is made of nonconforming characteristics. For example, a pelvis may be described as a female type with male features at the outlet.

We prefer the classification of Caldwell and Malloy:

INLET

	Gynecoid	Android	Anthropoid	Platypelloid
Sex Type	Normal female	Male	Ape-like	Flat female
Incidence	50 percent	20 percent	25 percent	5 percent
Shape	Round or transverse oval Transverse diameter is a little longer than the anteroposterior	Heart or wedge-shaped	Long anteroposterior oval	Transverse oval
Anteroposterior Diameter	Adequate	Adequate	Long	Short
Transverse Diameter	Adequate	Adequate	Adequate, but relatively short	Long
Posterior Sagittal Diameter	Adequate	Very short and inadequate	Very long	Very short
Anterior Sagittal Diameter	Adequate	Long	Long	Short
Posterior Segment	Broad, deep, roomy	Shallow The sacral promontory indents the inlet and reduces its capacity	Deep	Shallow
Anterior Segment	Well rounded forepelvis	Narrow and sharply angulated forepelvis	Deep	Shallow

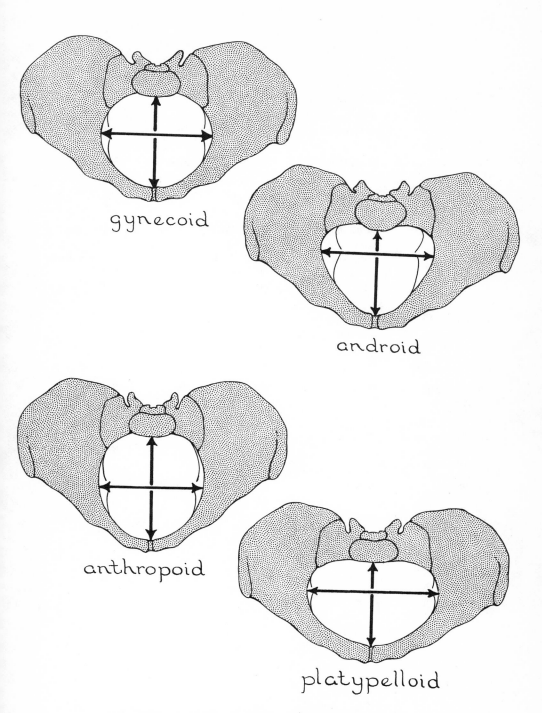

gynecoid

android

anthropoid

platypelloid

Fig. 9. The pelvic inlet (Caldwell–Moloy classification).

THE PELVIC CAVITY: THE MID PELVIS

	Gynecoid	Android	Anthropoid	Platypelloid
Anteroposterior Diameter	Adequate	Reduced	Long	Shortened
Transverse Diameter	Adequate	Reduced	Adequate	Wide
Posterior Sagittal Diameter	Adequate	Reduced	Adequate	Shortened
Anterior Sagittal Diameter	Adequate	Reduced	Adequate	Short
Sacrum	Wide deep curve. Short, slopes backward, light bone	Flat. Inclined forward. Long, narrow, heavy	Inclined backward Narrow, long	Wide deep curve—often sharply angulated with enlarged sacral bossa
Sidewalls	Parallel, straight	Convergent Funnel pelvis	Straight	Parallel
Ischial spines	Not prominent	Prominent	Variable	Variable
Sacrosciatic Notch	Wide and short	Narrow, long, high arch	Wide	Short
Depth: Iliopectineal eminence to tuberosities	Average	Long	Long	Short
Capacity	Adequate	Reduced in all diameters	Adequate	Reduced

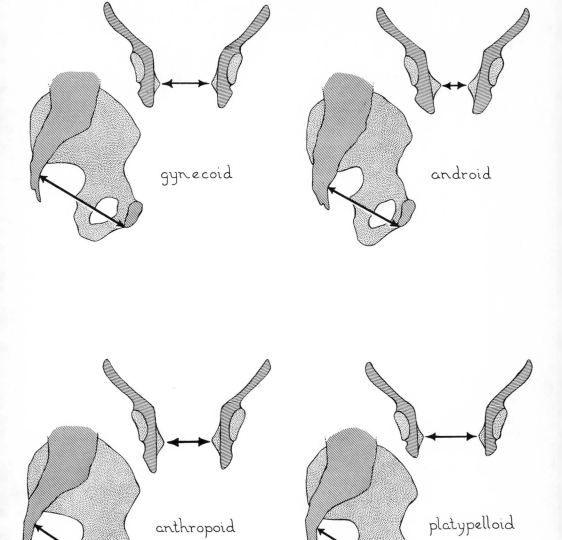

gynecoid

android

anthropoid

platypelloid

Fig. 10. The mid pelvis (Caldwell–Moloy classification).

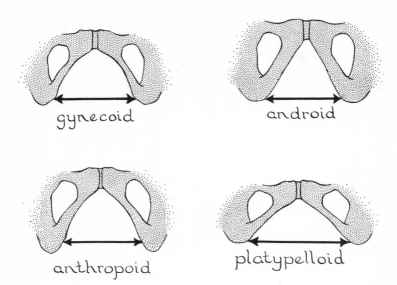

Fig. 11.   The pelvic outlet (Caldwell-Moloy classification).

OUTLET

	Gynecoid	Android	Anthropoid	Platypelloid
Anteroposterior Diameter	Long	Short	Long	Short
Transverse Diameter (Bituberous)	Adequate	Narrow	Adequate	Wide
Pubic Arch	Wide and round 90 degrees	Narrow and deep 70 degrees	Normal or relatively narrow	Very wide
Inferior Pubic Rami	Short and concave inward	Straight and long	Long and relatively narrow	Straight and short
Capacity	Adequate	Reduced	Adequate	Inadequate

EFFECT ON LABOR

	Gynecoid	Android	Anthropoid	Platypelloid
Fetal Head	Engages in transverse or oblique diameter in slight asynclitism Good flexion OA is common	Engages in transverse or posterior diameter in asynclitism Extreme molding	Engages in anteroposterior or oblique. Often occiput posterior	Engages in transverse diameter with marked asynclitism
Labor	Good uterine function Early and complete internal rotation Spontaneous delivery Wide pubic arch reduces perineal tears	Deep transverse arrest is common Arrest as OP with failure of rotation Delivery is often by difficult forceps application, rotation, and extraction The narrow pubic arch may lead to major perineal tears	Delivery and labor is usually easy Birth face to pubis is common	Delay at inlet
Prognosis	Good	Poor	Good	Poor Disproportion Delay at inlet Labor often terminated by cesarean section

BIBLIOGRAPHY

Caldwell, W. E., and Moloy, H. C. Anatomical variations in the female pelvis
    and their effect on labor with a suggested classification. Amer. J. Obstet.
    Gynec., 26:479, 1933.
Eastman, N. J., and Hellman, L. M. Williams Obstetrics, 13th ed. New
    York, Appleton-Century-Crofts, 1965.
Smout, C. F. V., and Jacoby, F. Gynaecological and Obstetrical Anatomy and
    Functional Histology, 3rd ed. Baltimore, The Williams & Wilkins Co.,
    1953.
Thoms, H. The Obstetric Pelvis. Baltimore, The Williams & Wilkins Co.,
    1935.
_____ Foote, W. R., and Friedman, I. The clinical significance of pelvic
    variations. Amer. J. Obstet. Gynec., 38:634, 1939.
_____ and Greulich, W. W. A comparative study of male and female pelves.
    Amer. J. Obstet. Gynec., 39:56, 1940.

6   The Passenger: The Fetus

GENERAL DATA

1. Resemblance to the adult human form may be perceptible at the end of 8 weeks and is obvious at the end of 12 weeks.
2. By the end of 12 weeks, and sometimes sooner, the sexual differences in the external genitalia may be recognized in abortuses.
3. Growth is greatest during the sixth and seventh months of intrauterine life.
4. Quickening (the perception by the pregnant woman of fetal movements in utero) occurs between the sixteenth and twentieth weeks of pregnancy. The time of quickening is too variable to be of value in determining the expected date of confinement or when term has been reached. Active intestinal peristalsis is the most common phenomenon mistaken for quickening.
5. The fetal heart is audible by the eighteenth or twentieth week.
6. The average length of the fetus at term is 50 cm.
7. Within wide variations the average male (7 1/2 pounds or 3,400 g) is a little heavier at birth than the female (7 pounds or 3,150 g).
8. In premature babies the circumference of the head is relatively large as compared with the shoulders. As the fetus matures the body grows faster than the head, so that at term the circumferences of the head and the shoulders are nearly the same.

THE FETAL OVOIDS

In its passage through the pelvis the fetus presents two oval shaped parts, movable on each other at the neck. The oval of the head is longer in its antero-posterior diameter, while that of the shoulders and body is longer transversely. Thus the two ovoids are perpendicular to each other.

THE FETAL HEAD

From the obstetric standpoint this is the most important part of the fetus. It is the largest, the least compressible, and the most frequently presenting part of the baby. Once the head has been born, rarely is there delay or difficulty with the remainder of the body.

Base of the Skull

The bones of this part are large, ossified, firmly united, and not compressible. Their function is to protect the vital centers in the brain stem.

The Vault of the Skull: the Cranium

The cranium is made up of several bones. Important ones are: 1, the occipital bone posteriorly; 2, the two parietal bones on the sides; and 3, the two temporal and the two frontal bones anteriorly. The bones of the cranial vault are laid down in membrane. At birth they are thin, poorly ossified, easily compressible, and are joined only by membrane. This looseness of union of the bones (actually there are spaces between them) permits their overlapping under pressure. In this way the head can change its shape to fit the maternal pelvis, an important function known as molding. The top of the skull is wider posteriorly (biparietal diameter) than anteriorly (bitemporal).

Sutures of the Skull

Sutures are membrane occupied spaces between the bones. They are useful in two ways:

1. Their presence makes molding possible.
2. By identifying the sutures on vaginal examination, the position of the baby's head can be diagnosed. The important sutures are:

The Sagittal Suture

The sagittal suture lies between the parietal bones. It runs in an antero-posterior direction between the fontanelles, and divides the head into left and right halves.

The Lambdoidal Sutures

The lambdoidal sutures extend transversely from the posterior fontanelle and separate the occipital bone from the two parietals.

The Coronal Sutures

The coronal sutures extend transversely from the anterior fontanelle and lie between the parietal and the frontal bones.

The Frontal Suture

The frontal suture is between the two frontal bones and is an anterior continuation of the sagittal suture. It extends from the glabella to the bregma.

The Fontanelles

Where the sutures intersect are the membrane filled spaces known as fontanelles. Two are important: the anterior and the posterior. These areas are useful clinically in two ways:

1. Their identification helps in diagnosing the position of the fetal head in the pelvis.
2. The large fontanelle is examined in assessing the condition of the child after birth. In dehydrated infants the fontanelle is depressed below the surface of the bony skull. When the intracranial pressure is elevated, the fontanelle is bulging, tense, and raised above the level of the skull.

The Anterior Fontanelle

The anterior fontanelle (bregma) is at the junction of the sagittal, frontal, and coronal sutures. It is by far the larger of the two, measuring about 3 x 2 cm, and is diamond-shaped. It becomes ossified by 18 months of age. The anterior fontanelle facilitates molding. By remaining patent long after birth it plays a part in accommodating the remarkable growth of the brain.

The Posterior Fontanelle

The posterior fontanelle (lambda) is located where the sagittal suture meets the two lambdoidals. The skull is not truly deficient at this point, and the area is a meeting point of the sutures rather than a true fontanelle. It is much smaller than the anterior one. The intersection of the sutures makes a Y with the sagittal suture as the base and the lambdoidals as the arms. This fontanelle closes at 6 to 8 weeks of age.

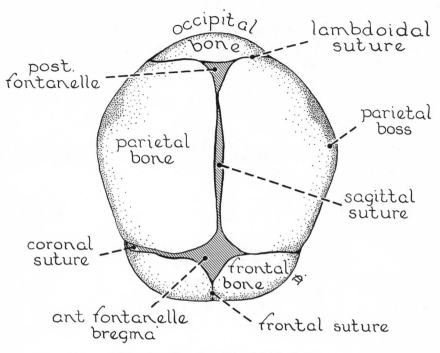

Fig. 1. Superior view of fetal skull.

Fig. 2. Transverse diameters of fetal skull.

Landmarks of the Skull

From posterior to anterior certain areas are identified:

1. The occiput: The area of the back of the head occupied by the occipital bone. It is behind and inferior to the posterior fontanelle and the lambdoidal sutures.
2. The posterior fontanelle
3. The vertex: The area between the two fontanelles. It is the top of the skull and is bounded laterally by the parietal bosses.
4. The bregma or large anterior fontanelle
5. The sinciput (or brow): The region bounded superiorly by the bregma and the coronal sutures, and inferiorly by the glabella and the orbital ridges
6. The glabella: The elevated area between the orbital ridges
7. The nasion: The root of the nose
8. The parietal bosses: Two eminences, one on the side of each parietal bone. The distance between them is the widest transverse diameter of the fetal head.

Diameters of the Fetal Skull

These are distances between given points on the fetal skull. Their size varies, and the particular anteroposterior diameter which presents to the maternal pelvis depends on the degree of flexion or extension of the fetal head.

1. The biparietal diameter is between the parietal bosses. It is the largest transverse diameter and measures 9.5 cm.
2. The bitemporal diameter lies between the temporal bones. It is 8.0 cm in length and is the shortest transverse diameter.
3. The suboccipitobregmatic diameter extends from the under surface of the occipital bone, where it meets the neck, to the center of the bregma. It is 9.5 cm long. It is the anteroposterior diameter which presents when the head is flexed well.
4. The occipitofrontal diameter presents in the military attitude, neither flexion nor extension. It extends from the external occipital protuberance to the glabella and is 11.0 cm long.
5. The verticomental diameter is involved in brow presentations (halfway extension of the head). It runs from the vertex to the chin, measures 13.5 cm, and is the longest anteroposterior diameter of the head.
6. The submentobregmatic is the diameter in face presentations (complete extension of the head). Reaching from the junction of the neck and lower jaw to the center of the bregma, it is 9.5 cm long.

Circumferences of the Fetal Skull

1. In the occipitofrontal plane the circumference of the head is 34.5 cm.
2. In the suboccipitobregmatic plane it is from 32 to 34 cm.
3. At term the bisacromial diameter of the shoulders is from 33 to 34 cm.

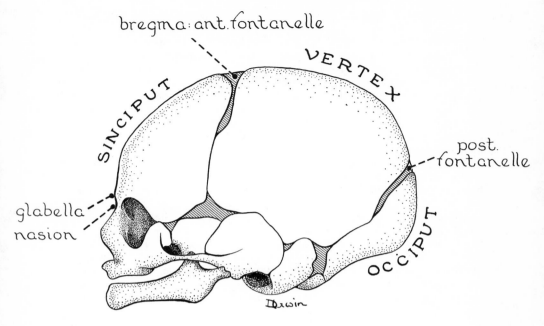

Fig. 3. Lateral view of fetal skull.

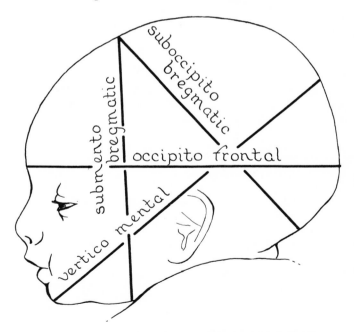

Fig. 4. Antero-posterior diameters of fetal skull.

Molding

Molding is the ability of the fetal head to change its shape and so adapt it-self to the unyielding maternal pelvis. This property is of the greatest value in the progress of labor and the descent of the head through the birth canal.

The fetal bones are joined loosely by membranes so that actual spaces ex-ist between the edges of the bones. This permits the bones to alter their rela-tionships to each other as pressure is exerted on the head by the bony pelvis. The bones can come closer to each other, or move apart. The side to side re-lationships of the bones are changeable, and one bone is able to override the other. When overlapping of the bones takes place, the frontal and occipital bones pass under the parietal bones. The posterior parietal bone is subjected to greater pressure by the sacral promontory; therefore it passes beneath the anterior parietal bone. A contributing factor to molding is the softness of the bones.

Compression in one direction is accompanied by expansion in another, and hence the actual volume of the skull is not reduced. Providing that molding is not excessive and that it takes place slowly, no damage is done to the brain.

The alteration of the shape of the head is produced by compression of the presenting diameter, with resultant bulging of the diameter which is at right angles. For example, in the occipitoanterior position the suboccipitobregmatic is the presenting diameter. The head, therefore, is elongated in the vertico-mental diameter, with bulging behind and above.

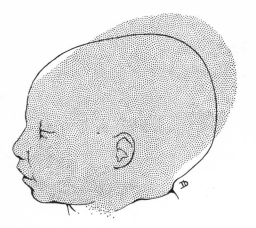

Fig. 5. Molding: Left Occiput Anterior.

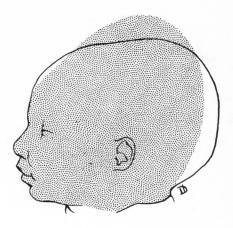

Fig. 6. Molding: Right Occiput Posterior.

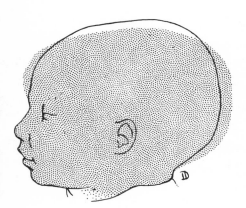

Fig. 7. Molding: face presentation.

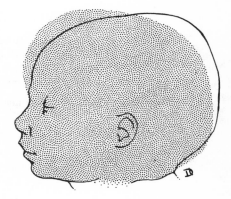

Fig. 8. Molding: brow presentation.

The Caput Succedaneum

The caput succedaneum is a localized swelling of the scalp formed by the effusion of serum. Pressure of the cervical ring causes obstruction of the venous return, so that the part of the scalp which lies within the cervix becomes edematous. The caput forms during labor and after the membranes have been ruptured. It will be absent if the baby is dead, the contractions poor, or the cervix not applied closely to the head.

The location of the caput varies with the position of the head. In occipito-anterior positions the caput forms on the vertex, to the right of the sagittal suture in LOA, and to the left in ROA. As flexion becomes more pronounced during labor, the posterior part of the vertex becomes the presenting part, and the caput is found in that region, a little to the right or left as before. Thus, when the position is LOA the caput is on the posterior part of the right parietal bone, and in ROA, on the posterior part of the left parietal bone.

The size of the caput succedaneum is an indication of the amount of pressure which has been exerted against the head. A large one suggests strong pressure from above and resistance from below. A small caput is present when the contractions have been weak or the resistance feeble. The largest are found in contracted pelves after long hard labor. In the presence of prolonged labor a large caput suggests disproportion or occipitoposterior position, while a small one indicates uterine inertia.

In performing rectal or vaginal examinations during labor, one must take care to distinguish between the station of the caput and the station of the skull. The enlarging caput may make the accoucheur believe that the head is descending, when in reality it means that the advancement of the head had become delayed or arrested. A growing caput is an indication for reassessment of the situation.

The caput is present at birth, begins to disappear immediately after birth, and is usually gone after 24 to 36 hours.

Cephalhematoma

A cephalhematoma is a hemorrhage under the periosteum of one or more of the bones of the skull. It is situated on one, and rarely both, parietal bones and is similar in appearance to a caput succedaneum. A cephalhematoma is caused by trauma to the skull, including:

1. Prolonged pressure of the head against the cervix, perineum, or pubic bones

Fig. 9. Formation of caput succedaneum.

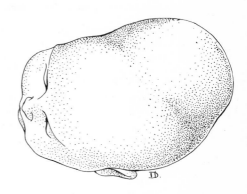

Fig. 10. Caput succedaneum: Left Occiput Anterior.

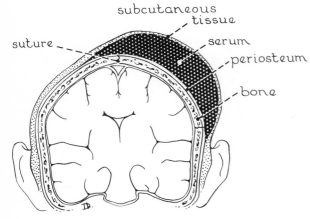

subcutaneous tissue

suture

serum

periosteum

bone

Fig. 11. Coronal section of skull: caput succedaneum.

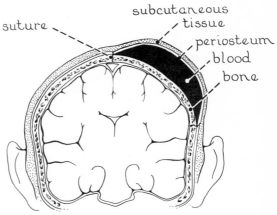

suture

subcutaneous tissue

periosteum

blood

bone

Fig. 12. Coronal section of skull: cephalhematoma.

2. Damage from forceps blades
3. Difficult manual rotation of the head
4. Rapid compression and relaxation of the forces which act on the fetal head, as in precipitate births
5. This injury may occur during normal spontaneous delivery.

Since the hemorrhage is under the periosteum, the swelling is limited to the affected bone, and does not cross the suture lines; this is one way of distinguishing it from a caput succedaneum. The swelling appears within a few hours of birth, and, since absorption is slow, it takes 6 to 12 weeks to disappear. The blood clots early at the edges and remains fluid in the center. Rarely, ossification takes place in the clot and may cause a permanent deformity of the skull. The health of the child is not affected, and the brain is not damaged.

The prognosis is good. No local treatment is indicated. Vitamin K may be given to reduce further bleeding. The area should be protected from injury. No attempt is made to evacuate the blood. Rarely, infection will set in and an abscess will form. This must be drained.

Caput Succedaneum	Cephalhematoma
Present at birth	May not appear for several hours
Soft, pits on pressure	Soft, does not pit
Diffuse swelling	Sharply circumscribed
Lies over and crosses the sutures	Limited to individual bones, does not cross suture lines
Movable on skull, seeks dependent portions	Fixed to original site
Is largest at birth and immediately begins to grow smaller, disappearing in a few hours	Appears after a few hours, grows larger for a time, and disappears only after weeks or months

Meningocele

A meningocele is a hernial protrusion of the meninges. It is a serious congenital deformity and must be distinguished from the caput succedaneum and the cephalhematoma. The meningocele always lies over a suture or a fontanelle, and becomes tense when the baby cries.

BIBLIOGRAPHY

Kraus, G. W., and Hendricks, C. H. Significance of the quickening date in determining duration of pregnancy. Obstet. Gynec., 24:178, 1964.

7 Fetopelvic Relationships

To understand the situation of the fetus in the uterus and pelvis, the descriptive terminology must be defined and clarified.

Lie: The relationship of the long axis of the fetus to the long axis of the mother

Presentation: Refers to the part of the fetus which lies over the inlet. The three main presentations are cephalic (head first), breech (pelvis first), and shoulder.

The Presenting Part: This is the most dependent part of the fetus and lies nearest the cervix. During vaginal or rectal examination it is the area with which the finger makes contact first.

Attitude: The relation of the fetal parts to each other. The basic attitudes are flexion and extension. The fetal head is in flexion when the chin approaches the chest, and in extension when the occiput nears the back. The typical fetal attitude in the uterus is flexion, with the head bent in front of the chest, the arms and legs folded in front of the body, and the back curved forward slightly.

The Denominator: An arbitrarily chosen point on the presenting part of the fetus used in describing position. Each presentation has its own denominator.

Position: The relationship of the denominator to the front, back, or sides of the maternal pelvis.

LIE

The two lies are:

1. Longitudinal, when the long axes of the fetus and mother are parallel
2. Transverse, or oblique, when the long axis of the fetus is perpendicular or oblique to the long axis of the mother

All terms as to direction refer to the mother in the standing position. Upper means toward the maternal head, and lower toward the feet. Anterior and posterior, right and left, refer to the mother's front, back, right, and left, respectively.

Lie	Presentation		Attitude	Presenting Part	Denominator
Longitudinal 99.5%	Cephalic (Head) 96 to 97%		Flexion	Vertex (Posterior part)	Occiput (O)
			Military	Vertex (Median part)	Occiput (O)
			Partial Extension	Brow	Forehead (Frontum) (Fr)
			Complete Extension	Face	Chin (Mentum) (M)
	Breech 3 to 4% (Pelvic)	Complete	Flexed Hips & Knees	Buttocks	Sacrum (S)
		Frank	Flexed Hips Extended Knees	Buttocks	Sacrum (S)
		Footling Single Double	Extended Hips & Knees	Feet	Sacrum (S)
		Kneeling Single Double	Extended Hips Flexed Knees	Knees	Sacrum (S)
Transverse or Oblique 0.5%	Shoulder		Variable	Shoulder Arm Trunk	Scapula (Sc)

Fig. 1.   Flexion of head.

Fig. 2.   Military attitude.

Fig. 3.   Brow presentation:
partial extension.

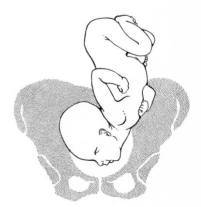

Fig. 4.   Face presentation:
complete extension.

Longitudinal Lies

Longitudinal lies are grouped into:

1. Cephalic, when the head comes first
2. Breech, when the buttocks or lower limbs lead the way

Cephalic Presentations

Cephalic presentations are subdivided, according to the attitude of the fetal head, into 4 main groups:

1. Flexion is present when the baby's chin is near its chest. The posterior part of the vertex is the presenting part, and the occiput is the denominator.
2. When there is neither flexion nor extension we have the military attitude or the median vertex presentation. The vertex (area between the 2 fontanelles) presents, and the occiput is the denominator.
3. In brow presentation there is halfway extension. The frontum (forehead) leads the way and is also the denominator.
4. When extension is complete the presenting part is the face, and the denominator is the mentum (chin).

Breech Presentations

Breech or pelvic presentations are classified according to the attitudes at the hips and knees:

1. The breech is complete when there is flexion at both hips and knees. The buttocks are the presenting part.
2. Flexion at the hips and extension at the knees change it to a frank breech. The lower limbs lie anterior to the baby's abdomen. The buttocks lead the way.
3. When there is extension both at the hips and at the knees we have a footling breech, single if one foot is presenting, and double if both feet are down.
4. Extension at the hips and flexion at the knees make it a kneeling breech, single or double. Here the knees present.

In all variations of breech presentation the sacrum is the denominator.

Transverse or Oblique Lie

Transverse or oblique lie exists when the long axis of the fetus is perpendicular or oblique to the long axis of the mother. Most often the shoulder is the presenting part, but it may be an arm, or some part of the trunk, such as the back, abdomen, or side. The scapula is the denominator. The position is anterior or posterior depending on the situation of the scapulas, and right or left according to the location of the head.

Fig. 5. Complete breech.

Fig. 6. Frank breech.

Fig. 7. Footling breech.

Fig. 8. Kneeling breech.

Fig. 9. Transverse lie.

POSITION

Position is the relationship of the denominator to the front, back, or sides of the mother's pelvis. The pelvic girdle has a circumference of 360 degrees. The denominator can occupy any part of the circumference. In practice 8 points, 45 degrees from each other, are demarcated, and the position of the fetus is described as the relationship between the denominator and one of these landmarks.

Three terms are used to describe position: 1, the denominator; 2, right or left, depending on which side of the maternal pelvis the denominator is in; 3, anterior, posterior, or transverse, according to whether the denominator is in the front, the back, or at the side of the pelvis.

With the patient lying in the lithotomy position, the pubic symphysis is anterior and the sacrum is posterior. Starting at the symphysis, and moving in a clockwise direction, 8 positions are described in succession, each 45 degrees from the preceding one.

1. Denominator Anterior: DA The denominator is situated directly under the pubic symphysis.
2. Left Denominator Anterior: LDA The denominator is in the anterior part of the pelvis, 45 degrees to the left of the midline.
3. Left Denominator Transverse: LDT The denominator is on the left side of the pelvis, 90 degrees from the midline, at 3 o'clock.
4. Left Denominator Posterior: LDP The denominator is now in the posterior segment of the pelvis, and is 45 degrees to the left of the midline.
5. Denominator Posterior: DP The denominator has rotated a total of 180 degrees and is now in the posterior part of the pelvis, directly in the midline, and directly above the sacrum.
6. Right Denominator Posterior: RDP The denominator is in the posterior part of the pelvis, 45 degrees to the right of the midline.
7. Right Denominator Transverse: RDT The denominator is on the right side of the pelvis, 90 degrees from the midline, at 9 o'clock.
8. Right Denominator Anterior: RDA The denominator is in the anterior segment of the pelvis, 45 degrees to the right of the midline.

Further rotation of 45 degrees will complete the circle of 360 degrees, and the denominator will be back under the symphysis pubis in the denominator anterior position.

This method of describing position is used for every presentation. Each presentation has its own denominator, but the basic descriptive terminology is the same.

The illustration demonstrates the various positions in which the vertex is the presenting part. The occiput (back of the head) is the denominator, and the 8 positions (moving clockwise) are: OA—LOA—LOT—LOP—OP—ROP—ROT—ROA—OA

In face presentations the chin (mentum) is the denominator, and the sequence of positions is: MA—LMA—LMT—LMP—MP—RMP—RMT—RMA—MA

A further example would be in breech presentations where the sacrum is the denominator. Here the 8 positions are: SA—LSA—LST—LSP—SP—RSP—RST—RSA—SA

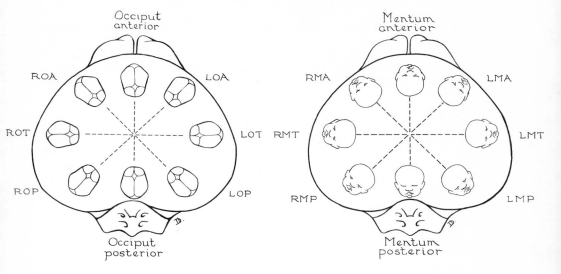

Fig. 10. Positions of the occiput.

Fig. 11. Positions of the face.

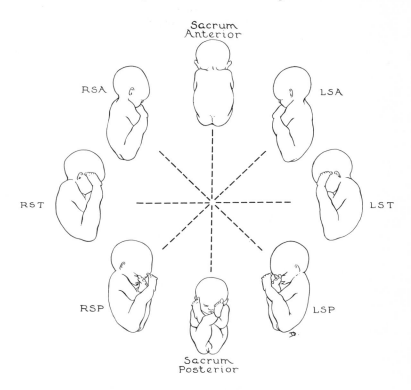

Fig. 12. Positions of the breech.

THE CEPHALIC PROMINENCE

The cephalic prominence is produced by flexion or extension. When the
head is well flexed, the occiput is lower than the sinciput, and the forehead is
the cephalic prominence. When there is extension the occiput is higher than the
sinciput, and the occiput or back of the head will be the cephalic prominence.
The cephalic prominence can be palpated through the abdomen by placing both
hands on the sides of the lower part of the uterus, and moving them gently toward the pelvis. When there is a cephalic prominence, the fingers will abut
against it on that side, and the fingers on the other side will meet little or no
resistance. The location of the cephalic prominence aids in diagnosing attitude.
When the cephalic prominence and the back are on opposite sides, the attitude
is flexion. When the cephalic prominence and the back are on the same side,
there is extension. When no cephalic prominence is palpable there is neither
flexion nor extension, and the head is in the military attitude.

Fig. 13. Cephalic prominence: flexion.

Fig. 14. Cephalic prominence: extension.

LIGHTENING

Lightening is the subjective sensation felt by the patient as the presenting part descends in the latter weeks of pregnancy. It is not synonymous with engagement, although both may take place at the same time. Lightening is caused by the tonus of the uterine and abdominal muscles and is a part of the adaptation of the presenting part to the lower uterine segment and to the pelvis. Symptoms include:

1. Less dyspnea
2. Decreased epigastric pressure
3. A feeling that the child is lower
4. Increased pressure in the pelvis
5. Low backache
6. Urinary frequency
7. Constipation
8. Initial appearance or aggravation of already present hemorrhoids and varicose veins of the lower limbs
9. Edema of the legs and feet
10. More difficulty in walking

GRAVIDITY AND PARITY

Gravidity

1. A gravida is a pregnant woman.
2. The word gravida refers to a pregnancy regardless of its duration.
3. A woman's gravidity relates to the total number of her pregnancies, regardless of their duration.
4. A primigravida is a woman pregnant for the first time.
5. A secundagravida is a woman pregnant for the second time.
6. A multigravida is a woman who has been pregnant several times.

Parity

1. The word para alludes to past pregnancies that have reached viability.
2. Parity refers to the number of past pregnancies that have gone to viability and have been delivered, regardless of the number of children involved. The birth of triplets increases the parity by only one.
3. A primipara is a woman who has delivered one pregnancy where the child has reached viability, without regard to the child's being alive or dead at the time of birth. Some authors consider that the designation of primipara includes women in the process of giving birth to their first child.
4. A multipara is a woman who has had two or more pregnancies terminate at the stage when the children were viable.
5. A parturient is a woman in labor.

Gravida and Para

1. A woman pregnant for the first time is a primigravida, and is described as Gravida 1 and Para 0.
2. If she aborts before viability she remains Gravida 1 and Para 0.
3. If she delivers a fetus which has reached viability she becomes a primipara, regardless of whether the child is alive or dead. She is now Gravida 1 and Para 1.
4. During a second pregnancy she is Gravida 2 and Para 1.
5. After she delivers the second child she is Gravida 2 and Para 2.
6. A patient with two abortions and no viable children is Gravida 2 and Para 0. When she becomes pregnant again she is Gravida 3 and Para 0. When she delivers a viable child she is Gravida 3 and Para 1.
7. Multiple births do not affect the parity by more than one. A woman who has viable triplets in her first pregnancy is Gravida 1 and Para 1.

8 Engagement, Synclitism, and Asynclitism

Engagement: By definition engagement has taken place when the widest diameter of the presenting part has passed through the inlet. In cephalic presentations, this diameter is the biparietal, between the parietal bosses. In breech presentation it is the intertrochanteric.

In most women, once the head is engaged, the bony presenting part (not the caput succedaneum) will be at, or nearly at, the level of the ischial spines. Radiologic studies have shown that this relationship is not constant and that in women with deep pelves the presenting part may be as much as a centimeter above the spines even though engagement has occurred.

The presence or absence of engagement is determined by abdominal, vaginal, or rectal examination. In primigravidas engagement usually takes place two to three weeks before term. In multiparas engagement may occur any time before or after the onset of labor. Engagement tells us that the pelvic inlet is adequate. It gives no information as to the midpelvis or the outlet. Lack of engagement in a primigravida is an indication for investigation to rule out disproportion, abnormal position, or some condition blocking the birth canal. The occurrence of engagement in normal cases is influenced by the tonus of the uterine and abdominal muscles.

Floating: The presenting part is entirely out of the pelvis, and is freely movable above the inlet.

Dipping: The presenting part has passed through the plane of the inlet, but engagement has not occurred.

Fig. 1. Floating.

Fig. 2. Dipping.

Fig. 3. Engaged.

STATION

Station is the relationship of the presenting part to an imaginary line drawn between the ischial spines. The location of the buttocks in breech presentations, or the bony skull (not the caput succedaneum) in cephalic presentations, at the level of the spines indicates that the station is zero. Above the spines the station is minus one, minus two, and so forth, depending on how many centimeters above the spines the presenting part is. At spines minus five it is at the inlet. Below the spines it is plus one, plus two, and so forth.

Relationships between station and the progress of labor include:

1. In nulliparas entering labor with the fetal head well below the spines, further descent is often delayed until the cervix is fully dilated.
2. In nulliparas beginning labor with the head deep in the pelvis, descent beyond the spines often takes place during the first stage of labor.
3. An unengaged head in a nullipara at the onset of labor may indicate disproportion, and warrants investigation. However, this condition is not rare, and in many cases descent and vaginal delivery will take place.
4. The incidence of disproportion is more common when the head is high at the onset of labor.
5. Patients who start labor with high fetal heads usually have lesser degrees of cervical dilatation. There is a tendency for lower stations to be associated with cervices which are more effaced and dilated, both at the onset of labor and in the beginning of the active phase.
6. Other factors being equal, the higher the station the longer the labor.
7. Dysfunctional labor is more frequent when the station is high.
8. The high head which descends rapidly is usually not associated with abnormal labor.

Fig. 4A. Antero-posterior view.

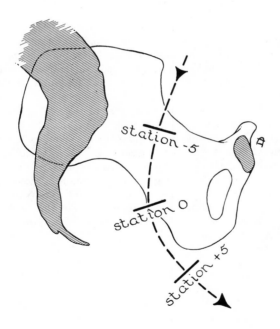

Fig. 4B. Lateral view.

SYNCLITISM AND ASYNCLITISM

Engagement in Synclitism

In cephalic presentations engagement has occurred when the biparietal diameter has passed through the inlet of the pelvis.   The fetal head engages most frequently with its sagittal suture (the anteroposterior diameter) in the transverse diameter of the pelvis.   Left occiput transverse is the commonest position at engagement.

When the biparietal diameter of the fetal head is parallel to the planes of the pelvis, the head is in synclitism. The sagittal suture is midway between the front and the back of the pelvis. When this relationship does not obtain, the head is in asynclitism.

Engagement in synclitism takes place when the uterus is perpendicular to the inlet and the pelvis is roomy. The head enters the pelvis with the plane of the biparietal diameter parallel to the plane of the inlet, the sagittal suture lies midway between the pubic symphysis and the sacral promontory, and the parietal bosses enter the pelvis at the same time.

Posterior Asynclitism (Litzmann's Obliquity)

In most women the abdominal wall maintains the pregnant uterus in an upright position, and prevents it from lying perpendicular to the plane of the pelvic inlet. As the head approaches the pelvis the posterior parietal bone is lower than the anterior parietal bone, the sagittal suture is nearer to the symphysis pubis than to the promontory of the sacrum, and the biparietal diameter of the head is in an oblique relationship to the plane of the inlet. This is posterior asynclitism. It is the usual mechanism in normal women, and is more common than engagement in synclitism or anterior asynclitism.

As the head enters the pelvis, the posterior parietal bone leads the way, and the posterior parietal boss (eminence) descends past the sacral promontory. At this point the anterior parietal boss is still above the pubic symphysis and has not entered the pelvis.   Uterine contractions force the head downward and into a movement of lateral flexion.   The posterior parietal bone pivots against the promontory, the sagittal suture moves posteriorly toward the sacrum, and the anterior parietal boss descends past the symphysis and into the pelvis. This brings the sagittal suture midway between the front and the back of the pelvis, and the head is now in synclitism.

Fig. 5. Synclitism at the inlet.

Fig. 6. Posterior asynclitism.

Anterior Asynclitism (Naegele's Obliquity)

Where the woman's abdominal muscles are lax and the abdomen is pendulous, so that the uterus and baby fall forward, or where the pelvis is abnormal and prevents the more common posterior asynclitism, the head enters the pelvis by anterior asynclitism. In this mechanism the anterior parietal bone descends first, the anterior parietal boss passes by the pubic symphysis into the pelvis, and the sagittal suture lies nearer to the sacral promontory than to the pubic symphysis. When the anterior parietal bone becomes relatively fixed behind the symphysis, a movement of lateral flexion takes place so that the sagittal suture moves anteriorly toward the symphysis, and the posterior parietal boss squeezes by the sacral promontory and into the pelvis. The mechanism of engagement in anterior asynclitism is the reverse of that of posterior asynclitism.

There is a mechanical advantage to the head's entering the pelvis in asynclitism. When the two parietal bosses enter the pelvic inlet at the same time (synclitism), the presenting diameter is the biparietal of 9.5 cm. In asynclitism the bosses come into the pelvis one at a time, and the diameter is the sub-superparietal of 8.75 cm. Thus engagement in asynclitism enables a larger head to pass through the inlet than would be possible if the head entered with its biparietal diameter parallel to the plane of the inlet.

Fig. 7. Anterior asynclitism.

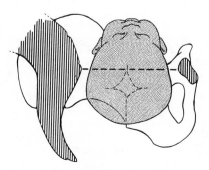

Fig. 8. Synclitism in the pelvis.

Whenever there is a small pelvis or a large head, asynclitism plays an important part in enabling engagement to take place.   Marked and persistent asynclitism, however, is abnormal.   When asynclitism is maintained until the head is deeply in the pelvis, it may prevent normal internal rotation.

BIBLIOGRAPHY

Friedman, E. A., and Sachtleben, M. R.   Station of the fetal presenting part. Amer. J. Obstet. Gynec., 93:522, 1965.

9 The Examination of the Patient

ABDOMINAL INSPECTION AND PALPATION

To ascertain how the baby is lying in utero the maternal abdomen is inspected and palpated to obtain the answers to these questions:

1. Is the lie longitudinal, transverse, or oblique?
2. What presents at or in the pelvic inlet?
3. Where is the back?
4. Where are the small parts?
5. What is in the uterine fundus?
6. On which side is the cephalic prominence?
7. Has engagement taken place?
8. How high in the abdomen is the uterine fundus?
9. How big is the baby?

Fig. 1. Position of the patient for abdominal palpation.

The patient lies on her back with the abdomen uncovered. In order to help relax the abdominal wall muscles the shoulders are raised a little and the knees are drawn up slightly. If the patient is in labor the examination is carried out between contractions.

First Maneuver

The examiner stands at the patient's side and grasps the lower uterine segment between the thumb and fingers of one hand to feel the presenting part. The other hand may be placed on the fundus to steady the uterus. This maneuver should be performed first. Since the head is the part of the fetus that can be identified with the most certainty, and since it is at or in the pelvis in 90 percent of cases, the logical thing to do first is to look for the head in its most frequent location. Once it has been established that the head is at the inlet, two important facts are known: 1, that the lie is longitudinal; and 2, that the presentation is cephalic.

An attempt is made to move the head from side to side to see if it is outside of the pelvis and free (floating), or if it is in the pelvis and fixed (engaged). In contrast to the breech the head is harder, smoother, more globular, and easier to move. A groove representing the neck may be felt between the head and the shoulders. The head can be moved laterally without an accompanying movement of the body. When the head is in the fundus and when there is sufficient amniotic fluid the head can be ballotted. When a floating rubber ball is forced under water, it returns to the surface as soon as it is released. So the fetal head can be pushed posteriorly in the amniotic fluid, but as soon as the pressure on it is relaxed it rises back and abuts against the examining fingers.

Second Maneuver

The examiner stands at the patient's side facing her head. The hands are placed on the sides of the abdomen, using one hand to steady the uterus, while the other hand palpates the fetus. The location of the back and the small parts is determined.

The side on which the back is located feels firmer, smoother, and forms a gradual convex arch. Resistance to the palpating fingers (as pressure is exerted toward the umbilicus) is even in all regions.

On the other side the resistance to pressure is uneven, the fingers sinking deeper in some areas than they do in others. The discovery of moving limbs is diagnostic.

Fig. 2. First maneuver.

Fig. 3. Second maneuver.

Third Maneuver

The hands are moved up the sides of the uterus and the fundus is palpated. In most cases the breech is here. It is a less definite structure than the head and is not identified as easily. The breech is softer, more irregular, less globular, and not as mobile as the head. It is continuous with the back, there being no intervening groove. When the breech is moved laterally the body moves as well. The finding of moving small parts in the vicinity of the breech strengthens the diagnosis.

Fourth Maneuver

The examiner turns and faces the patient's feet. Gently the fingers are moved down the sides of the uterus toward the pubis. The cephalic prominence is felt on the side where there is greater resistance to the descent of the fingers into the pelvis. In attitudes of flexion the forehead is the cephalic prominence. It is on the opposite side from the back. In extension attitudes the occiput is the cephalic prominence, and is on the same side as the back. In addition it is noted whether the head is free and floating or fixed and engaged.

Relationship of the Head to the Pelvis

1. The floating head lies entirely above the symphysis pubis, so that the examining fingers can be placed between the head and the pubis. The head is freely movable from side to side.
2. When the head is engaged the biparietal diameter has passed the inlet, and only a small part of the head may be palpable above the symphysis. The head is fixed and cannot be moved laterally. Sometimes the head is so low in the pelvis that it can barely be felt through the abdomen.
3. The head may be midway between the previous two locations. Part of it is felt easily above the symphysis. It is not freely movable, but it is not fixed. It is not engaged. The head is described as lying in the brim of the pelvis, or "dipping."

See Chapter 8, pages 58 and 59.

Fig. 4.   Third maneuver.

Fig. 5.   Fourth maneuver.

AUSCULTATION OF THE FETAL HEART

The fetal heart should be auscultated every 15 minutes during the first stage of labor, and every 3 to 5 minutes in the second stage. It is heard best by using a fetoscope. Information gained by listening to the fetal heart falls into two main groups. It tells us something about: 1, the general health of the baby in utero and 2, the presentation and position of the fetus.

Fig. 6. Auscultation of the fetal heart beat.

General Health of the Fetus

The general health of the fetus can be estimated by observing the rate and rhythm of its heart.

1. The presence of the fetal heart sound indicates that the baby is alive.
2. The normal heart rate is between 120 and 160 beats per minute. The fetal heart becomes slower at the height of a uterine contraction, and speeds up after the contraction has worn off. A fetal heart rate of less than 100 or more than 160 per minute, with the uterus at rest, suggests fetal distress. A slow rate has greater significance than a rapid one.
3. The rhythm is regular and of a tic toc quality. An irregularity is a sign of fetal embarrassment.
4. The loudness of the fetal heart, contrary to popular belief, is not a sign of fetal vigor. It depends upon the following:
   a. The relationship between the fetal back and the mother's abdomen. When the baby's back is near the anterior abdominal wall, the fetal heart is strong and near. This is so in anterior positions. In posterior positions, on the other hand, the fetal heart gives the impression of being far away.

    b. In obese women with thick abdominal walls the fetal heart is not heard
       clearly.
    c. An excessive amount of amniotic fluid muffles the fetal heart tones.
5. Other sounds which may be heard include:
    a. The funic souffle, which is synchronous with the fetal heart, is caused
       by the blood rushing through the umbilical arteries.
    b. The uterine (maternal) souffle pulses at the same speed as the maternal
       pulse, and results from the blood passing through the large blood ves-
       sels of the uterus.
6. Failure to hear the fetal heart may result from one of the following:
    a. Too early in the pregnancy. The fetal heart is heard only rarely before
       the eighteenth week.
    b. Fetal death. Inability to hear the baby's heart in a patient where it has
       been audible previously is a suggestion of fetal death. Usually fetal ac-
       tivity has ceased.
    c. Maternal obesity
    d. Polyhydramnios, an excessive amount of amniotic fluid
    e. A loud maternal souffle which obscures the fetal heart tones, and makes
       it difficult or impossible to identify them
    f. Posterior position of the occiput, where the fetal back is away from the
       anterior abdominal wall
    g. At the height of a strong uterine contraction
    h. Defective stethoscope
    i. An excessive amount of noise in the room

In some instances one observer is unable to find the fetal heart tones, while
another listener can hear them clearly.

Presentation and Position

    In most cases there is a constant relationship between the location of the
baby's heart and the fetal position in the uterus. In attitudes of flexion the fetal
heart is transmitted through the scapula and the back of the shoulder. It will,
therefore, be heard loudest in that area of the mother's abdomen to which the
fetal back is closest. In attitudes of extension the fetal heart is transmitted
through the anterior chest wall of the baby.

    In cephalic presentations the fetal heart is heard loudest below the umbili-
cus; in anterior positions, it is clearest in one or the other lower quadrant of
the mother's abdomen. The relationship of the fetal back and the fetal heart to
the midline of the maternal abdomen is similar. As the one comes nearer to,
or moves away from, the midline, so does the other. In posterior positions
the fetal heart is loudest in the maternal flank on the side to which the back is
related. In breech presentation the point of maximum intensity of the baby's
heart is above the umbilicus.

    The position of the fetal heart changes with descent and rotation. As the
baby descends, so does the fetal heart. One can follow the anterior rotation of
an occipitoposterior position by listening to the fetal heart as it moves gradually from the maternal flank toward the midline of the abdomen.

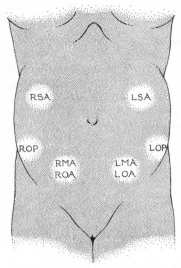

Fig. 7.   Location of the fetal
heart beat in relation to the various
positions.

The location of the fetal heart may be used to check, but should not be relied upon to make, the diagnosis of presentation and position. Occasionally the
point of maximum intensity of the fetal heart will not be in the expected location
for a given position. For example, it is not unusual in breech presentations for
the fetal heart to be heard loudest below the umbilicus, instead of above it. The
diagnosis made by careful abdominal palpation is the more reliable finding. The
finding of the fetal heart sound in an unexpected place is an indication for reexamination. If the findings on palpation are confirmed the fetal heart sound
should be disregarded.

Fetal Electrocardiography

There are two methods of obtaining the fetal electrocardiogram. 1, The
electrodes are placed on the mother's abdomen. It is difficult to eliminate the
maternal signal, and the tracings obtained in this fashion contain both a maternal and a fetal complex. 2, The electrodes are placed directly on the fetal buttocks or scalp, being introduced either through the maternal abdomen and uterus, or through the dilated cervix. In these tracings most, if not all, of the maternal electrocardiogram is eliminated.

Uses of this technic include:

1. Fetal life can be diagnosed 2 to 4 weeks before the fetal heart can be aus-
    cultated.
2. A positive fetal electrocardiogram establishes fetal life when there is a
    question of intrauterine fetal death.
3. The diagnosis of multiple pregnancy can be made safely.
4. Probably the greatest value is in the monitoring of the fetal heart in prob-
    lem cases, so that variations in the heart rate can be observed immediately.
5. While changes in the electrocardiographic complexes have been noted, their
    significance has not been established. This technic has only limited value
    in the diagnosis of congenital abnormalities.

RECTAL EXAMINATION

Because some obstetricians believe that there is danger of infection during vaginal examinations, the course of labor in normally progressing cases is followed by rectal examinations. During pregnancy, and especially during labor, the muscles of the pelvic floor soften and are more dilatable, so that rectal examination is easier to perform. However, rectal examination is painful, and should be done only as often as is necessary for the safe conduct of labor.

Rectal examination during labor has several drawbacks:

1. It is less accurate than vaginal examination, and is not to be relied on in problem cases.
2. The condition and dilatation of the cervix is often difficult to determine, especially when a bag of waters is present.
3. The caput succedaneum may be mistaken for the skull, resulting in erroneous diagnoses of station.
4. It is unreliable in breech presentation.
5. During examination the posterior wall of the vagina is pushed against the cervix, bringing the vaginal bacteria into direct contact with the cervix.
6. Rectal examination is painful and aggravates hemorrhoids.

VAGINAL EXAMINATION

Several recent studies have demonstrated that there is no greater danger of infection with vaginal than with rectal examination. Points in favor of the vaginal examination in the management of labor include:

1. Vaginal examination is more accurate than rectal examination in determining the condition and dilatation of the cervix, the station and position of the presenting part, and the relationship of the fetus to the pelvis.
2. Vaginal examination takes less time, requires less manipulation, and gives more information than the rectal approach.
3. Cultures, taken during the puerperium from women whose vaginas were sterile on admittance to hospital, showed no higher incidence of positive results in those who had vaginal examinations during labor than those who had only rectals. The same results were obtained after rupture of the membranes.
4. Clinical studies have shown that maternal morbidity is no higher following vaginal than following rectal examinations.
5. Vaginal examination causes less pain.
6. Vaginaphobia leads to the dangerous attitude of always waiting a little longer before doing a necessary vaginal examination during labor.
7. Prolapse of the umbilical cord can be diagnosed early, as can compound presentations.
8. It is important to remember that a clean or sterile glove is different from the contaminated finger of Semmelweiss' time.

The examination must be done gently, carefully, thoroughly, and under aseptic conditions. Some authors feel that rectal gloves are clean enough. Others suggest using sterile gloves, believing that they are safer and that their use will prevent a careless attitude developing in the case room. As for position, we prefer the lithotomy or dorsal position, finding the examination and orientation easier. It is the best position for determining proportion between the presenting part and the pelvis.

Palpation of the Cervix

1. Is the cervix soft or hard?
2. Is it thin and effaced, or thick and long?
3. Is it easily dilatable or resistant?
4. Is it closed or open? If it is open, estimate the length of the diameter of the cervical ring.

The Presentation

1. What is the presentation? Breech, cephalic, shoulder?
2. Is there a caput succedaneum, and is it small or extensive?
3. What is the station? What is the relationship of the presenting part (not the caput succedaneum) to a line between the ischial spines? If it is above the spines it is -1, -2, or -3 cm. If it is below the spines it is +1, +2, or +3 cm.

The Position

1. If it is a breech, where is the sacrum, and are the legs flexed or extended?
2. With a cephalic presentation, identify the sagittal suture. What is its direction? Is it in the anteroposterior, oblique, or transverse diameter of the pelvis?
3. Is the sagittal suture midway between the pubis and the sacrum (synclitism); is it near the sacral promontory (anterior asynclitism); or is it near the pubic symphysis (posterior asynclitism)?
4. Is the bregma right or left, anterior or posterior? It is diamond-shaped, and is the meeting point of four sutures.
5. Where is the posterior fontanelle? It is Y shaped and has three sutures.
6. Is the head in flexion (occiput lower than sinciput), or is there extension (sinciput lower than occiput)?
7. In cases where there is difficulty in identifying the sutures, the palpation of an ear will help establish the direction of the sagittal suture and thus the anteroposterior diameter of the long axis of the head. The tragus points to the face.

The Membranes

Feeling the bag of waters is evidence that the membranes are intact. The drainage of fluid, the passage of meconium, and the grasping of fetal hair in a clamp indicate that the membranes have ruptured.

Fig. 8. Determining the station and palpation of the sagittal suture. (From Douglas and Stromme. Operative Obstetrics, Appleton–Century–Crofts, 1957.)

Fig. 9. Identification of the posterior fontanelle. (From Douglas and Stromme. Operative Obstetrics, Appleton–Century–Crofts, 1957.)

Fig. 10. Identification of the anterior fontanelle. (From Douglas and Stromme. Operative Obstetrics, Appleton–Century–Crofts, 1957.)

Fig. 11. Palpation of the posterior ear. (From Douglas and Stromme. Operative Obstetrics, Appleton–Century–Crofts, 1957.)

General Assessment of the Pelvis

1. Can the sacral promontory be reached? The diagonal conjugate can be measured clinically. It extends from the inferior margin of the pubic symphysis to the middle of the sacral promontory, and its average length is 12.5 cm. During the vaginal examination the promontory is palpated. When the distal end of the finger reaches the middle of the promontory, the point where the proximal part of the finger makes contact with the subpubic angle is marked. The fingers are withdrawn from the vagina, and the distance between these two points is measured. By deducting 1.5 cm from the diagonal conjugate, the approximate length of the obstetric conjugate can be obtained. In many women the promontory cannot be reached, and this is accepted as evidence that the anteroposterior diameter of the inlet is adequate. If the promontory can be felt and the obstetric conjugate is thought to be short, x-ray pelvimetry should be carried out.
2. Is the pelvic brim symmetrical?
3. Are the ischial spines prominent and posterior?
4. Is the sacrum long and straight, or short and concave?
5. Are the sidewalls parallel or convergent?
6. Is the sacrosciatic notch wide or narrow?
7. Is there any bony or soft tissue encroachment into the cavity of the pelvis?
8. How wide is the subpubic angle? The distance between the ischial tuberosities (average 10.5 cm) can be measured roughly by placing a fist between them. If this can be done, the transverse diameter of the outlet is considered to be adequate.
9. Are the soft tissues and the perineum relaxed and elastic, or hard and rigid?

Fetopelvic Relationship

1. How does the presenting part fit the pelvis?
2. If engagement has not taken place can the presenting part be pushed into the pelvis by fundal and suprapubic pressure?
3. Does the presenting part ride over the pubic symphysis?

Fig. 12. Vaginal examination.

Fig. 13. Rectal examination.

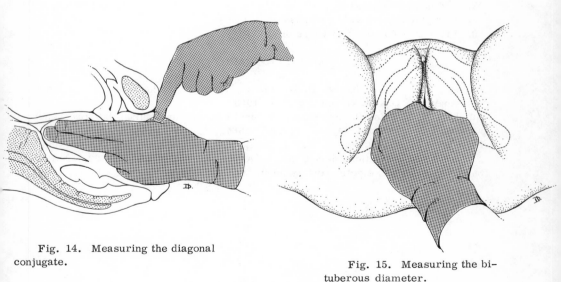

Fig. 14. Measuring the diagonal conjugate.

Fig. 15. Measuring the bi-tuberous diameter.

X-RAY EXAMINATION

In problem cases radiologic pelvimetry is invaluable in providing information about the following:

1. The shape and type of pelvis
2. The internal measurements of the pelvis
3. The presentation, position, and station of the fetus
4. The relationship of the fetus to the pelvis
5. An estimate of the fetal size
6. The maturity of the fetus can be judged by the ossification of certain bones. The most important is the lower femoral epiphysis, which is ossified at 36 to 40 weeks. Its presence suggests that the baby is 36 weeks or more. Its absence is not as significant, since in 17 percent, the ossification of the lower femoral epiphysis is not seen until term or past term.

Indications for x-ray pelvimetry include:

1. Clinical suspicion of a small or abnormal pelvis, including such findings as a diagonal conjugate under 11.5 cm, or a bituberous diameter less than 8.5 cm
2. Floating head near term in a primigravida
3. Suspicion of a large baby
4. History of previous difficult labor and delivery
5. Cases with history of bony pelvic injury or disease
6. Breech presentation in a primigravida
7. Attitudes of extension
8. Unexplained arrest of progress
9. Primigravidas over 35 years of age

BIBLIOGRAPHY

Bertelsen, H., and Johnson, B. D. Routine vaginal examinations during labor. Amer. J. Obstet. Gynec., 85:527, 1963.

Gunther, R. E., and Harer, W. B. Vaginal examinations during late pregnancy and labor. Obstet. Gynec., 24:695, 1964.

Peterson, W. F., Stauch, J. E., Toth, B. N., and Robinson, L. M. Routine vaginal examinations during labor. Amer. J. Obstet. Gynec., 92:310, 1965.

Shenker, L. Fetal electrocardiography. Obstet. Gynec. Survey, 21:367, 1966.

10 Anterior Positions of the Occiput and the Normal Mechanism of Labor

LEFT OCCIPUT ANTERIOR: LOA

LOA is a common longitudinal cephalic presentation. The attitude is flexion, the presenting part is the posterior part of the vertex and the posterior fontanelle, and the denominator is the occiput (O).

Diagnosis of Position: LOA

Abdominal Examination

1. The lie is longitudinal. The long axis of the fetus is parallel to the long axis of the mother.
2. The head is at, or in, the pelvis.
3. The back is on the left and anterior. It is palpated easily, except in obese women.
4. The small parts are on the right and are not felt clearly.
5. The breech is in the fundus of the uterus.
6. The cephalic prominence (in this case the forehead) is on the right. When the attitude is flexion, the cephalic prominence and the back are on opposite sides. The reverse is true in attitudes of extension.

Fetal Heart

The fetal heart is heard loudest in the left lower quadrant of the mother's abdomen. In attitudes of flexion the fetal heart rate is transmitted through the baby's back. The point of maximum intensity varies with the degree of rotation. As the child's back approaches the midline of the maternal abdomen, so does the point where the fetal heart is heard most strongly. Therefore, in a left anterior position, it will be heard below the umbilicus and somewhere to the left of the midline, depending on the exact situation of the back.

Vaginal Examination

1. The station of the head is noted, whether it is above, at, or below the ischial spines.
2. If the cervix is dilated, the suture lines and the fontanelles of the baby's head can be felt. In the LOA position the sagittal suture is in the right oblique diameter of the pelvis.
3. The small posterior fontanelle is anterior and to the mother's left.
4. The bregma is posterior and to the right.
5. Since the head is probably flexed, the occiput is a little lower than the brow.

X-ray Examination

In problem cases the position and station of the presenting part, as well as the adequacy of the pelvis in relation to the fetus, may be determined by radiologic methods.

Fig. 1A. Abdominal view.

Fig. 1B. Vaginal view.

The Normal Mechanism of Labor: LOA

The mechanism of labor as we know it today was described first by William Smellie in the eighteenth century. It is the way the baby adapts itself to, and passes through, the maternal pelvis. There are six movements with considerable overlapping. The following description is for left anterior positions of the occiput.

Descent

Descent, which includes engagement in the right oblique diameter of the pelvis, continues throughout normal labor as the baby passes through the birth canal. The other movements are superimposed on it. In primigravidas considerable descent should have taken place before the onset of labor in the process of engagement, provided there is no disproportion and the lower uterine segment is well formed. In multiparas engagement may not take place until good labor has set in. Descent is brought about by the downward pressure of the uterine contractions, aided in the second stage by the bearing-down efforts of the patient and to a minimal extent by gravity.

Flexion

Partial flexion exists before the onset of labor, since this is the natural attitude of the fetus in utero. Resistance to descent leads to increased flexion. The occiput descends in advance of the sinciput, the posterior fontanelle is lower than the bregma, and the baby's chin approaches its chest. This usually takes place at the inlet, but it may not be complete until the presenting part reaches the pelvic floor. The effect of flexion is to change the presenting diameter from the occipitofrontal of 11.0 cm to the smaller and rounder suboccipitobregmatic of 9.5 cm. Since the fit between fetal head and maternal pelvis may be snug, the reduction of 1.5 cm in the presenting diameter is important.

A. Vaginal view.

B. Lateral view.

Fig. 2. L.O.A.: onset of labor.

A. Vaginal view.

B. Lateral view.

Fig. 3. L.O.A.: descent and flexion of the head.

Internal Rotation

In the majority of pelves the inlet is a transverse oval. The anteroposterior diameter of the midpelvis is a little longer than the transverse diameter. The outlet is an anteroposterior oval. The fetal head is an anteroposterior oval. The long axis of the fetal head must fit into the long axis of the maternal pelvis. Hence, the head, which entered the pelvis in the transverse or oblique diameter, must rotate internally to the anteroposterior diameter in order that it can be born. This is the purpose of internal rotation.

The occiput now leads the way to the midpelvis, where it makes contact with the pelvic floor (the levator ani muscles and fascia). Here the occiput rotates 45 degrees to the right (toward the midline). The sagittal suture turns from the right oblique diameter to the anteroposterior diameter of the pelvis: LOA to OA. The occiput comes to lie near the pubic symphysis and the sinciput near the sacrum.

The head rotates from the right oblique diameter to the anteroposterior diameter of the pelvis. The shoulders, however, remain in the left oblique diameter. Thus, the normal relationship of the long axis of the head to the long axis of the shoulders is changed, and the neck undergoes a twist of 45 degrees. This situation is maintained as long as the head is in the pelvis.

We do not know accurately why the fetal head which entered the pelvis in the transverse or oblique diameter rotates so that the occiput turns anteriorly in the great majority of cases, and posteriorly in so few. One explanation is based on pelvic architecture. Both the bones and the soft tissues play a part. The ischial spines extend into the pelvic cavity. The sidewalls of the pelvis anterior to the spines curve forward, downward, and medially. The pelvic floor, made up of the levator ani muscles and fascia, slopes downward, forward, and medially. The part of the head that reaches the pelvic floor and ischial spines first is rotated anteriorly by these structures. In most cases the head is well flexed when it reaches the pelvic floor, and the occiput is lower than the sinciput. Hence the occiput strikes the pelvic floor first and is rotated anteriorly under the pubic symphysis.

This does not explain why some well-flexed heads in the LOT and ROT positions (proved by x-ray) do rotate posteriorly. Nor do the theories based upon pelvic architecture explain the situation where, in the same patient, the head will rotate anteriorly in one labor and posteriorly in another. In truth we do not know the exact reasons for internal rotation taking place in the way that it does. In most labors internal rotation is complete when the head reaches the pelvic floor, or soon after. Early internal rotation is frequent in multiparas and in patients having efficient uterine contractions. Internal rotation takes place mainly in the second stage of labor.

Fig. 4B. Lateral view.

Fig. 4A. Vaginal view.

Fig. 4C. Antero-posterior view.

Extension

Extension is basically the result of two forces: 1, the uterine contractions exerting downward pressure; and 2, the pelvic floor offering resistance. It must be pointed out that the anterior wall of the pelvis (the pubis) is only 4 to 5 cm long, while the posterior wall (the sacrum) is 10 to 15 cm in length. Hence, the sinciput has a greater distance to travel than the occiput. As the flexed head continues its descent there is bulging of the perineum followed by crowning. The occiput passes through the outlet slowly and the nape of the neck pivots in the subpubic angle. Then by a rapid process of extension, the sinciput sweeps along the sacrum, and the bregma, forehead, nose, mouth, and chin are born in succession over the perineum.

Fig. 5A. Vaginal view.

Fig. 5B. Lateral view.

Restitution

When the head reaches the pelvic floor the shoulders enter the pelvis. Since the shoulders remain in the oblique diameter while the head rotates anteriorly, the neck becomes twisted. Once the head is born and free of the pelvis, the neck untwists and the head restitutes back 45 degrees (OA to LOA) to resume the normal relationship with the shoulders and its original position in the pelvis.

Fig. 6B. Lateral view.

Fig. 6A. Vaginal view.

Fig. 6C. Antero-posterior view.

External Rotation

External rotation of the head is really the outward manifestation of internal rotation of the shoulders. As the shoulders reach the pelvic floor the lower anterior shoulder is rotated forward under the symphysis, and the bisacromial diameter turns from the left oblique to the anteroposterior diameter of the pelvis. In this way the long diameter of the shoulders can fit the long diameter of the outlet. The head, which had already restituted 45 degrees to resume its normal relationship to the shoulders, now rotates another 45 degrees to maintain it: LOA to LOT.

Fig. 7B.   Lateral view.

Fig. 7A.   Vaginal view.

Fig. 7C.   Antero-posterior view.

Fig. 8A. Onset of labor.

Fig. 8B. Descent and flexion.

Fig. 8C. Internal rotation: L.O.A. to O.A.

Fig. 9A. Extension.

Fig. 9B. Restitution: O.A. to L.O.A.

Fig. 9C. External rotation: L.O.A. to L.O.T.

Mechanism of the Shoulders

When the head appears at the outlet, the shoulders enter the inlet. The shoulders engage in the oblique diameter opposite to that of the head. For example, in LOA, when the head engages in the right oblique diameter of the inlet, the shoulders engage in the left oblique.

The uterine contractions and the bearing–down efforts of the mother force the baby downward. The anterior shoulder reaches the pelvic floor first and rotates anteriorly under the symphysis. Anterior rotation of the shoulders takes place in a direction opposite to the direction of anterior rotation of the head. The anterior shoulder is born under the pubic symphysis and pivots there. Then the posterior shoulder slides over the perineum by a movement of lateral flexion.

Birth of the Trunk and Extremities

Once the shoulders have been born the rest of the child is delivered by the mother's forcing down, with no special mechanism, and with no difficulty.

Molding

In LOA the presenting suboccipitobregmatic diameter is diminished, and the head is elongated in the verticomental diameter.

Fig. 10.   Birth of anterior shoulder.

Fig. 11.   Birth of posterior shoulder.

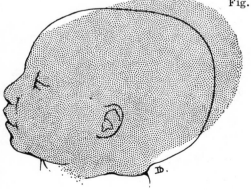

Fig. 12.   Molding: L.O.A.

THE BIRTH OF THE PLACENTA

Separation of the Placenta

Within a few minutes of the delivery of the child the uterine contractions begin again. Because the fetus is no longer in the uterus, the extent of the retraction of the upper segment is larger than in the first and second stages. This retraction decreases greatly the area of the site of placental attachment. The size of the placenta itself, however, is not reducible. The resultant disparity between the size of the placenta and its area of attachment leads to a cleavage in the spongy layer of the decidua, and in this way the placenta is separated from the wall of the uterus. During the process of separation blood accumulates between the placenta and uterus. When the detachment is complete the blood is released and gushes from the vagina.

Expulsion of the Placenta

Soon after the placenta has separated it is expelled into the vagina by the uterine contractions. From here it is delivered by the bearing–down efforts of the patient. Two methods of expulsion of the placenta have been described. In the Duncan method the lower edge of the placenta comes out first, with the maternal and fetal surfaces appearing together, and the rest of the organ slides down. In the Schultze method the placenta comes out like an inverted umbrella, the shiny fetal side appearing first, and the membranes trailing after. Although the Schultze mechanism suggests fundal implantation, while the Duncan method intimates that the placenta was attached to the wall of the uterus, the exact mechanism of birth of the placenta is of little practical significance.

Control of Hemorrhage

The blood vessels which pass through the myometrium are tortuous and angular. The muscle fibers are arranged in an interlacing network through which the blood vessels pass. After the placenta has separated, retraction leads to a permanent shortening of the uterine muscle fibers. This compresses, kinks, twists, and closes the arterioles and venules in the manner of living ligatures. The blood supply to the placental site is effectively shut off, and bleeding is controlled. If the uterus is atonic and fails to retract properly after the separation of the placenta, the vessels will not be closed off, and a severe postpartum hemorrhage may take place.

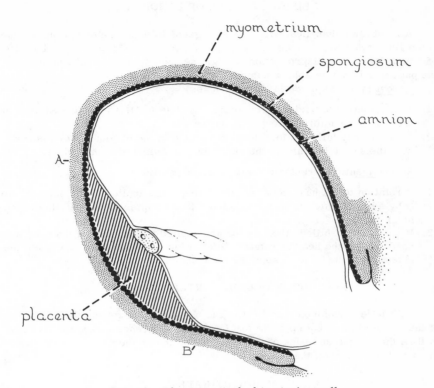

Fig. 13.   Placenta attached to uterine wall.

Fig. 14.   Placenta separated from uterine wall.

CLINICAL COURSE OF LABOR: LOA

Almost always an LOA will turn 45 degrees to bring the occiput under the pubic arch, whence spontaneous delivery takes place. Occasionally, because of minor degrees of disproportion, a rigid perineum, or generalized fatigue, the patient may not be able to complete the second stage.

Arrest may take place in two positions:

1. After rotation to occiput anterior is complete (OA), so that the sagittal suture is in the anteroposterior diameter
2. Rotation may fail, the fetal head remaining in the original LOA position, with the sagittal suture in the right oblique diameter of the pelvis.

Management of arrested occipitoanterior positions:

1. If rotation to OA has occurred, the forceps are applied to the sides of the baby's head, which is then extracted. (See Chapter 25 for details of technic.)
2. If rotation has failed, the forceps are applied to the sides of the baby's head. First the head is rotated with the forceps from LOA to OA and then it is extracted. (See Chapter 25 for technic.)

RIGHT OCCIPUT ANTERIOR: ROA

ROA is less common than LOA. The physical findings and the mechanism of labor are similar but opposite to LOA. The difference lies in the fact that in ROA the occiput and back of the fetus are on the mother's right side, while the small parts are on the left.

BIBLIOGRAPHY

Caldwell, W. E., Moloy, H. C., and D'Esopo, D. A. A roentgenologic study of the mechanism of engagement of the fetal head. Amer. J. Obstet. Gynec., 28:824, 1934.

Calkins, L. A. The etiology of occiput presentations. Amer. J. Obstet. Gynec., 37:618, 1939.

_____ The second stage of labor; internal rotation. Amer. J. Obstet. Gynec., 53:488, 1947.

_____ The second stage of labor. Amer. J. Obstet. Gynec., 57:106, 1949.

Glaister, J. Doctor William Smellie and His Contemporaries. Glasgow, J. MacLehose, 1894.

Javert, C. T., and Steele, K. B. The transverse position and the mechanism of labor. Int. Abstr. Surg., 75:507, 1942.

Johnstone, R. W. William Smellie, the Master of British Midwifery. Edinburgh & London, E. & S. Livingstone Ltd., 1952.

Oxorn, H. William Smellie and the mechanism of labor. Amer. J. Obstet. Gynec., 77:41, 1959.

Smellie, W. Smellie's Treatise on the Theory and Practice of Midwifery. London, New Sydenham Society, 1876-1878.

11 Clinical Course of Normal Labor

DEFINITIONS

Labor: A function of the female by which the products of conception (fetus, amniotic fluid, placenta, and membranes) are separated and expelled from the uterus, through the vagina, and into the outside world.

Abortion: The interruption of the pregnancy before the fetus is viable (capable of existence outside the uterus). A child is believed to reach viability at 26 weeks, or when it has reached 1,000 g in weight.

Premature Labor: The termination of pregnancy after viability but before term. A baby weighing between 1,000 g and 2,499 g is considered to be premature.

Eutocia: Normal labor. A labor is considered to be normal when the child presents by the vertex of the head, when there are no complications, and when the labor is completed by the natural efforts of the mother. It should take no longer than 24 hours.

Prolonged Labor: Labor that lasts over 24 hours.

Dystocia: Abnormal labor.

Expected Date of Confinement: An estimate can be made of this day by going back three months from the first day of the last normal menstrual period and then adding seven days.

THE ONSET OF LABOR

Causes of the Onset of Labor

We do not know the exact reason for the onset of labor, nor why it takes place at about 40 weeks gestation. Several theories have been evolved to explain this phenomenon:

1. It is suggested that when the uterus is stretched to a certain degree, labor begins. The early onset of labor in twins and polyhydramnios is explained in this way.
2. Pressure of the presenting part on the cervix and the lower uterine segment, as well as on the nerve plexuses around the cervix and the vagina, stimulates labor to begin.

101

3. The menstrual cycle recurs every four weeks, and labor usually comes on at the end of 40 weeks or 10 menstrual cycles.
4. Once the uterus has reached term, any emotional or physical factor can set it into labor. Such stimuli include falls, intestinal events such as diarrhea, enemata, and castor oil, or mental shocks.
5. Some believe that a special hormone, produced by the placenta when it has reached term, is responsible for labor's beginning.
6. Placental aging resulting in the drop of the blood levels of estrogen and progesterone is believed by some to cause labor to begin. This has its parallel in the menstrual cycle. With the death of the corpus luteum, the blood levels of estrogen and progesterone drop, and menstruation begins a few days later.

Phenomena Preliminary to the Onset of Labor

1. Lightening occurs two or three weeks before, and is the subjective sensation felt by the mother as the baby settles into the lower uterine segment.
2. Engagement takes place two to three weeks before term in primigravidas.
3. The vaginal secretions increase in amount.
4. Loss of weight is caused by the excretion of body water.
5. The mucous plug is discharged from the cervix.
6. Bloody show is noted.
7. The cervix becomes soft and effaced.
8. Persistent backache is present.
9. False labor pains occur with variable frequency.

TRUE AND FALSE LABOR

The Signs of True Labor

1. The uterine contractions occur at regular intervals. Coming every 20 or 30 minutes at the beginning, the contractions get closer together. As labor proceeds the contractions increase in duration and severity.
2. The uterine systoles are painful.
3. The hardening of the uterus is palpable.
4. Pain is felt both in the back and in the front of the abdomen.
5. True labor is effective in dilating the cervix.
6. The presenting part descends.
7. The head is fixed between pains.
8. Bulging of the membranes is a frequent result.

False Labor Pains

These are inefficient contractions of the uterus or painful spasms of the intestines, bladder, and abdominal wall muscles. They appear a few days to a month before term. They are sometimes brought on by a digestive upset or a strong laxative. Usually they start on their own. They are irregular and short, and are felt more in the front than in the back.

There may be either no accompanying uterine contraction at all, or one that lasts only a few seconds. The uterus does not become stony hard, and can be indented with the finger. These contractions are inefficient in pushing down the presenting part, and do not bring about progressive effacement and dilatation of the cervix.

False labor pains can have the harmful effect of tiring out the patient, so that when true labor does come on she is in poor condition, both mentally and physically. Treatment is directed to the cause if there is one, or the physician can prescribe an efficient sedative which will stop the false labor pains, but will not interfere with true labor.

True Labor	False Labor
Pains occur at regular intervals	Irregular
Intervals gradually shorten	No change
Duration and severity increase	No change
Pain starts in back and moves to the front	Pain is mainly in the front
Walking increases the intensity	No change
Association between the degree of uterine hardening and intensity of pain	No relationship
Bloody show is present often	No show
Cervix becomes effaced and dilated	No change in cervix
Descent of presenting part	No descent
Head is fixed between pains	Head remains free
Sedation will not stop true labor	An efficient sedative will stop false labor pains

THE STAGES OF LABOR

First stage: From the onset of true labor to complete dilatation of the cervix. It lasts from 6 to 18 hours in a primigravida, and from 2 to 10 hours in a multipara.

Second stage: From the complete dilatation of the cervix to the birth of the baby. It takes 30 minutes to 3 hours in a primigravida, and 5 to 30 minutes in the multipara. The median duration is slightly under 20 minutes in multiparas, and just under 50 minutes for primigravidas.

Third stage: From the birth of the baby to the delivery of the placenta. It takes 5 to 30 minutes.

Fourth stage: From the birth of the placenta until the postpartum condition of the patient has become stabilized.

FIRST STAGE OF LABOR

The first stage of labor lasts from the onset of true labor to full dilatation of the cervix. The contractions are intermittent and painful, and the hardening of the uterus is felt easily by a hand on the abdomen. The pains become more frequent and more severe as labor proceeds. As a rule they begin in the back and pass to the front of the abdomen and the upper thighs.

Dilatation of the Cervix

During pregnancy the cervix is of normal length. Toward the end of pregnancy, the cervix begins to be effaced, becoming shorter, and the internal os starts to disappear as the cervical canal becomes part of the lower uterine segment. Ideally the cervix should be ripe at the onset of labor. A ripe cervix is one that is soft, less than half an inch in length, admits a finger easily, and is dilatable. When the cervix is ripe, it is a sign that the uterus is ready to begin labor. When these conditions are present induction of labor is feasible. During labor the cervix shortens further, and the external os dilates. When the os has opened enough (average 10 cm) to permit the passage of the fetal head it is said to be fully dilated.

Fig. 1.   Cervix thick and closed.   Fig. 2.   Cervix effaced.

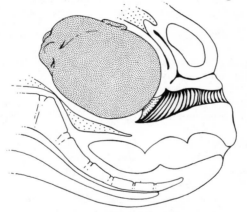

Fig. 3.   Cervix effaced and dilated 2 to 3 cm.

Fig. 4.   Cervix half open.   Fig. 5.   Cervix fully dilated and
retracted.

The Bag of Waters: The Membranes

The fetus lies in a sac with an inner layer of amnion and an outer covering of chorion. The sac is filled with the amniotic fluid. As labor proceeds and the internal os becomes effaced and opens, the membranes separate from the lower uterine segment. The lower pole of the membranes bulges a little with each contraction and may adopt various shapes:

1. The protruding part may have the shape of a watch glass containing a small amount of amniotic fluid. This is called the "forewaters."
2. In other cases the membranes point into the cervix like a cone.
3. Still again, the bag may hang into the vagina.
4. In some cases the membranes are applied so tightly to the fetal head that no bag forms.

Frequently the membranes rupture near the end of the second stage, but this event can take place at any time during or before labor. When the membranes rupture the fluid may come away with a gush, or it may dribble away. On occasion it is difficult to know whether the membranes are ruptured or intact.

Methods of diagnosing whether the bag of waters has ruptured include:

1. Seeing the fluid escaping from the vagina spontaneously or by pressure on the fundus
2. Putting a speculum in the vagina and seeing whether fluid is coming from the cervix. The amount may be increased by pressure on the fundus of the uterus.
3. Grasping the fetal scalp with a forceps. If hair is seen in the forceps, it is proof that the membranes have ruptured.
4. The passage of meconium
5. Use of Nitrazine paper to determine the pH of the vaginal fluid. The vagina, normally acid in pH, becomes neutral or alkaline when contaminated with alkaline amniotic fluid. Hence, an alkaline pH in the vagina suggests that the membranes are ruptured.
6. Use of special staining of vaginal fluid, followed by microscopic search for components of amniotic fluid, including lanugo hairs, fetal squamous cells, and fat. Quinaldine blue stains fetal cells only faintly, while vaginal squamous cells become dark.
7. The arborization test depends on the property of dried amniotic fluid to form crystals in an arborization pattern. A few drops of vaginal fluid are aspirated from the vagina by a bulb syringe, and are placed on a clean, dry glass slide. After waiting for 5 to 7 minutes for drying to take place, the slide is examined under the low power microscope for identification of the arborization pattern.

A bag of waters which hangs into the vagina is of little or no help in dilating the cervix; it may impede labor by filling the vagina and preventing the descent of the fetal head. The intact bag of amniotic fluid does little to help labor progress. In normal cases after the membranes have ruptured (spontaneously or artificially) the uterine contractions are more efficient and labor progresses faster. However, in dysfunctional labor, or in the presence of an unripe cervix (one that is thick, hard, and closed), amniotomy is ineffectual in shortening labor, and may complicate the situation by introducing an irreversible factor.

Fig. 6. Forewaters: watch glass shape.

Fig. 7. Forewaters: cone into the cervix.

Fig. 8. Bag of waters in the vagina.

Fig. 9. No forewaters.

Management of the First Stage of Labor

1. As long as the patient is healthy, the presentation normal, the presenting part well engaged, and the fetus in good condition, the parturient woman may walk about or be in bed as she wishes.
2. The patient's condition and progress is checked periodically. The pulse, temperature, and blood pressure are measured every 4 hours, or more often if necessary.
3. The fetal heart is auscultated every 15 minutes if normal, and more frequently if irregular or slow.
4. The progress of labor is followed by abdominal, rectal, or vaginal examination to note the position of the baby, the station of the presenting part, and the dilatation of the cervix. These examinations should be done only often enough to ensure the safe conduct of labor.
5. The patient is given an enema. This has the effect of cleaning the rectum and of stimulating the contractions.
6. Overdistension of the bladder is obviated by urging the patient to pass urine every few hours. If she is not able to do so catheterization may be necessary, since a full bladder impedes progress.
7. Adequate amounts of fluids and nourishment are essential. In most normal labors sugared drinks or clear soups can be taken by mouth. Since solid foods remain in the stomach during labor, tend to be vomited, and increase the danger of aspiration, they should not be given. If the patient is unable to take enough orally, an intravenous infusion of glucose in water is given.
8. The patient must rest and she must maintain her self-restraint. This is important, for lost control is difficult to regain. The attendants can help the patient by continual reassurance, frequent encouragement, and judicious sedation. This has the effect of helping the patient to rest, assisting her to keep control, and accelerating the progress of labor by the patient's relaxing. When the pains are severe an analgesic preparation may be given (see Chapter   ). Since there is a limit to the amount of drugs which can be administered without harming the baby or interfering with labor, these must be given in logical dosage and sequence. It has been said that the best sedative for a woman in labor is to see her doctor at the side of the bed.
9. During the first stage the patient is impressed continually with the importance of relaxing with the contractions. Bearing down must be avoided. It does nothing to improve progress. Bearing down comes into its own when the cervix is fully dilated, and not before. It has only bad effects:
   a. It delays cervical dilatation.
   b. It tires out the patient needlessly.
   c. It forces down the uterus and stretches the supporting ligaments, predisposing to later prolapse.

10. Measures to improve the character and the efficiency of the contractions
    include:
    a. A hot soap suds enema
    b. Walking, which increases stimulation of the cervix and reflexly intensi-
       fies the uterine contractions
    c. Artificial rupture of the membranes
    d. Oxytocin (see Chapter 36)
11. While the setting up of an intravenous infusion of 5 percent glucose in water
    is often useful in normal labor, it is mandatory in the complicated case,
    and for these reasons:
    a. Fluids and nourishment can be given without provoking emesis. The pa-
       tient who cannot take adequate fluids by mouth, and the woman who is
       nauseated or is vomiting, can be maintained in a state of good hydration.
    b. Analgesics in small amounts can be administered for rapid effect.
    c. When the uterine action is inefficient pitocin added to the solution will
       improve the labor.
    d. When there is excessive bleeding in the third or fourth stages, oxytocic
       agents can be given quickly.
    e. Blood and plasma expanders may be infused without delay.
    f. Once hypotension has occurred the veins often collapse and it is difficult
       to insert a needle. Having an infusion going obviates this problem.

Passage of Meconium in Cephalic Presentations

The passage per vaginam of meconium or meconium stained amniotic fluid
in a cephalic presentation is a sign of fetal distress. It is believed to result
from the relaxation of the rectal sphincter and increased peristalsis as a con-
sequence of anoxia. Etiologic factors include cord entanglements, prolonged
labor, and toxemia of pregnancy. In most cases no cause is found.

The incidence of meconium staining is around 5 percent. The occurrence
of stillbirth, when this is the only sign, is low, but the number of newborn requiring resuscitation is higher than the overall incidence.

When meconium is passed, the fetal heart must be observed closely.
Should there be a significant alteration in the rate and rhythm of the fetal heart,
immediate delivery may be needed to save the child. Operative delivery is not
indicated on the basis of meconium staining alone.

In breech presentations the passage of meconium is caused by the pressure
of the uterine contractions on the fetal intestines, and is not accepted as a sign
of anoxia or fetal distress.

SECOND STAGE OF LABOR

The second stage of labor lasts from the end of the first stage, when the cervix has reached full dilatation, to the birth of the baby. As the patient passes through the end of the first stage and into the second stage, the contractions become more frequent and are accompanied by some of the worst pain of the whole labor. Once the second stage is achieved the discomfort is less.

Indications that the second stage has started:

1. There is an increase in bloody show.
2. The patient wants to bear down with each contraction.
3. She feels pressure on the rectum accompanied by the desire to defecate.
4. Nausea and retching occur frequently as the cervix reaches full dilatation.

These signs are not infallible and the condition of the cervix and the station of the presenting part must be confirmed by rectal examination.

Position for Delivery

The Left Lateral or Sims Position

The left lateral or Sims position is best when the delivery is being conducted at home in the patient's bed. The advantages of this include the following:

1. Comfort for the patient and lack of restraint while awaiting delivery
2. Release of pressure of the pregnant uterus on the inferior vena cava (a situation which sometimes results in the supine hypotensive syndrome)
3. If the patient vomits, drainage from the pharynx is facilitated.
4. The bearing-down efforts are under better control, allowing slow delivery of the head, and less perineal lacerations.

This is, however, not a good position in which to handle difficult forceps deliveries. The management of the third stage is awkward, and vaginal and cervical lacerations are not accessible for repair.

The Dorsal Position

In the dorsal position the patient lies on her back on the table or in bed, with the knees flexed. This position approaches the primitive squatting position, and enables the woman to bear down harder.

The Lithotomy Position

The lithotomy position is the best. Here the patient lies with her legs in stirrups, and her buttocks close to the lower edge of the table. The patient is in the ideal position for the attendant to deal with any complications which may arise.

Fig. 10.   Sims' left lateral position.

Fig. 11.   Dorsal position.

Fig. 12.   Lithotomy position.

Bearing Down by the Patient

During the first stage, labor will progress faster, and the patient will feel less pain, if she breathes slowly and deeply during each uterine contraction, and avoids bearing down. The more effective the relaxation, the more rapid will be the cervical dilatation. In the second stage, on the other hand, the patient has to work hard. She must force down with each contraction, and rest between them. The more effectively she bears down, the shorter will be the second stage. In the early part of the second stage the abdominal muscles, which are responsible for the bearing-down efforts, are under the patient's complete control. Later on she sometimes finds it impossible to stop bearing down even if she wants to. This action will be more efficient if the patient braces herself against a solid object. On delivery tables hand bars are provided. When the contraction comes on the patient takes one or two deep breaths and then holds her breath to fix the diaphragm. She then pulls on the hand bars, and at the same time bears down as hard, and for as long a period, as she can. With each contraction the pressure on the perineum and rectum stimulates the patient to move toward the head of the table and out of the best position. Shoulder braces will prevent this.

Descent, Crowning, and Spontaneous Birth of the Head

With each contraction the head advances and then recedes as the uterus relaxes. Each time a little ground is gained. The introitus becomes an anteroposterior slit, then an oval, and finally a circular opening. The pressure of the head thins out the perineum. Feces may be forced out of the rectum. As the anus opens, the anterior wall of the rectum bulges through. With descent the occiput comes to lie under the pubic symphysis. The head continues to advance and recede with the contractions, until a strong one forces the largest diameter of the head through the vulva (crowning). Once this has occurred there is no going back, and by a process of extension the head is born, as the bregma, forehead, nose, mouth, and chin appear over the perineum. At the stage where the head is passing through the introitus the patient has the sensation of being torn apart. Laceration of the vulva sometimes occurs.

The head then falls back toward the anus. Once it is out of the vagina it restitutes as the neck untwists. After a few moments, external rotation takes place as the shoulders move from the oblique to the anteroposterior diameter of the pelvis.

DILATATION OF THE INTROITUS

Fig. 13. Introitus: antero-posterior slit.

Fig. 14. Introitus: oval opening.

Fig. 15. Introitus: circular shape.

BIRTH OF THE HEAD

Fig. 16. Crowning.

Fig. 17. Extension.

Fig. 18. Birth.

Fig. 19. Restitution.

Fig. 20. External rotation.

Assisted Delivery of the Head

Many women can deliver their babies spontaneously, in bed, and without assistance. The advantages of having an accoucheur in attendance and the patient on a delivery table are: 1, should an unexpected complication arise, immediate action can be carried out; 2, the obstetrician is able to assist the patient so that the incidence of large and uncontrolled lacerations is reduced.

Controlled Birth of the Head

Procedures designed to promote the leisurely egress of the fetal head should be performed. The slow and gradual birth of the head will reduce the incidence of lacerations. The attendant must guard against a sudden bursting out of the head, as this leads to large and jagged lacerations, which in the extreme may extend through the anal sphincter and into the rectum.

1. Management of bearing-down efforts: The correct management of the bearing-down efforts of the parturient is important. The two forces responsible for the birth of the child are uterine contractions and bearing-down forces. The uterine contractions are involuntary, but the bearing-down forces can be controlled. During the first part of the second stage the patient must bear down during the uterine contractions to expedite progress. However, during the actual delivery, the too rapid emergence of the fetal head can be slowed by the patient's ceasing to bear down. This is accomplished best by the patient's panting rapidly through the open mouth during the contraction. When the patient breathes in and out rapidly, the diaphragm moves, making it impossible for effective intra-abdominal pressure to be built up, and so the power to bear down is lost.

2. Manual pressure: In most cases, by gentle manual pressure against the baby's head, the speed of delivery can be reduced. Occasionally the propulsive force is so great that it is impossible, or even dangerous, to try and slow down the birth. The head should never be held back forcibly.

3. The Ritgen maneuver: The objective of this maneuver is to encourage extension of the fetal head, and thus expedite its birth. This procedure is performed ideally between uterine contractions. During this interval the head can be delivered slowly, gradually, and under the obstetrician's complete control. Further, the soft tissues are more relaxed and tissue damage is less. The maneuver cannot be carried out before the occiput has come under the symphysis. It is done when the suboccipitofrontal diameter is ready to be born.

    The operator's hand, covered with a towel or a pad, is placed so that the fingers are behind the maternal anus. Extension of the fetal head is furthered by pressing against the baby's face, preferably the chin, through the rectum. The bregma, forehead, and face are born in that order. The other hand is placed against the baby's head to control the speed of its delivery. Sometimes fundal pressure is needed to deliver the head, or if the patient is awake she can bear down gently.

Fig. 21. Ritgen maneuver.

Fig. 22. Hooking out the chin.

4. Hooking out the chin: Occasionally the chin gets stuck against the perineum. It is extracted by inserting the fingers into the vagina, over the cheek and under the chin, which is then brought out over the perineum.

5. Episiotomy: When large lacerations seem inevitable it is better to make an incision into the perineum (episiotomy). In this way the direction and size of the cut can be controlled, and tears into the rectum can be obviated.

Following Delivery of the Head

1. The head should be supported as it restitutes and rotates externally.
2. The face should be wiped gently and mucus aspirated from the mouth and throat by a small soft rubber bulb syringe.
3. The region of the neck is explored for coils of umbilical cord. If the cord is around the neck loosely it can be slipped over the head. If it is coiled around the neck tightly, it must be clamped doubly, cut between the clamps, and then unwound.

Birth of the Body

Birth of the Shoulders

By the time the shoulders are ready for delivery, restitution has occurred and external rotation is taking place. During a uterine contraction the patient is asked to bear down. If the patient is anesthetized, or unable to force down, pressure is exerted by an attendant on the fundus of the uterus. At the same time the head is grasped with the hands on the parietal bones, or with one hand over the face and the other on the occiput; the head is then depressed toward the rectum. This enables the anterior shoulder to emerge under the symphysis pubis. When this has been achieved the head is raised so that the posterior shoulder can be born over the perineum. It must be emphasized that the operator merely lowers and lifts the baby's head to facilitate the birth of the shoulders. He does not exert great traction, as this carries with it the danger of damaging the nerve plexus in the neck. The force which actually pushes out the shoulder is provided by the bearing-down efforts of the mother if she is awake, and by pressure on the fundus by an assistant if the patient is asleep.

Birth of the Trunk and Lower Limbs

Once the head and shoulders have been delivered, the rest of the body slips out easily, usually with a gush of amniotic fluid.

Fig. 23.   Lowering of the fetal head.

Fig. 24.   Delivery of anterior shoulder.

Fig. 25.   Delivery of posterior shoulder.

Fig. 26. Holding the baby.

Immediate Care of the Baby

Once the infant is born it should be held head down for a few moments to promote drainage of mucus. The best way of holding the baby is to place it with the back on the attendant's forearm; one leg is tucked between the doctor's arm and his side to prevent the infant from rolling off; the neck is between the third and fourth fingers; the shoulders rest on the palmar surfaces of the fingers; and the baby's head is below the operator's hand. The advantages of this method are:

1. The infant is held securely and cannot slip between the fingers.
2. The head is maintained in slight extension which straightens the trachea and helps drainage.
3. The baby is held in a fixed position so that the trachea can be milked down, the mucus aspirated from the mouth and throat, and any other needed procedure can be carried out without the infant's swinging like a pendulum, which it does when it is held by the ankles.

The baby is then placed on the mother's abdomen. Further suction is carried out as needed. The umbilical cord is then tied doubly with cord tapes, or special mechanical ties may be employed. Some prefer to delay the tying of the cord until it stops pulsating so that the baby can get an additional supply of blood. If this is the belief, the baby must be held lower than the placenta or the blood will not reach it.

The infant is then weighed and placed in its cot. The eyes are treated with silver nitrate or an antibiotic ointment to prevent ophthalmia neonatorum.

THIRD STAGE OF LABOR

The Birth of the Placenta

The delivery of the placenta occurs in two stages: 1, separation of the placenta from the wall of the uterus and into the lower uterine segment and/or the vagina; and 2, the actual expulsion of the placenta out of the birth canal.

Separation of the Placenta

Placental separation takes place, as a rule, within 5 minutes of the end of the second stage. Signs which suggest that detachment has taken place include:

1. A gush of blood from the vagina
2. A lengthening of the umbilical cord outside the vulva
3. A rising of the uterine fundus in the abdomen as the placenta passes from the uterus into the vagina
4. The uterus becoming firm and globular

Expulsion of the Placenta

When these signs have appeared the placenta is ready for expression. If the patient is awake she is asked to bear down while gentle traction is exerted on the cord. If she is asleep or unable to bear down, pressure is made on the uterine fundus and the placenta is delivered in this way. It is wise to avoid rough manipulations of the uterus before separation of the placenta has taken place. This will not hasten delivery of the placenta, but may lead to excessive bleeding.

The actual birth of the placenta takes place in one of two ways:

1. The Duncan method (Dirty Duncan): When the rough maternal edge comes first
2. The Schultze mechanism (Shiny Schultze): When the placenta comes out like an inverted umbrella with the glistening fetal membranes leading the way

Examination of the Delivered Placenta

Examination of the delivered placenta is performed to see that no parts are missing, and hence, left in the uterus. The finding of torn blood vessels along the edge suggests that an accessory lobe may have remained in the uterus. Some obstetricians feel that examination of the placenta does not ensure that fragments have not been left behind, and they explore the uterine cavity manually after each delivery.

Delayed Separation and Delivery of the Placenta

Delayed separation and delivery of the placenta may be the result of:

1. Placenta separated but trapped in the uterus by the cervix
2. Placenta separated incompletely
3. Placenta not separated at all
4. Placenta accreta, where the decidua is deficient, and the chorionic villi have grown into the myometrium.

Manual Removal of the Placenta

At one time invasion of the postpartum uterus was believed to be so dangerous a procedure that a placenta which did not deliver spontaneously was left in situ even for days. Today we feel that prolonged retention of the afterbirth increases the danger of infection and hemorrhage. Current practice is to remove the placenta manually if it does not deliver within 30 minutes of the birth of the baby, provided bleeding is not excessive. If hemorrhage is profuse, the placenta must be removed immediately (see Chapter 38). The average blood loss in the third stage is from 200 to 250 ml.

Manual Exploration of the Uterus

Manual exploration of the uterus is mandatory:

1. When examination of the placenta is inconclusive or there is suspicion that something has been left in the uterus
2. After a traumatic delivery to rule out lacerations of the uterus and cervix
3. When there is excessive postpartum bleeding
4. When a congenital anomaly of the uterus is suspected

The most common cause of excessive bleeding is the mismanagement of the third stage. The most frequent fault is to try to hasten the delivery of the placenta before it has separated. Kneading or massaging the uterus roughly when it is not ready to contract may cause partial separation of the placenta, and result in a postpartum hemorrhage.

Oxytocics in the Placental Stage

These are drugs which stimulate the uterus to contract. Posterior pituitary extract causes clonic rhythmic contractions. The ergot alkaloids bring on a tonic type of contraction. The purpose of using these substances is to hasten placental delivery and so to reduce uterine blood loss.

Many clinics use these drugs routinely. However, a recent study has shown that, while patients who were not given oxytocic drugs in the placental stage had a higher incidence of hemorrhage and required additional treatment in the form of an oxytocic agent, 88 percent of this group had no difficulty in the fourth stage of labor. On the other hand, 5 percent of those who did receive an oxytocic drug developed uterine atony in spite of the preventive treatment.

Pitocin and Syntocinon

Pitocin was originally the trade name for posterior pituitary extract which had been purified by removing the vasopressor substances almost completely. Today both Pitocin and Syntocinon are trade names for synthetic oxytocin. These substances may be given in several ways:

1. 10 units intramuscularly after the birth of the baby
2. 10 units intramuscularly after delivery of the placenta
3. As an intravenous infusion using 5 or 10 units of oxytocin per liter of 5 percent glucose in water, and given either before or after placental separation.

Ergometrine

Ergometrine is given most commonly after the end of the third stage, either intramuscularly in the amount of 0.5 mg, or intravenously in the dosage of 0.125 or 0.25 mg. A popular method of using ergometrine is to give 0.125 mg intravenously when the anterior shoulder has come out under the symphysis pubis and the rest of the baby can be delivered at will. The birth of the rest of the baby is delayed for 10 or 15 seconds. This gives the ergometrine time to reach the uterus and to stimulate it to contract. The baby's buttocks are still in the uterine cervix, and will hold it open, so that the placenta will be expelled from the uterus literally on the baby's heels. The aim of this technic is to speed expulsion of the placenta and to reduce bleeding. Before employing this method the presence of twins must be ruled out. A rare complication is spasm of the cervix trapping the placenta. In such a case one has to wait for the spasm to wear off.

Repair of Lacerations

The cervix, vagina, and perineum must be examined carefully, lacerations repaired, and bleeding controlled.

FOURTH STAGE OF LABOR

The patient is kept in the delivery suite for one hour postpartum under close observation. She is checked for bleeding, the blood pressure is measured, and the pulse is counted. The third stage and the hour after delivery are more dangerous to the mother than any other time.

Before the doctor leaves the patient he must do the following:

1. Feel the uterus through the abdomen to be sure it is firm and not filling with blood
2. Look at the introitus to see that there is no hemorrhage
3. See that the mother's vital signs are normal and that she is in good condition
4. Examine the baby to be certain that it is breathing well and that the color and tone are normal

ASEPSIS AND ANTISEPSIS

Anatomic Factors

The birth passage is divided into three parts:

1. The vulva and vaginal orifice which are loaded with bacteria of all kinds
2. The vagina which contains some vaginal bacteria with their acid secretion, a few fungi, and a number of leukocytes
3. The uterine cavity which is separated from the vagina by the mucous plug. Here there are no organisms.

Natural Safeguards

1. In the first and second stages there is an increase in the vaginal secretion which cleans the passage.
2. When the membranes rupture the amniotic fluid flushes out the vagina.
3. As the baby passes through the vagina it distends the walls. Usually the birth of the baby is accompanied by another discharge of amniotic fluid, and this helps to wash out the vagina.
4. As the membranes and placenta pass through the vagina they also exert a cleaning, mop-like action.

Cleansing Procedures

The patient is given a bath, the vulva is shaved and washed, the rectum is cleaned by an enema, and the bladder is prevented from overfilling.

Personal Care by the Attendants

All who come in contact with the patient in labor should:

1. Wash hands carefully
2. Wear gloves
3. Wear sterile masks to prevent passing bacteria from the nose and throat
4. Wear sterile gowns when delivering the patient
5. Avoid contact with infected cases

BIBLIOGRAPHY

Friedman, E. A., and Sachtleben, M. Amniotomy and the course of labor. Obstet. Gynec., 22:755, 1963.

Howard, W. F., McFadden, P. R., and Keetel, W. C. Oxytocic drugs in the fourth stage of labor. J. A. M. A., 189:411, 1964.

Jones, R. F., Warren, B. L., and Thorton, W. N. Planned postpartum exploration of uterus, cervix, and vagina. Obstet. Gynec., 27:699, 1966.

Leonard, J. L. The significance of meconium stained amniotic fluid in cephalic presentation. Obstet. Gynec., 20:320, 1962.

Tricomi, V., Hall, J. E., Bittar, A., and Chambers, D. Arborization test for the detection of ruptured fetal membranes. Obstet. Gynec., 27:275, 1966.

Van Praagh, I., and Hendricks, C. H. The effect of amniotomy during labor in multiparas. Obstet. Gynec., 24:258, 1964.

12 Transverse Positions of the Occiput

Engagement is more frequent in the transverse diameter of the inlet than in the oblique, and LOT is the most common position at the onset of labor.

Diagnosis of Position: LOT

Abdominal Examination

1. The lie is longitudinal
2. The head is at, or in, the pelvis.
3. The back is on the left and toward the mother's flank.
4. The small parts are on the right, and sometimes they can be felt clearly.
5. The breech is in the fundus of the uterus.
6. The cephalic prominence (forehead) is on the right.

Fetal Heart

The fetal heart is heard loudest in the left lower quadrant of the mother's abdomen.

Vaginal Examination

1. The sagittal suture is in the transverse diameter of the pelvis. If the head is in synclitism the sagittal suture will be midway between the symphysis pubis and the promontory of the sacrum. If there is anterior asynclitism the sagittal suture will be nearer the sacral promontory, while with posterior asynclitism it will be closer to the pubic symphysis.
2. The small posterior fontanelle is toward the mother's left, at 3 o'clock.
3. The bregma is on the right, at 9 o'clock.
4. If there is flexion the occiput is lower than the brow. If flexion is poor the occiput and brow are almost at the same level in the pelvis.

Fig. 1.   Left Occiput Transverse.

Fig. 2.   L. O. T.: synclitism.

Fig. 3.   L. O. T.: posterior asynclitism.

Fig. 4.   L. O. T.: anterior asynclitism.

The Mechanism of Labor: LOT

Descent

Descent includes engagement, which may have taken place before labor. Descent continues throughout labor.

Flexion

Resistance to descent causes the head to flex so that the chin approaches the chest. This reduces the presenting diameter by 1.5 cm. The occipitofrontal diameter of 11.0 cm is replaced by the suboccipitobregmatic diameter of 9.5 cm.

Internal Rotation

The head enters the pelvis with the sagittal suture in the transverse diameter of the inlet and the occiput at 3 o'clock. The occiput then rotates 90 degrees to arrive under the pubic symphysis. The sinciput comes to lie anterior to the sacrum. The sequence is LOT to LOA to OA. The shoulders lag behind 45 degrees so that when the sagittal suture of the head is in the anteroposterior diameter of the pelvis, the shoulders are in the left oblique. Thus the neck is twisted.

Fig. 5. L.O.T.: onset of labor.

Fig. 6. Descent and flexion.

Fig. 7. Internal rotation:
L.O.T. to L.O.A.

Fig. 8. Internal rotation:
L.O.A. to O.A.

Extension

Birth is by extension. The nape of the neck pivots under the pubis, while the vertex, bregma, forehead, face, and chin are born over the perineum.

Restitution

When the head has made its exit the neck untwists, and the head turns back 45 degrees to the left, resuming the normal relationship with the shoulders (OA to LOA).

External Rotation

The shoulders now rotate 45 degrees to the left to bring their bisacromial diameter into the anteroposterior diameter of the pelvis. The head follows the shoulders and rotates externally another 45 degrees to the left (LOA to LOT).

Birth of the Shoulders, Trunk, and Placenta

Birth of the Shoulders, trunk, and placenta is the same as described in Chapter 10, Anterior Positions of the Occiput.

Fig. 9. Extension beginning.

Fig. 10. Extension complete.

Fig. 11. Restitution: O.A. to
L.O.A.

Fig. 12. External rotation:
L.O.A. to L.O.T.

CLINICAL COURSE OF LABOR: LOT

Most fetuses which begin labor in the LOT position rotate the head 90 degrees (LOT to LOA to OA) to bring the occiput under the pubic symphysis, whence spontaneous delivery takes place.

Arrest of Progress

Arrest of progress can occur in any of these situations:

1. Anterior rotation of 90 degrees to the OA position, but spontaneous delivery does not take place
2. Anterior rotation of 45 degrees, with cessation of progress in the LOA position
3. No rotation occurs. The head is arrested with the sagittal suture in the transverse diameter of the pelvis. This is known as transverse arrest.
4. In the rare case posterior rotation takes place, LOT to LOP. The mechanism of labor then becomes that of occipitoposterior positions.

Management of Arrested Cases

Providing the prerequisites for operative vaginal delivery are present, the following treatment is carried out:

1. Arrest in OA position: Forceps are applied to the sides of the fetal head, which is then extracted (see Ch. 25 for technical details).
2. Arrest as LOA: Forceps are applied to the fetal head, which is then rotated 45 degrees to the OA position, and extracted (see Ch. 25 for technical details).
3. Transverse arrest: LOT: Two operative technics are available.
   a. Manual rotation, 90 degrees, LOT to LOA to OA, followed by forceps extraction (see Ch. 26 for technic).
   b. Application of the forceps to the sides of the baby's head, rotation by the forceps of 90 degrees, LOT to LOA to OA, and then extraction by the forceps (see Ch. 26 for technic).
4. Arrest as an occiput posterior is treated like other occiput posterior deliveries (see Ch. 13).

RIGHT OCCIPUT TRANSVERSE: ROT

ROT is similar to LOT. The difference is that the back and occiput are on the mother's right, and the limbs are on her left.

BIBLIOGRAPHY

Javert, C. T., and Steele, K. B. The transverse position and the mechanism of labor. Int. Abstr. Surg., 75:507, 1942.

Fig. 13A. At onset of labor.

Fig. 13B. Descent and flexion.

Fig. 13C. Internal rotation:
L. O. T. to L. O. A.

Fig. 13D. Internal rotation:
L. O. A. to O. A.

Fig. 13E. Extension beginning.

Fig. 13F. Extension complete.

Fig. 13G. Restitution: O. A. to
L. O. A.

Fig. 13H. External rotation:
L. O. A. to L. O. T.

13 Posterior Positions of the Occiput

Definition: The occiput and the small posterior fontanelle are in the rear segment of the maternal pelvis, and the brow and bregma are in the anterior segment.

Incidence: The incidence of this position is from 15 to 30 percent. The exact incidence of posterior positions is difficult to ascertain, since most of them rotate anteriorly and are considered erroneously as being originally occipitoanterior. The posterior positions which rotate anteriorly with no difficulty are often not diagnosed, and only the persistent posteriors are recognized regularly. Right occiput posterior (ROP) is five times as common as left occiput posterior (LOP).

Etiology: The etiology of posterior positions of the occiput is the same as the etiology of other abnormal positions. Cephalopelvic disproportion is a frequent and serious complicating factor which must be considered at all times. The shape of the pelvic inlet influences the position of the occiput. Where the forepelvis is narrow there is a tendency for the back of the head with its long biparietal diameter to be pushed to the rear, so that the front of the head with its short bitemporal diameter can be accommodated by the small forepelvis. Hence, posterior positions of the occiput are found often in android and anthropoid pelves.

Fig. 1A. Abdominal view.

Fig. 1B. Vaginal view.

RIGHT OCCIPUT POSTERIOR: ROP

Diagnosis of Position: ROP

Abdominal Examination

1. The lie is vertical. The long axis of the fetus is parallel to the long axis of the mother.
2. The head is at or in the pelvis.
3. The fetal back is in the right maternal flank. In most cases it cannot be outlined clearly.
4. The small parts are felt easily anteriorly on the left side. The maternal abdomen has been described as being alive with little hands and feet.
5. The breech is in the fundus of the uterus.
6. The cephalic prominence is on the left. It is not felt as easily as in anterior positions, because flexion is less marked.

Fetal Heart

The fetal heart tones are transmitted through the scapula, and, hence, are heard in the right maternal flank, on the same side as the baby's back. Frequently the fetal heart sounds are indistinct. The heart sounds can be transmitted through the baby's chest, and in some cases they are heard loudest in the left anterior lower quadrant of the abdomen. The location of the fetal heart sounds is not a reliable sign in determining how the baby is placed, and, hence, a carefully made diagnosis of posterior position should not be changed because of the situation of the fetal heart. As the back rotates anteriorly the fetal heart tones approach the midline of the abdomen.

Vaginal Examination

1. The sagittal suture is in the right oblique diameter of the pelvis.
2. The small posterior fontanelle is in the right posterior segment of the pelvis.
3. The bregma is anterior, and to the left of the symphysis pubis.
4. Since flexion is imperfect, the fontanelles may be close to the same level in the pelvis.
5. Where there is difficulty in diagnosis, the pinna (auricle) of the ear will be found pointing to the occiput.

X-ray Examination

X-ray examination is important where diagnosis of fetal position or pelvic adequacy is in doubt.

Mechanism of Labor: ROP

Rotation of varying degree and direction can take place:

1. Anterior rotation
   a. The long arc rotation of 135 degrees, ROP to ROT to ROA to OA. This occurs in 90 percent of occipitoposterior positions. The baby is born as an occipitoanterior.
   b. Rotation of 90 degrees, ROP to ROT to ROA
   c. Rotation of 45 degrees, ROP to ROT. The result is deep transverse arrest.
2. No rotation; the position remains ROP.
3. Posterior rotation of 45 degrees, ROP to OP, with the occiput turning into the hollow of the sacrum

Spontaneous delivery can take place after:

1. Anterior rotation to OA with normal birth
2. Posterior rotation to OP with face-to-pubis delivery

Arrest can occur:

1. High in the pelvis, with failure to engage. These are often problems of disproportion.
2. In the midpelvis, with complete or partial failure of rotation
   a. Deep transverse arrest, ROT
   b. Arrest with the sagittal suture in the right oblique diameter of the pelvis, ROP
   c. Arrest with the occiput in the hollow of the sacrum, OP
3. Arrest at the outlet

Long Arc Rotation: 135 Degrees to the Anterior

Descent

The head enters the inlet with the sagittal suture in the right oblique diameter, and unless obstruction is encountered, descent continues throughout labor. Engagement may be delayed, and the entire labor may take longer than in normal anterior positions.

Flexion

Flexion is imperfect and often is not complete until the head reaches the pelvic floor. The partial flexion and the resulting larger diameter of the presenting part contribute to the labor's being longer and harder for both mother and child.

Internal Rotation

The occiput rotates 135 degrees anteriorly under the symphysis pubis (ROP to ROT to ROA to OA).

Fig. 4. Internal rotation:
R.O.P. to R.O.T.

Fig. 2. R.O.P.: onset of labor.

Fig. 5. Internal rotation:
R.O.T. to R.O.A.

Fig. 3. Descent and flexion.

Fig. 6. Internal rotation:
R.O.A. to O.A.

Extension

The nape of the neck pivots in the subpubic angle, and the head is born by extension. The bregma, forehead, nose, mouth, and chin pass over the perineum in order.

Restitution

Restitution (OA to ROA) takes place to the right. The extent of restitution depends on how far the shoulders have followed the head during internal rotation. In most cases the shoulders turn with the head, lagging behind only 45 degrees, and restitution will be the usual 45 degrees. Occasionally the shoulders may lag behind more or may swing back. The head will then restitute 90 degrees, or even 135 degrees.

External Rotation

The anterior shoulder strikes the pelvic floor and rotates 45 degrees toward the pubic symphysis so that the bisacromial diameter of the shoulders is in the anteroposterior diameter of the outlet. The head follows the shoulders, and the occiput rotates 45 degrees to the right transverse position (ROA to ROT).

Fig. 7. Extension beginning.

Fig. 8. Extension complete.

Fig. 9. Restitution: O.A. to R.O.A.

Fig. 10. External rotation: R.O.A. to R.O.T.

Mechanism of Labor: ROP

Short Arc Rotation: 45 Degrees to the Posterior

Descent

The head enters the inlet with the sagittal suture in the right oblique.   Descent continues throughout labor.

Flexion

Flexion is imperfect, resulting in a longer presenting diameter.

Internal Rotation

The occiput turns posteriorly 45 degrees (ROP to OP) into the hollow of the sacrum.   The sagittal suture is in the anteroposterior diameter of the pelvis. The bregma is behind the pubis.

Fig. 11. R.O.P.: onset of labor.

Fig. 12. Descent and flexion.

Fig. 13. Internal rotation: R.O.P. to O.P.

<u>Birth of the head</u> is by a combination of flexion and extension.

Flexion

There are two mechanisms:

1. Where there is good flexion the area anterior to the bregma pivots under the symphysis pubis. The presenting diameter is the suboccipitofrontal of 10.5 cm. The bregma, vertex, small fontanelle, and occiput are born by further flexion.
2. Where flexion is incomplete the root of the nose pivots under the symphysis. The presenting diameter is the larger occipitofrontal of 11.5 cm. This bigger diameter is more traumatic than the smaller one. By flexion, the forehead, bregma, vertex, and occiput are born over the perineum.

Fig. 14. O.P.: birth by flexion.

Fig. 15. O.P.: crowning.

Fig. 16. O.P.: flexion beginning.

Fig. 17. O.P.: flexion complete.

Extension

Once the top and back of the head have been born by flexion, the occiput falls back toward the anus, and the nose, mouth, and chin are born under the symphysis pubis by extension.

Restitution

Restitution of the occiput is 45 degrees to the right oblique (OP to ROP) to resume the normal relationship of the head to the shoulders.

External Rotation

The anterior shoulder strikes the pelvic floor and rotates 45 degrees toward the symphysis pubis, to bring the bisacromial diameter of the shoulders into the anteroposterior diameter of the pelvis. The head follows, and the occiput rotates 45 degrees to the right transverse position (ROP to ROT).

Molding

In persistent occipitoposterior positions the head is shortened in the occipitofrontal, and lengthened in the suboccipitobregmatic and mentobregmatic diameters. The head rises steeply in front and in back. The caput succedaneum is located over the bregma. Molding and extensive edema of the scalp make accurate identification of the sutures and fontanelles difficult, and this obscures the diagnosis.

A. Vaginal view.

B. Lateral view.

Fig. 18. Extension.

Fig. 19. Restitution: O.P. to R.O.P.

Fig. 20. External rotation: R.O.P. to R.O.T.

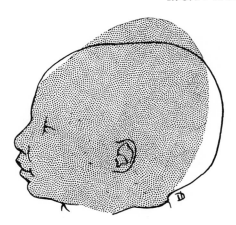

Fig. 21. Molding: R.O.P.

SUMMARY OF LONG ARC ROTATION: R.O.P. TO O.A.

Fig. 22A. R.O.P.: onset of labor.

Fig. 22B. Descent and flexion.

Fig. 22C. Internal rotation: R.O.P. to R.O.T.

Fig. 22D. Internal rotation: R.O.T. to R.O.A.

Fig. 22E. Internal rotation: R.O.A. to O.A.

Fig. 22F. Extension.

Fig. 22G. Restitution. O.A. to R.O.A.

Fig. 22H. External rotation: R.O.A. to R.O.T.

Fig. 23A. R.O.P.: onset of labor.

Fig. 23B. Descent and flexion.

Fig. 23C. Internal rotation: R.O.P. to O.P.

Fig. 23D. Birth by flexion.

Fig. 23E. Birth by extension.

Fig. 23F. Restitution: O.P. to R.O.P.

Fig. 23G. External rotation: R.O.P. to R.O.T.

Management of the Progressive Case

1. Expectant observation is the best policy. Given sufficient time, most posterior positions of the occiput will rotate anteriorly, and the baby will be delivered spontaneously or by low forceps. Thus, as long as the fetus and mother are in good condition and labor is progressing, there is no justification for hasty interference. The safe and wise rule is to leave occipitoposterior positions to nature, supplying only supportive measures, until there is a definite indication for active intervention.
2. While it is believed that anterior rotation is helped by the patient's lying on the same side as the fetal limbs, most patients will remain in the position of greatest comfort.
3. Because the labor may be long and difficult for mother and child, care must be exercised to insure the adequate intake of fluids and nourishment. More judicious use of analgesia and sedation is required than in normal occipitoanterior positions.
4. When the head is delivered in the posterior position (face to pubis) the large back part of the head (biparietal diameter of 9.5 cm) causes greater streching and more lacerations of the perineum than does the narrow anterior part of the head (bitemporal of 8.0 cm). For this reason a large episiotomy is indicated. Frequently there is arrest at the perineum, and low forceps is the management of choice to save the mother and child from the effects of a prolonged period of bearing down.

Indications for Interference

Maternal Distress

Maternal distress is fatigue or exhaustion of the laboring woman and is accompanied by the following signs:

1. Pulse above 100
2. Temperature above 100
3. Dehydration, dry tongue, dry skin, concentrated urine
4. Loss of emotional stability

Fetal Distress

Fetal distress is shown by:

1. Irregular fetal heart rate
2. Fetal heart rate below 100 or over 160 per minute between uterine contractions
3. The passage of meconium in a vertex presentation

Lack of Progress

The cessation of descent and/or rotation indicates that labor has become arrested and that interference is mandatory. Reasons for failure of descent and rotation include:

1. Cephalopelvic disproportion
2. Android midpelvis
3. Ineffective uterine contractions
4. Deflexion of the head
5. Uterine contraction ring preventing the shoulders from rotating anteriorly
6. Multiparity, pendulous abdomen, poor abdominal and uterine tone
7. A weak pelvic floor fails to guide the occiput anteriorly.

While the basic strategy of nonintervention is, up to a point, a wise one, it is not safe to wait too long, and fine judgment is needed to decide the point at which further delay is undesirable or even harmful. Where the standard signs of fetal or maternal distress are present, the decision to interfere is based on clear-cut grounds. However, when the contractions are long, strong, and too frequent, the risk of intracranial damage is present, and operative therapy must be instituted sooner, even though the fetal heart sounds are normal and no meconium has been passed.

In competent hands a wait of 2 hours in the second stage is sufficient. If, however, the attendant is not skilled in operative obstetrics, it may be safer to wait longer, but only if the baby and mother are in good condition.

Methods of Operative Vaginal Delivery in Arrested Occipitoposterior

While vaginal delivery is hoped for in all patients, operative intervention via the birth canal should not be undertaken before the following prerequisites have been fulfilled:

1. The fetal head must be engaged, i.e., the biparietal diameter has passed through the inlet, and the bony presenting part has reached the level of the ischial spines.
2. There can be no gross fetopelvic disproportion.
3. The cervix must be dilated fully.
4. The membranes should have ruptured.
5. The patient has to be in good labor with strong, regular uterine contractions.

Under these conditions the arrest of progress for approximately two hours in a primigravida and one hour in a multipara calls for the consideration of operative delivery. The presence of fetal or maternal distress is, of course, an indication for earlier interference.

If the prerequisites are not present, operative vaginal delivery cannot be carried out at that time, and other therapeutic measures must be instituted.

There are many ways of management. We shall describe only a few. Their purpose is to rotate the head to a more favorable position, and to extract the baby. (For more detailed description of technics, see Ch. 27.)

Delivery of the Head in the Posterior Position

The forceps are applied to the sides of the baby's head, an episiotomy is performed, and the head is extracted face to pubis.

Manual Rotation to the Anterior and Forceps Extraction

Pomeroy Maneuver: The head is disengaged so that the operator's hand can grasp the shoulder. The shoulder is rotated along with the head to the anterior position. The head is then extracted in the OA position with forceps.

Manual Rotation of the Head: The head is grasped with the hand in the vagina and rotated 135 degrees, ROP to OA. Forceps are then used to extract the head in the OA position. To prevent the head from turning back to ROP, some obstetricians overrotate the head from ROP to LOA before applying the forceps.

Forceps Rotation

Scanzoni Maneuver: This is a double application of forceps. The forceps are applied to the baby's head in the ROP position. The head is then rotated by the forceps from ROP to OA. The forceps are now upside down, so they are removed, turned right side up, and reapplied to the fetal head, which is then extracted.

The Maughan Maneuver: One blade of the forceps is used to rotate the head from ROP to ROT. Then the other blade is applied, the rotation completed, ROT to OA, and the head extracted.

The Key in Lock Maneuver of De Lee: This is a multiple application method, whereby the head is rotated anteriorly 5 or 10 degrees each time, until the occiput is anterior. The head is then extracted.

Failed Forceps

When the above procedures are not successful in effecting delivery, the following may be considered:

Cesarean Section: Even in the second stage it is better for both mother and child if cesarean section is performed than if the baby is dragged through the pelvis by brute force.

Internal Podalic Version and Extraction: Internal podalic version and extraction as a breech, though once a popular method, is used rarely today. The risk of uterine rupture and fetal injury or death is too great.

Destructive Operation: Destructive operation on the fetus is performed only when the baby is dead or the contraindications to other means of treatment are absolute.

Management when Conditions for Immediate
Vaginal Delivery Are not Present

We have described several methods of operative vaginal delivery of arrested occipitoposterior positions, employable, however, only when certain
prerequisites have been fulfilled. When these conditions are not present, extraction by forceps cannot be carried out, and other methods of management are
utilized.

Fetopelvic Disproportion

If there has been no progress in the face of good contractions, and vaginal
and X-ray examinations demonstrate gross fetopelvic disproportion, cesarean
section should be performed.

Intact Membranes

Intact membranes do not always help labor, but seem, often, to retard it.
Therefore, before the progress of labor can be considered as halted the membranes should be ruptured artificially and the patient given a further trial of labor. Frequently the patient will make good progress in rotation and descent,
and spontaneous delivery will take place.

Ineffective Uterine Contractions

Ineffective uterine contractions result in slow advance, or none at all.
There are two main groups of cases:

1. Myometrial fatigue resulting from long labor
2. Inefficient uterine action, a condition which is frequently associated with
   posterior positions of the occiput, as well as with other malpresentations

Two types of therapy are available: 1, the uterus can be rested; or 2, it
can be stimulated. Since, in most cases, the patient is weary, she should be
helped to rest. Ten milligrams of morphine sulphate or 100 mg of Demerol
will give the patient an hour or two of sleep, and an infusion of a liter (or more
if needed) of 5 percent glucose in water will improve her state of hydration. In
many instances good labor will set in soon after the patient awakens.

If effective labor does not begin the uterus may be stimulated. The best
method of doing this is to add 5 units of oxytocin to a liter of 5 percent glucose
in water and to give this as an intravenous infusion. The drip is started slowly,
at a rate of about 10 drops per minute, and the effect on the contractions and
the fetal heart is observed. The subsequent speed is governed by the effect.
The aim is to achieve good uterine contractions every 2 to 3 minutes, lasting
45 to 60 seconds (see Ch. 36).

Undilated Cervix

The causes and management of failure of the cervix to dilate fully or to progress beyond 4 or 5 cm fall into several groups (see Ch. 31).

1. When the basic etiology is cephalopelvic disproportion, treatment by cesarean section is best for mother and child.
2. Artificial rupture of the bag of waters, by bringing the presenting part into closer apposition with the cervix, will bring about more rapid dilatation in many instances.
3. When inefficient uterine action will not open the cervix, treatment is instituted to correct the defective contractions.
4. When some intrinsic disease of the cervix prevents it from dilating, cesarean section has to be performed.

There is a special group of cases where vaginal delivery is indicated. All the prerequisites are present except that the cervix, although well effaced, is only three fourths dilated.

1. The anterior lip of the cervix is caught between the head of the fetus and the pubic symphysis. During a contraction, and with the patient bearing down, the anterior rim can be pushed back over the head, using two fingers in the vagina. In the absence of other obstructing factors, good progress is the common result.
2. In other instances there is a thin rim of cervix all around the head. This too can be pushed back during a contraction.
3. The forceps can be applied inside the cervix and the head pulled through slowly. Cervical lacerations are almost inevitable, and must be repaired carefully (see Ch. 38).
4. Dührssen's incisions can be made. Under direct vision the cervix is incised at 2, 6, and 10 o'clock. The baby is delivered with forceps and the incisions repaired. These sites of incision are chosen because their extension will result in the least serious damage. It must be emphasized that deliveries through an incompletely dilated cervix or through Dührssen's incisions are done only when the cervix is thin and near full dilatation and never when the cervix is thick or less than half open. These procedures are performed rarely today. Better methods of therapy are available (see Ch. 38).

BIBLIOGRAPHY

Bill, A. H.   The treatment of the vertex occipito posterior position.   Amer. J. Obstet. Gynec., 22:615, 1931.

Calkins, L. A.   Occiput posterior.   Amer. J. Obstet. Gynec., 38:993, 1939.

———   Occiput posterior presentation.   Obstet Gynec., 1:466, 1953.

Danforth, W. C.   The treatment of occipito posterior positions with especial reference to manual rotation.   Amer. J. Obstet. Gynec., 23:360, 1932.

DeLee, J. B.   The treatment of obstinate occipito-posterior positions. J. A. M. A., 75:145, 1920.

King, E. L. , Herring, J. S. , Dyer, I. , and King, J. A. The modification of
  the Scanzoni rotation in the management of persistent occipito posterior
  positions. Amer. J. Obstet. Gynec. , 61:872, 1951.
Maughan, G. B. The safe and simple delivery of persistent posterior and
  transverse positions. Amer. J. Obstet. Gynec. , 71:741, 1956.
Melhado, G. C. The occipito posterior position. Amer. J. Obstet. Gynec. ,
  26:696, 1933.
Reddoch, J. W. The management of occipito posterior positions with special
  reference to the Scanzoni maneuver. Southern Med. J. , 27:615, 1934.

14 Malpresentations

<u>General Etiologic Factors</u>

Accidental

No cause discoverable

Maternal and Uterine

1. Contracted pelvis. This is the most important factor.
2. A pendulous maternal abdomen. By permitting the uterus and fetus to fall forward, there may be difficulty in engagement.
3. Neoplasms. Uterine fibromyomata or ovarian cysts can block the entry to the pelvis.
4. Uterine anomalies. In a bicornuate uterus the nonpregnant horn may obstruct labor in the pregnant one.
5. Abnormalities of placental size or location. Conditions such as placenta previa are associated with unfavorable positions of the fetus.

Fetal

1. Large baby
2. Errors in fetal polarity, such as breech presentation and transverse lie
3. Abnormal internal rotation. The occiput rotates posteriorly or fails to rotate at all.
4. Fetal attitude. Extension in place of normal flexion
5. Multiple pregnancy
6. Fetal anomalies, including hydrocephaly and anencephaly
7. Polyhydramnios. An excessive amount of amniotic fluid allows the baby freedom of activity, and it may assume abnormal positions.

Effects of Malpresentations

Effects on Labor

The less symmetrical adaptation of the presenting part to the cervix and to the pelvis plays a part in reducing the efficiency of labor.

1. The incidence of fetopelvic disproportion is higher.
2. Inefficient uterine action is common. The contractions tend to be weak and irregular.
3. Prolonged labor is seen frequently.
4. Pathologic retraction rings can develop, and rupture of the lower uterine segment may be the end result.
5. The cervix often dilates slowly and incompletely.
6. The presenting part stays high.
7. Premature rupture of the membranes occurs often.
8. The need for operative delivery is increased.

Effects on the Mother

1. Because greater uterine and intraabdominal muscular effort is required, and because labor is often prolonged with attendant lack of rest and inadequate nourishment, maternal exhaustion is common.
2. There is more stretching of the perineum and soft parts, and there are more lacerations.
3. Bleeding is more profuse, resulting from:
   a. Tears of the uterus, cervix, and vagina
   b. The placental site, maternal exhaustion leading to uterine atony
4. There is a greater incidence of infection. This is caused by:
   a. Early rupture of the membranes
   b. Excessive blood loss
   c. Tissue damage
   d. Frequent rectal and vaginal examinations
5. The patient's discomfort seems out of proportion to the strength of the uterine contractions. She complains bitterly of pain before the uterus is felt to harden, and continues to feel the pain after the uterus has relaxed.
6. Paresis of the bowel and bladder add to the patient's suffering.

Effects on the Fetus

1. The fetus fits the pelvis less perfectly, making it more difficult for it to pass through the pelvis and leading to excessive molding.
2. The long labor is harder on the baby, with a greater incidence of anoxia, brain damage, asphyxia, and intrauterine death.
3. There is a higher incidence of operative delivery, increasing the danger of trauma to the baby.
4. Prolapse of the umbilical cord is more common than in normal positions.

15   Face Presentation

Definition: The lie is longitudinal, the presentation is cephalic, the presenting part is the face, the attitude is one of complete extension, the chin (mentum; M) is the denominator and leading pole, and the presenting diameter is the submentobregmatic of 9.5 cm. In face presentations the part between the glabella and chin presents. In brow presentations it is the part between the glabella and bregma. However, positions between these are seen often.

Incidence: The incidence is less than 1 percent (one in 250), and is higher in multiparas than primigravidas. Primary face presentations are present before the onset of labor and are rare. Most face presentations are secondary, extensions taking place during labor, generally at the pelvic inlet. About 70 percent of face presentations are anterior or transverse, while 30 percent are posterior.

Etiology: Anything which delays engagement in flexion can contribute to the etiology of attitudes of extension. There is an association between attitudes of extension and cephalopelvic disproportion, and since this is a serious combination, the presence of a small pelvis or a large head must be ruled out carefully. Rare causes of extension include thyroid neoplasms which act by pushing the head back, multiple coils of cord around the neck which prevent flexion, and monsters. Anencephalic fetuses present by the face frequently, and there is an increased incidence of prematurity.

In many cases no causal factor can be found.

ANTERIOR FACE PRESENTATIONS
LEFT MENTUM ANTERIOR: LMA

Diagnosis of Position: LMA

Abdominal Examination

1. The long axes of the fetus and mother are parallel.
2. The head is at the pelvis. Early in labor the head is not engaged.
3. The back is on the right side of the mother's abdomen, but since it is posterior, it is often felt indistinctly. The small parts are on the left and anterior. The extension of the spine causes the chest to be thrown out and the back to be hollowed.
4. The breech is in the fundus.
5. The cephalic prominence (the occiput) is on the right. An important diagnostic sign of extension attitudes is that the back and the cephalic prominence are on the same side. When flexion is present, the cephalic prominence and the back are on opposite sides.
6. It must be kept in mind that in anterior face presentations the baby's back and occiput are posterior. When the chin is posterior, on the other hand, the back and occiput are anterior.

Fetal Heart

The fetal heart tones are transmitted through the anterior chest wall of the fetus, and are heard loudest in the left lower quadrant of the maternal abdomen, on the same side as the small parts.

Vaginal Examination

1. The clue to diagnosis is a negative finding, namely the absence of the round, even, hard vertex. In place of the dome of the skull with its identifying suture lines and fontanelles, there is a softer and irregular presenting part. One suspects face or breech. Identification of the various parts of the face clinches the diagnosis. After prolonged labor marked edema may confuse the picture.
2. The long axis of the face is in the right oblique diameter of the pelvis.
3. The chin is in the left anterior quadrant of the maternal pelvis.
4. The forehead is in the right posterior quadrant of the pelvis.
5. Vaginal examination must be performed gently to avoid injury to the eyes.

Radiologic Examination

Radiologic examination is helpful both in diagnosis of position and in estimation of pelvic capacity.

Late diagnosis: Because most face presentations make good progress, the diagnosis may not be made until the face has reached the floor of the pelvis, or until advance has ceased.

LEFT MENTUM ANTERIOR

Fig. 1A. Abdominal view.

Fig. 1B. Vaginal view.

Mechanism of Labor: LMA

Extension

For some reason the head does not flex. Instead it extends, so that in place of an LOP or ROP we have an RMA or an LMA. The baby enters the pelvis chin first. The presenting diameter in face presentations (submentobregmatic) and in well-flexed head presentations (suboccipitobregmatic) is 9.5 cm in each case. This is one of the reasons why most anterior face presentations come to spontaneous delivery.

Descent

With the chin as the leading part, engagement takes place in the right oblique diameter of the pelvis. Descent is slower than in flexed attitudes. The face is low in the pelvis before the biparietal diameter has passed the brim.

When the forward leading edge of the presenting face is felt at the level of the ischial spines, the trachelobregmatic diameter is still above the inlet.

Internal Rotation

With descent and molding the chin reaches the pelvic floor where it is directed downward, forward, and medially. As it rotates 45 degrees anteriorly toward the symphysis (LMA to MA), the long axis of the face comes into the anteroposterior diameter of the pelvis. With further descent the chin escapes under the symphysis. The shoulders have remained in the oblique diameter, so the neck is twisted 45 degrees. An essential feature of internal rotation is that the chin must rotate anteriorly and under the symphysis, or spontaneous delivery is impossible. Anterior rotation does not take place until the face is well applied to the pelvic floor, and may be delayed until late in labor. The attendant must not give up hope too soon.

Fig. 2. L.M.A.: onset of labor.

Fig. 3. Extension and descent.

A. Vaginal view.

B. Lateral view.

Fig. 4. Internal rotation:
L.M.A. to M.A.

Flexion

The head is born by flexion. The submental region at the neck impinges under the symphysis pubis. With the head pivoting around this point, the mouth, nose, orbits, forehead, vertex, and occiput are born over the perineum by flexion. The head then falls back.

Fig. 6. Flexion beginning.

Fig. 5. Flexion.

Fig. 7. Flexion complete.

Fig. 8. Head falls back in extension: vaginal view.

Fig. 9. Head falls back in extension: lateral view.

Restitution

As the head is released from the vagina the neck untwists, and the chin turns 45 degrees back toward the original side.

External Rotation

The anterior shoulder reaches the pelvic floor and rotates toward the symphysis to bring the bisacromial diameter from the oblique to the anteroposterior diameter of the outlet. The chin rotates back another 45 degrees to maintain the head in its correct relationship to the shoulders.

Molding

Molding leads to an elongation of the head in its anteroposterior diameter, and flattening from above downward. The forehead and occiput protrude. The extension of the head on the trunk disappears after a few days.

Fig. 10. Restitution: M.A. to
L.M.A.

Fig. 11. External rotation:
L.M.A. to L.M.T.

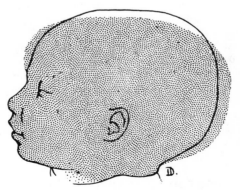

Fig. 12. Molding: face presentation.

Prognosis: Anterior Face Presentations

Labor: Because the face is a poor dilator, and because attitudes of extension are less favorable, labor takes longer than in normal occipitoanterior positions. The labor is conducted with this in mind. Delay takes place at the inlet, but once the face presentation and the labor are well established, steady progress is the rule.

Maternal: The mother has more work to do, suffers more pain, and receives greater lacerations than in normal positions.

Fetal: The baby does well in most cases, but the prognosis is less favorable than in normal presentations. The outlook for the child can be improved by early diagnosis, carefully conducted first and second stages of labor, and the restriction of operative vaginal deliveries to easily performed procedures. Cesarean section is preferable to complicated, difficult, and traumatic vaginal operations.

The membranes rupture early in labor, and the face takes the brunt of the punishment, so that it becomes badly swollen and misshapen. Its appearance is a great worry to the parents. The edema disappears gradually and the infant takes on a more normal appearance. Edema of the larynx may result from prolonged pressure of the hyoid region of the neck against the pubic bone. For the first 24 hours the baby must be watched carefully to detect any difficulty in breathing.

Management of Anterior Face Presentations

X-ray pelvimetry helps to establish the diagnosis and to assess the pelvic capacity.

1. Disproportion: Disproportion, shown by pelvic and radiologic examinations, is treated by cesarean section.
2. Normal pelvis: In a normal pelvis, anterior face presentations are left alone, for these reasons:
   a. Most will deliver spontaneously or with the aid of low forceps.
   b. Should conversion (flexion) be successful, the anterior face will be replaced by an occipitoposterior (LMA to ROP or RMA to LOP). This does not improve the situation, but may make it worse.
   c. If conversion is partially successful, the face is changed to a brow presentation. In this case a face presentation which usually delivers spontaneously is replaced by a brow which cannot.
3. Arrest: Arrest below the spines is treated best by extraction with low forceps (see Ch. 28 for details). Arrest high in the pelvis is treated by cesarean section.

RIGHT MENTUM ANTERIOR: RMA

The mechanism is similar to LMA except that the chin, small parts, and fetal heart are on the right side, while the back and cephalic prominence are on the left.

SUMMARY OF MECHANISM OF LABOR: L.M.A.

Fig. 13A. L.M.A.: onset of labor.

Fig. 13B. Extension and descent.

Fig. 13C. Internal rotation: L.M.A. to M.A.

Fig. 13D. Flexion.

Fig. 13E. Extension.

Fig. 13F. Restitution: M.A. to L.M.A.

Fig. 13G. External rotation: L.M.A. to L.M.T.

TRANSVERSE FACE PRESENTATIONS

The long axis of the face is in the transverse diameter of the pelvis, with the chin on one side and the forehead on the other.

LEFT MENTUM TRANSVERSE: LMT

Diagnosis of Position: LMT

Abdominal Examination

1. The long axis of the fetus is parallel to that of the mother.
2. The head is at the pelvis.
3. The back is on the right, toward the maternal flank. The small parts are on the left side.
4. The breech is in the fundus.
5. The cephalic prominence (the occiput) is on the right, the same side as the back.

Fetal Heart

The fetal heart is heard loudest in the left lower quadrant of the mother's abdomen.

Vaginal Examination

1. The long axis of the face is in the transverse diameter of the pelvis.
2. The chin is to the left, at 3 o'clock.
3. The forehead is to the right, at 9 o'clock.

Fig. 14A. Abdominal view.

Fig. 14B. Vaginal view.

Mechanism of Labor: LMT

Extension

   Extension to LMT occurs instead of flexion to ROT.

Descent

   Engagement takes place in the transverse diameter of the pelvis. Descent
is slow.

Internal Rotation

   The chin rotates 90 degrees anteriorly to the midline (LMT to LMA to MA).
The chin comes under the symphysis.

Flexion

   The submental region of the neck impinges in the subpubic angle. Birth is
by flexion, after which the head falls backward.

Restitution

   As the neck untwists, the head turns back 45 degrees.

External Rotation

   The shoulders turn from the oblique into the anteroposterior diameter of
the pelvis, and the head rotates back another 45 degrees.

Clinical Course of Labor and Management of Left Mentum Transverse

1. Anterior rotation takes place in the majority of cases, LMT to LMA to MA.
   The treatment is the same as LMA. Delivery is spontaneous or assisted
   by low forceps.
2. Arrest as LMT low in the pelvis is treated by rotation of the face (LMT to
   LMA to MA), either manually or by forceps. Once rotation has been
   achieved, the head is extracted with forceps.
3. Arrest as LMT high in the pelvis is treated by cesarean section.

RIGHT MENTUM TRANSVERSE: RMT

   The mechanism of labor is the same as LMT except that the chin, small
parts, and fetal heart are on the right, while the back and cephalic prominence
are on the left.

Fig. 15. L.M.T.: onset of labor.

Fig. 16. Descent.

Fig. 17. Internal rotation: L.M.T. to L.M.A.

Fig. 18. Internal rotation: L.M.A. to M.A.

Fig. 19. Birth by flexion.

Fig. 20. Extension.

Fig. 21. Restitution: M.A. to L.M.A.

Fig. 22. External rotation: L.M.A. to L.M.T.

POSTERIOR FACE PRESENTATIONS

Some 30 percent of face presentations are posterior. Most of these rotate anteriorly. The flexed counterpart of the posterior face is the anterior occiput. Thus LMP flexes to ROA and RMP to LOA. Persistent posterior face presentations become arrested, as they cannot deliver spontaneously.

LEFT MENTUM POSTERIOR: LMP

Diagnosis of Position: LMP

Abdominal Examination

1. The long axis of the fetus is parallel to the long axis of the mother.
2. The head is at the pelvis.
3. The back is anterior and to the right. The small parts are on the left and posterior.
4. The breech is in the fundus of the uterus.
5. The cephalic prominence (occiput) is to the right and anterior. It is on the same side as the back.

Fetal Heart

The fetal heart tones, transmitted through the anterior shoulder, are heard loudest in the left lower quadrant of the mother's abdomen.

Vaginal Examination

1. The long diameter of the face is in the left oblique diameter of the pelvis.
2. The chin is in the left posterior quadrant of the pelvis.
3. The forehead is in the right anterior quadrant.

Fig. 23A. Abdominal view.

Fig. 23B. Vaginal view.

Mechanism of Labor: LMP

There are two basic mechanisms:

1. Long arc rotation, with the chin rotating 135 degrees to the anterior. About two thirds of posterior face presentations do this and deliver spontaneously or with the aid of low forceps.
2. Short arc rotation of 45 degrees to the posterior, with the chin ending up in the hollow of the sacrum. These cases become arrested as persistent posterior face presentations.

Long Arc Rotation: 135 Degrees to the Anterior

Extension

Extension to LMP occurs instead of flexion to ROA.

Descent

Descent is slow. The presenting part remains high while the essential molding takes place. Without extreme molding the vertex cannot pass under the anterior part of the pelvic inlet.

Internal Rotation

The slow descent continues, the marked molding enables the chin to reach the pelvic floor, where it rotates 135 degrees to the anterior, and comes to lie under the symphysis. Since the original position was LMP, the sequence is LMP to LMT to LMA to MA in rotations of 45 degrees between each step.

Flexion

The submental area pivots under the symphysis and the head is born by flexion. The head then falls backward.

Restitution

The chin rotates back 45 degrees as the neck untwists.

External Rotation

With the rotation of the shoulders from the oblique into the anteroposterior diameter of the pelvis, the chin turns back another 45 degrees.

Fig. 24. L.M.P.: descent.

Fig. 25. Internal rotation: L.M.P. to L.M.T.

Fig. 26. Internal rotation: L.M.T. to L.M.A.

Fig. 27. Internal rotation: L.M.A. to M.A.

Fig. 28. Birth by flexion.

Fig. 29. Head falls back in extension.

Fig. 30. Restitution: M.A. to L.M.A.

Fig. 31. External rotation: L.M.A. to L.M.T.

Short Arc Rotation: 45 Degrees to the Posterior

Extension

Extension to LMP takes place.

Descent

Descent occurs with the help of extreme molding.

Internal Rotation

The chin rotates 45 degrees posteriorly into the hollow of the sacrum (LMP to MP). Impaction follows. The sacrum is 12 to 15 cm in length while the fetal neck is only 5 cm. Flexion is impossible and further advancement cannot take place unless the baby is so small that the shoulders and head can enter the pelvis together. This is rarely feasible, and arrest of progress results.

Fig. 32. L. M. P. : onset of labor.   Fig. 33. Descent.

A. Vaginal view.

B. Lateral view.

Fig. 34. Internal rotation:
L. M. P. to M. P.

Prognosis: Posterior Face Positions

The prolonged labor and the difficult rotation are traumatic to both the baby and the mother. When the chin rotates posteriorly the prognosis is poor unless the situation is corrected. Maternal morbidity is directly proportional to the degree of difficulty of the birth. High forceps or version and extraction carry with them the most morbid postpartum courses.

Management of Posterior Face Presentations

X-ray pelvimetry is useful in establishing the diagnosis and in assessing pelvic adequacy.

1. Disproportion: Disproportion, as revealed by pelvic and radiologic examinations, or arrest of progress high in the pelvis, is treated best by cesarean section.
2. Normal pelvis: Since two thirds of posterior faces rotate anteriorly and deliver spontaneously, the patient should be given plenty of time to accomplish this rotation. Internal rotation may not take place until late in labor when the face is distending the pelvic floor. Hence, interference must not be rash.
3. Persistent posterior face—multipara with normal pelvis: Since persistent mentum posteriors cannot deliver spontaneously, operative interference is necessary. Several procedures are available.
   a. Flexion (conversion) from mentoposterior to occipitoanterior is the best treatment. One method of accomplishing this is by the Thorn maneuver. The cervix must be fully dilated. With the vaginal hand the operator flexes the fetal head. Through the maternal abdomen he uses the other hand to flex the body by pushing on the breech. At the same time an assistant presses against the baby's thorax or abdomen to try and jackknife the infant's body. This procedure is performed under anesthesia, and must be done soon after the rupture of the membranes. If the amniotic fluid has drained away, the dry uterine cavity and the snug fit of the uterus around the baby will make it difficult or impossible to carry out this treatment. Once flexion has been accomplished, the head is pushed into the pelvis and held in place.
   b. Rotation to a mentum anterior can sometimes be achieved by manual rotation, but in most cases forceps are required.
   c. Cesarean section is employed if the above maneuvers fail.
   d. Version and extraction, although once popular, has no place in the modern management of face presentations, except in the occasional case of a second twin.
   e. Destructive operation on the baby may be necessary if nothing else can be done and the baby is dead.
4. Persistent posterior face—primigravida with normal pelvis: Cesarean section will give the best results in most cases. Some authorities feel that flexion to occiput anterior or rotation to mentum anterior should be attempted before cesarean section is carried out.

Fig. 35. Thorn maneuver.

BIBLIOGRAPHY

Dede, J. A. , and Friedman, E. A. Face presentation. Amer. J. Obstet.
    Gynec. , 87:515, 1963.
Hellman, L. M. , Epperson, J. W. , and Connally, F. Face and brow presenta-
    tion. Amer. J. Obstet. Gynec. , 59:831, 1950.
Kenwick, A. Face and brow presentations. Amer. J. Obstet. Gynec. , 66:67,
    1953.

16 Brow Presentation

Definition: Brow presentation is an attitude of partial (halfway) extension, in contrast to face presentation where extension is complete. The presenting part is the area between the orbital ridges and the bregma. The denominator is the forehead (frontum: Fr). The presenting diameter is the verticomental, which, at 13.5 cm, is the longest anteroposterior diameter of the fetal head.

Incidence: The incidence is under 1 percent, ranging from 1/3,000 to 1/1,000. Primary brow presentations, those that occur before labor has started, are rare. The majority are secondary; that is, they occur after the onset of labor. Often the position is transitory, and the head will either flex to an occiput presentation, or will extend completely and become a face presentation.

Etiology: The causes are the same as for face presentation, and include anything that interferes with engagement in flexion. Care must be taken to rule out cephalopelvic disproportion.

LEFT FRONTUM ANTERIOR: LFrA

Diagnosis of Position: LFrA

Abdominal Examination

1. The lie is longitudinal.
2. The head is at the pelvis, but is not engaged.
3. The back is on the mother's right and posterior. It may be difficult to palpate. The small parts are on the left and anterior.
4. The breech is in the fundus of the uterus.
5. The cephalic prominence (occiput) and the back are on the same side, the right.

Fetal Heart

Fetal heart sounds are heard best in the left lower quadrant of the maternal abdomen.

Vaginal Examination

1. The anteroposterior diameter of the head is in the right oblique diameter of the pelvis.
2. The brow, the area between the nasion and the bregma, presents and is felt in the left anterior quadrant of the pelvis.
3. The vertex is in the right posterior quadrant.
4. The bregma (anterior fontanelle) is palpated easily.
5. The frontal suture is felt, but the sagittal is usually out of reach.
6. Identification of the supraorbital ridges is a key to diagnosis.

X-ray Examination

X-ray examination is helpful in diagnosing position and in assessing the pelvis.

Late and Failed Diagnosis: The difference, on vaginal examination, between the hard smooth dome of the skull and the soft irregular face is great enough to make diagnosis of the abnormal position, or at least suspicion of it, reasonably easy. On the other hand, the feel of the vertex and that of the forehead may be similar, and molding and edema add to the difficulty of differentiation. Hence, anything short of a most careful abdominal and vaginal examination with a high index of suspicion will fail to identify the malposition. A good rule is that whenever there is failure of progress, one should examine the patient thoroughly, keeping brow presentation in mind.

Fig. 1A. Abdominal view.

Fig. 1B. Vaginal view.

Mechanism of Labor: LFrA

The presenting diameter is the verticomental, measuring 13.5 cm. It is the longest anteroposterior diameter of the head. When engagement takes place it is accompanied by extensive molding, and progress, when it occurs, is slow.

The spontaneous mechanism of labor and delivery can take place when there is the combination of 1, a large pelvis; 2, strong uterine contractions; and 3, a small baby. In these cases the following mechanism of labor occurs.

Extension

The head extends and the verticomental diameter presents, with the forehead leading the way.

Descent

Descent is slow and late. Usually the head does not settle into the pelvis until the membranes have ruptured and the cervix has reached full dilatation.

Internal Rotation

The forehead rotates anteriorly 45 degrees so that the face comes to lie behind the pubic symphysis (LFrA to FrA). A considerable amount of internal rotation may take place between the ischial spines and the tuberosities.

Fig. 2.   L. Fr. A.: onset of labor.

Fig. 3.   Descent.

Fig. 4.   Internal rotation: L. Fr. A. to Fr. A.

Birth is by a combination of flexion and extension.

Flexion

The face impinges under the pubis and as the head pivots round this point, the bregma, vertex, and occiput are born over the perineum.

Extension

The head then falls back in extension, and the nose, mouth, and chin slip under the symphysis.

Fig. 5. Birth by flexion.

Fig. 6. Flexion beginning.

Fig. 7. Flexion complete.

A. Vaginal view.

B. Lateral view.

Fig. 8. Head falls back in extension.

Restitution

The neck untwists, and the head turns 45 degrees back to the original side.

External Rotation

As the shoulder rotates anteriorly from the oblique to the anteroposterior diameter of the pelvis, the head turns back another 45 degrees.

Molding

Molding is extreme. The verticomental diameter is compressed. The occipitofrontal diameter is elongated markedly, so that the forehead bulges greatly. The face is flattened, and the distance from the chin to the top of the head is long. This is exaggerated by the large caput succedaneum which forms on the forehead.

Fig. 9. Restitution: Fr. A. to L. Fr. A.

Fig. 10. External rotation: L. Fr. A. to L. Fr. T.

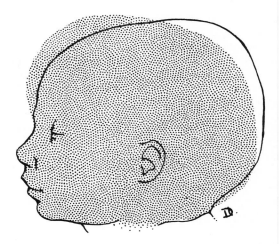

Fig. 11. Molding: brow presentation.

PROGNOSIS: BROW PRESENTATIONS

Labor: In many cases brow presentations do not deliver spontaneously. If the malposition is detected early in labor, and if appropriate therapeutic measures are undertaken, the fetal and maternal results are good.   Failure to recognize the problem leads to prolonged and traumatic labor.

Maternal: The passage of a brow through the pelvis is slower, harder, and more traumatic to the mother than any other presentation. Perineal laceration is inevitable, and may extend high into the vaginal fornices or into the rectum because of the large diameter offered to the outlet.

Fetal: Fetal mortality is high.   The excessive molding may cause irreparable damage to the brain.   Mistakes in diagnosis and treatment are the main causes of the poor fetal prognosis.

MANAGEMENT OF BROW PRESENTATIONS

X-ray pelvimetry will help in making the diagnosis and in assessing the pelvis.

1. Normal pelvis: Since brow presentation may be transitory, and since spontaneous delivery is possible, a trial of labor is permissible in the hope that flexion to an occiput presentation, complete extension to a face presentation, or progress as a brow presentation will take place.
2. Cephalopelvic disproportion: Disproportion, as shown by vaginal examination or x-ray, and arrest high in the pelvis, is treated best by cesarean section.
3. Persistent brow presentation—multipara with normal pelvis: Since most brow presentations do not deliver spontaneously, operative interference is necessary.
   a. The head should be flexed by the Thorn maneuver described in the section on posterior face presentation   This is done when the cervix is dilated and as soon as possible after the membranes rupture.
   b. Sometimes the head can be flexed by forceps. The forceps are applied biparietally, the head is pushed up just enough so that the brow can be rotated from one quadrant of the pelvis to the opposite one, and at the same time flexion is attempted.
   c. If the head cannot be flexed, an attempt is made to extend it to a face presentation.
   d. When these methods fail, cesarean section should be performed in the interests of both mother and child.
   e. Version and extraction is dangerous and is performed only in unusual situations, when other treatment is contraindicated.
   f. If the baby is dead, and other means of therapy are not possible, a destructive operation on the infant may be necessary.

4. Persistent brow presentation—primigravida with normal pelvis: Flexion or extension maneuvers may be attempted. Most authorities feel, however, that immediate cesarean section yields the best results and that no time should be wasted with other procedures.

BIBLIOGRAPHY

Hellman, L. M., Epperson, J. W., and Connally, F. Face and brow presentation. Amer. J. Obstet Gynec., 59:831, 1950.

Jacobson, L. J., and Johnson, C. E. Brow and face presentations. Amer. J. Obstet. Gynec., 84:1881, 1962.

Kenwick, A. Face and brow presentations. Amer. J. Obstet. Gynec., 66:67, 1953.

17 Median Vertex Presentation: The Military Attitude

Definition: There is neither flexion nor extension; the occiput and the brow are at the same level in the pelvis. The presenting part is the vertex. The denominator is the occiput. The presenting diameter is the occipitofrontal which, at 11.0 cm, is longer than the more favorable suboccipitobregmatic of 9.5 cm. Hence, progress is slower and arrest a little more frequent. In many cases the military attitude is transitory, and as it descends the head flexes. Occasionally extension to a brow or face takes place.

Diagnosis of Position: Median Vertex Presentation

Abdominal Examination

1. The long axes of fetus and mother are parallel.
2. The head is at or in the pelvic inlet.
3. The back is in one flank, the small parts on the opposite side.
4. The breech is in the fundus.
5. Since there is neither flexion nor extension there is no marked cephalic prominence on one side or the other.

Fetal Heart

The fetal heart tones are heard loudest in the lower quadrant of the mother's abdomen, on the same side as the fetal back.

Vaginal Examination

1. The sagittal suture is felt commonly in the transverse diameter of the pelvis, as LOT or ROT.
2. The two fontanelles are equally easy to palpate and identify. They are at the same level in the pelvis.

Radiologic Examination

Radiologic examination is helpful in diagnosing position and in assessing the pelvis.

Fig. 1A. Abdominal view.

Fig. 1B. Vaginal view.

Mechanism of Labor: Median Vertex Presentation

Engagement takes place most often in the transverse diameter of the inlet. The head descends slowly with the occiput and the brow at the same level (there is neither flexion nor extension), and with the sagittal suture in the transverse diameter of the pelvis, until the median vertex reaches the pelvic floor.   Now several terminations are possible:

1. Most often the head flexes, the occiput rotates to the anterior, and delivery takes place as an occipitoanterior position.
2. The head may become arrested in the transverse diameter of the pelvis. Operative assistance is necessary for deep transverse arrest.
3. The head may rotate posteriorly with or without flexion.   The occiput turns into the hollow of the sacrum and the forehead to the pubis.   The mechanism is that of persistent occipitoposterior positions.   Delivery may be spontaneous or by operative methods.
4. In rare instances delivery can occur with the sagittal suture in the transverse diameter.
5. Occasionally the head will extend, and the mechanism will be that of face or brow presentations.

Prognosis: Median Vertex Presentation

While labor is a little longer and harder on mother and child, the prognosis is reasonably good.   Many cases flex and proceed to normal delivery.

Management of Median Vertex Presentation

1. Since flexion occurs so frequently, there should be no interference as long as progress is being made.
2. When flexion takes place the management is that of occipitoanterior (see Ch. 10) or occipitoposterior (see Ch. 13) positions.
3. Cases in which the head extends are treated as face (see Ch. 15) or brow (see Ch. 16) presentations.
4. When arrest occurs in the normal pelvis with a persistent military attitude, vaginal delivery should be attempted by flexing the head, rotating the occiput to the anterior, and extracting the head by forceps (see Ch. 26).
5. Where disproportion is a complicating or etiologic factor, or where attempts at vaginal delivery fail, cesarean section should be performed.

18   Breech Presentation

Definition: Breech presentation is a longitudinal lie with a variation in polarity.   The fetal pelvis is the leading pole.   The denominator is the sacrum. A right sacrum anterior (RSA) is a breech presentation where the fetal sacrum is in the right anterior quadrant of the mother's pelvis, and the bitrochanteric diameter of the fetus is in the right oblique diameter of the pelvis.

Incidence: Breech presentation at delivery occurs in 3 to 4 percent of pregnancies.   The incidence decreases as term is reached, and it is increased by premature labor.

Etiology: Etiologic factors include prematurity, excess of amniotic fluid, multiple pregnancy, placenta previa, contracted pelvis, fibromyomata, hydrocephalus, and large baby.   Anything which interfered with the engagement of the fetal head plays a part in the etiology of breech presentation.   In many cases no reason can be found, and by exclusion the cause of the malposition is ascribed to pure chance.   On the other hand, there is the habitual breech.   Some women deliver all their children as breeches.   This suggests that the pelvis is so shaped that the breech fits better than the head.   Implantation of the placenta in the fundus or the cornu of the uterus tends to favor breech presentation.

NOTES AND COMMENTS ON BREECH PRESENTATION

1. The patient feels fetal movements in the lower abdomen and may complain of painful kicking against the rectum.
2. Engagement before the onset of labor is uncommon.   The patient experiences lightening rarely.
3. The uneven fit of breech to pelvis predisposes to early rupture of the membranes, with the danger of prolapse of the umbilical cord.   The incidence of prolapse of the umbilical cord, which is from 4 to 5 percent, is higher with footling breeches.   It is wise, therefore, when the bag of waters breaks, to make a sterile vaginal examination to determine the exact state of the cervix and to make certain that the cord has not prolapsed.
4. In theory the breech is a poor dilator in comparison with the well-flexed head, and labor, descent, and cervical dilatation are believed to take longer.   While this is true in some cases, the mean duration of labor of 9.2 hours in primigravidas and 6.1 hours in multiparas suggests that in the majority of cases labor is not prolonged.

195

5. In frank breeches the baby's lower limbs, which are flexed at the hips and extended at the knees, lie anterior to and against the baby's abdomen. This has the effect of a splint, and by decreasing the maneuverability of the baby may result in delay or arrest of progress.

6. One of the dangers to the fetus in breech presentation is that the largest and least compressible diameter comes last.

7. There is an added risk in premature infants because the head is relatively larger in proportion to the rest of the body than in full-term babies. Thus, while the small body slips through with no difficulty, it does not dilate the soft parts sufficiently to allow the head to pass easily.

8. On the one hand, the frank breech has the disadvantage of a large and less maneuverable presenting part and may have difficulty passing through the pelvis. On the other hand, it dilates the soft parts to the greatest degree and makes the most room for the head. The small footling breech slips through the pelvis easily, but makes less provision for the aftercoming head.

9. Since the posterior segment of the pelvis is roomier than the anterior segment, the posterior parts of the baby are usually born first.

10. Because of the rapid passage of the head through the pelvis there is no time for molding to take place. The fetal head is round and symmetrical.

11. The baby which lay in utero as a frank breech will lie with its hips flexed and the feet near its face for some time after birth.

12. A caput (edema of the lowest part) forms on the buttocks. The external genitalia are edematous.

13. The passage of meconium in a breech presentation does not have the same significance of fetal distress as in a vertex presentation. The meconium is squeezed out of the intestine by the uterine contractions pressing the lower part of the baby's body against the pelvis.

CLASSIFICATION

Complete: Flexion at thighs and knees

Frank: Flexion at thighs; extension at knees. This is the most common variety, and includes almost two thirds of breech presentations.

Footling: Single or double; extension at thighs and knees. The foot is the presenting part.

Kneeling: Single or double; extension at thighs, flexion at knees. The knee is the presenting part.

CLASSIFICATION OF BREECH

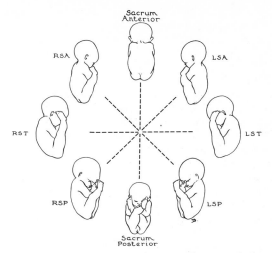

Fig. 1.   The positions of breech presentation.

Fig. 2.   Complete breech.

Fig. 3.   Frank breech.

Fig. 4.   Footling breech.

Fig. 5.   Kneeling breech.

RIGHT SACRUM ANTERIOR: RSA

Diagnosis of Position

Abdominal Examination

1. The lie is longitudinal.
2. A soft irregular mass is felt lying over the pelvis which does not feel like the head. One suspects breech. In a frank breech the muscles of the thighs are drawn taut over the underlying bones, giving an impression of hardness not unlike the head, and leading to diagnostic errors.
3. The back is on the right near the midline. The small parts are on the left, away from the midline, and posterior.
4. The head is felt in the fundus of the uterus. If the head is under the liver or the ribs it may be difficult to palpate. The head is harder and more globular than the breech, and sometimes it can be ballotted. Whenever a ballottable mass is felt in the fundus, breech presentation should be suspected.
5. There is no cephalic prominence and the breech is not ballottable.

Fetal Heart

The fetal heart tones are heard loudest at or above the umbilicus, and on the same side as the back. In RSA the fetal heart is heard best in the right upper quadrant of the maternal abdomen. Sometimes the fetal heart is heard below the umbilicus, and, hence, the diagnosis made by palpation should not be changed because of the location of the fetal heart.

Vaginal Examination

1. The presenting part is high.
2. The smooth regular, hard head with its suture lines and fontanelles is absent. This negative finding suggests a malpresentation.
3. The presenting part is soft and irregular. The anal orifice and the ischial tuberosities are in a straight line. The breech may be confused with a face.
4. Sometimes in frank breeches the sacrum is pulled down, and is felt by the examining finger. It may be mistaken for the head because of its bony hardness.
5. The sacrum is in the right anterior quadrant of the pelvis, and the bitrochanteric diameter is in the right oblique.
6. Sometimes a foot is felt. It must be distinguished from a hand.

X-ray Examination

The X-ray is valuable both in confirming the diagnosis and in estimating the size and configuration of the maternal pelvis. It should be carried out in all primigravidas and in multiparas who have had only small babies or difficult deliveries. The X-ray will show accurately the attitude and position of the fetus, as well as abnormalities such as hydrocephalus.

Fig. 6A. Abdominal view.

Fig. 6B. Vaginal view.

MECHANISMS OF LABOR: BREECH PRESENTATIONS

Cephalic and breech presentations are like triangles. When the head presents, the base of the triangle leads the way in that the largest and most unyielding part of the baby comes first, and the parts that follow are progressively smaller. When the breech presents, on the other hand, the apex of the triangle comes first and the succeeding parts are progressively bigger, with the relatively large head being last. In cases of cephalopelvic disproportion, by the time that it is realized that the head is too big for this pelvis, the rest of the baby has been born and vaginal delivery must be carried on, with sad results for the baby.

In breech presentations there are three mechanisms of labor:

1. The buttocks and lower limbs
2. The shoulders and arms
3. The head

Mechanism of Labor: Right Sacrum Anterior

The Buttocks and Lower Limbs

Descent: Engagement has been achieved when the bitrochanteric diameter has passed through the inlet of the pelvis. In RSA the sacrum is in the right anterior quadrant of the maternal pelvis, and the bitrochanteric diameter is in the right oblique diameter of the pelvis. Since the breech is a less efficient dilator than the head, descent is slow, and the breech may remain high until labor has been in progress for some time. In many instances the breech does not come down until the cervix is fully dilated and the membranes ruptured.

Flexion: In order to facilitate passage of the breech through the pelvis, lateral flexion takes place at the waist. The anterior hip becomes the leading part. Where the breech is frank, the baby's legs act as a splint along the body, and, by reducing lateral flexion and maneuverability, may prevent descent into the pelvis.

Internal Rotation of the Breech: The anterior hip meets the resistance of the pelvic floor and rotates forward, downward, and toward the midline. The bitrochanteric diameter rotates 45 degrees from the right oblique diameter of the pelvis to the anteroposterior. The sacrum turns away from the midline, from the right anterior quadrant to the right transverse (RSA to RST).

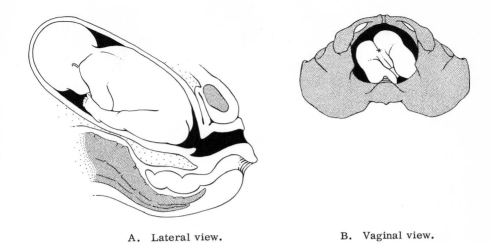

A. Lateral view.   B. Vaginal view.

Fig. 7. R.S.A.: onset of labor.

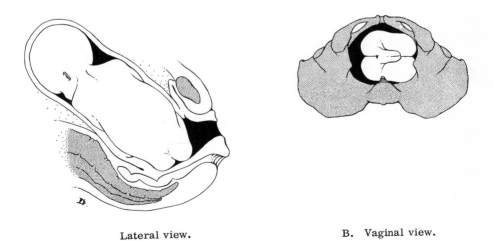

Lateral view.   B. Vaginal view.

Fig. 8. Descent and internal rotation of buttocks.

Birth of the Buttocks by Lateral Flexion: The anterior hip impinges under the pubic symphysis, lateral flexion occurs, the posterior hip rises and is born over the perineum.   The buttocks then fall toward the anus and the anterior hip slips out under the symphysis.

Fig. 9. Breech crowning.

Fig. 10. Birth of posterior buttock.

Fig. 11. Birth of anterior buttock.

The Shoulders and Arms

   Engagement: Engagement of the shoulders takes place in the right oblique diameter of the pelvis, as the sacrum rotates RST to RSA.

   Internal Rotation of the Shoulders: The anterior shoulder rotates under the symphysis, and the bisacromial diameter turns 45 degrees from the right oblique to the anteroposterior diameter of the outlet. The sacrum goes along, RSA to RST.

   Birth of the Shoulders by Lateral Flexion: The anterior shoulder impinges under the symphysis and the posterior shoulder and arm are born over the perineum as the baby's body is lifted upward. The baby is then lowered and the anterior shoulder and arms pass out under the symphysis.

Fig. 12. Feet born, shoulders engaging.

Fig. 13. Descent and internal rotation of shoulders.

Fig. 14. Posterior shoulder born; head has entered the pelvis.

The Head

Descent and Engagement: When the shoulders are at the outlet, the head is entering the pelvis. It enters the pelvis with the sagittal suture in the left oblique diameter. The occiput is in the right anterior quadrant of the pelvis.

Flexion: Flexion of the head will take place just as in any other presentation. It is important that flexion is maintained.

Internal Rotation: The head strikes the pelvic floor and rotates internally so that it comes to the outlet with the sagittal suture in the anteroposterior diameter, the brow in the hollow of the sacrum, and the occiput under the symphysis. The sacrum rotates toward the pubis, so that the back is anterior.

Birth of the Head by Flexion: The diameters are the same as in occipitoanterior positions but in reverse order. The nape of the neck pivots under the symphysis, and the chin, mouth, nose, forehead, bregma, and occiput are born over the perineum by a movement of flexion.

Mechanism of Labor: Sacrum Directly Anterior

Descent: Engagement takes place with the bitrochanteric diameter in the transverse diameter of the inlet. The sacrum is directly anterior, behind the symphysis pubis (SA).

Flexion: Flexion is the same as in RSA.

Internal Rotation: The bitrochanteric diameter rotates 90 degrees from the transverse diameter of the pelvis to the anteroposterior. The sacrum turns away from the midline to the transverse (SA to RST).

The rest of the mechanism of labor is the same as in RSA.

Fig. 15. Anterior shoulder born; descent of head.

Fig. 16. Internal rotation and beginning flexion of the head.

Fig. 17. Flexion of the head complete.

Mechanism of Labor: Sacrum Posterior

In the rare case, the sacrum and the head rotate posteriorly so that the occiput is in the hollow of the sacrum and the face is behind the pubis.

If the head is flexed, delivery occurs with the occiput posterior. The nasion pivots in the subpubic angle, and the nape of the neck, occiput, and vertex roll over the perineum. The face then emerges from behind the pubis. This method of delivery is helped by lifting up the child's body.

If the head is extended, the chin impinges behind the pubis, and the submental area of the neck pivots in the subpubic angle. For delivery to take place the infant's body must be raised by the accoucheur so that the occiput, vertex, and forehead can pass over the perineum in that order.

Delivery of the head from this position can be difficult. The best management of this complication lies in its prevention. Once the breech has been born, any tendency for the sacrum to rotate posteriorly must be restrained by the attendant, and the breech encouraged to turn with the sacrum anteriorly toward the symphysis pubis.

Mechanism of Labor in Footling and Kneeling Breech

The mechanism of labor is the same as has been described in RSA with the difference being that in complete and frank breech presentations the buttocks form the leading part. In footling presentations, it is one or both feet; and in kneeling breeches, it is the knees.

PROGNOSIS: BREECH PRESENTATIONS

Maternal

When spontaneous delivery takes place the maternal prognosis is good. Genital tract lacerations and hemorrhage may be caused by excessively rapid and forceful delivery of the baby through a pelvis which may be too small or in which the soft parts have not been dilated sufficiently.

Fetal

The gross mortality ranges between 10 and 20 percent. The main cause of fetal loss is prematurity (30 percent as contrasted with 10 percent in cephalic presentations). Congenital malformations are twice as common in breech as in cephalic presentations and contribute to fetal wastage.

Fig. 18. Sacrum posterior: head flexed.

Fig. 19. Sacrum posterior: head extended.

While the risk to the baby of breech presentation must be distinguished from the intrinsic danger of breech delivery, the risk to the infant of breech birth is higher than that of being born head first.   Excluding malformations incompatible with life, and intrauterine death before the onset of labor, the fetal mortality in mature infants (2,500 g and over) is between 1 and 2 percent in the hands of skilled obstetricians.   With inexperienced attendants the risk is higher.

Causes of Death or Damage to the Baby

1. Asphyxia
   a. Prolonged compression of the umbilical cord between the pelvis and the aftercoming head
   b. Actual prolapse of the cord
   c. Aspiration of amniotic fluid and vaginal contents caused by active breathing before the head has been born
   d. Prolonged and hard labor
2. Injury to brain and skull
   a. The aftercoming head passes through the pelvis rapidly.   Instead of gradual molding taking place over several hours, there is rapid, and sometimes excessive, compression and decompression occurring within a few minutes.   The ligaments of the brain are subjected to sudden and marked stretching, with the risk of lacerations and intracranial hemorrhage.   Injury to the brain may follow delivery through an incompletely dilated cervix or through a pelvis whose adequacy has been estimated incorrectly.
   b. Minute hemorrhages
   c. Fractures of the skull
3. Damage resulting from rough handling during the delivery
   a. Fractures of the neck, humerus, clavicle, and femur
   b. Cervical and brachial plexus paralyses
   c. Rupture of the liver caused by grasping the baby too tightly around the abdomen while extracting it
4. The size of the baby
   a. Large babies, over 8 pounds, give trouble in that they may be too big for the pelvis.
   b. Premature babies have small bodies in relation to their heads.   The little breech is not a good dilator and fails to make room for the head.
5. Congenital malformation: The incidence of congenital malformation such as hydrocephalus in breech presentations is close to 8 percent, and this makes prognosis less favorable.   Polyhydramnios is three times as common as in normal presentations.

6. Rupture of membranes: It has been shown that the fetal mortality is significantly higher if the interval from rupture of the membranes to delivery is
prolonged. The perinatal loss of mature infants was increased threefold if
more than 24 hours elapsed from the rupture of the bag of waters to delivery. If the latent period between rupture of membranes and onset of labor
was over 12 hours, the fetal loss was increased three times in primigravidas and fivefold in multiparas. These findings do not hold for premature
infants.

MANAGEMENT OF BREECH PRESENTATION

Classification of Breech Births

Vaginal

1. Spontaneous breech delivery: The entire infant is expelled by the natural
   forces of the mother, with no assistance other than support of the baby as
   it is being born.
2. Assisted breech (or partial breech extraction): The infant is delivered by
   the natural forces as far as the umbilicus. The remainder of the baby is
   extracted by the attendant. In normal cases, we believe this to be the best
   method.
3. Total breech extraction: The entire body of the infant is extracted by the
   attendant.

Cesarean Section

The incidence is about 10 percent.

Management of Breech Presentation in Late Pregnancy

External Version

There is disagreement as to the advisability of external version during
pregnancy. Since fetal mortality is higher in breech than in cephalic deliveries,
many authorities believe that external version (turning the breech to a cephalic
presentation) should be attempted in all cases (see Ch.   for technic). While
the incidence of breech presentation decreases as term is neared, in most pregnancies the fetus has assumed its final position by the thirty-fourth week. The
best time for external version is at 32 to 34 weeks gestation. The procedure
must be done gently and with no excessive force, since there is danger of placental separation or damage to the fetus. Version may succeed, may be unsuccessful, or may recur. Before attempting external version one must be certain
of the position to avoid turning a cephalic presentation to a breech.

On the other hand, because the fetal loss associated with external version
is about the same as that with breech delivery; because at 32 to 34 weeks around
20 percent of fetuses present by the breech, with all but 3 or 4 percent changing
spontaneously to cephalic presentations; and because experience in management
of breech deliveries must be obtained so that proper care can be taken of those
cases which persist as breeches (where external version fails, or where the

breech presentation recurs after successful version), many obstetricians believe that external version is unnecessary and inadvisable. External version is most difficult to perform in frank breeches (especially in the primigravida), and this is the commonest variety.

X-ray Pelvimetry

X-ray pelvimetry is indicated in all primigravidas and in multiparas who have had only small babies or difficult deliveries. This aids in deciding as to the method of delivery. If the pelvigram shows a poor pelvis, elective cesarean section is preferable. If the pelvis is adequate or borderline then a test of labor with probable vaginal delivery is the procedure of choice. The x-ray will help diagnose fetal anomalies such as hydrocephaly.

Management of Labor and Delivery in the Progressing Case

First Stage of Labor

1. Because most breech presentations progress to successful vaginal delivery, observant expectancy, supportive therapy, and absence of interference are the procedures of choice.
2. The patient is best in bed.
3. It is best to maintain intact membranes until the cervical dilatation is far advanced. Too frequent vaginal or rectal examinations, or any procedure which might contribute to premature rupture of the bag of waters, should be avoided.
4. When the membranes do rupture, vaginal examination is done to rule out prolapse of the umbilical cord and to determine the exact condition of the cervix.
5. Meconium is no cause for alarm as long as the fetal heart is normal.

Second Stage of Labor

Position for Delivery: Once the cervix is fully dilated the patient is placed on the delivery table. The firmness of the table and the handbars, which the patient uses to brace herself, increase the effectiveness of the bearing-down efforts, and so expedite progress.

When the breech begins to distend the perineum, the patient is placed in the lithotomy position, with the legs in stirrups, and the buttocks extending slightly past the end of the table. This is the best position in which to assist the birth and to handle complications.

During a contraction the pressure of the presenting part on the perineum stimulates the patient to move up the table and out of position. To prevent this shoulder braces are invaluable.

An assistant should be scrubbed and gowned for every delivery.

The patient's bladder is catheterized.

Intravenous Infusion: When the second stage has started, an intravenous infusion of 5 percent glucose in water should be set up. It is important for the successful delivery of a breech presentation that good uterine contractions continue and that the patient retains the ability, and uses it, to bear down. Should the contractions become weak or irregular during the actual delivery, oxytocin can be added quickly to the infusion, and the uterus stimulated to more effective activity.

Assisted Breech: The fetal heart is checked frequently. As long as the baby is in good condition spontaneous delivery is awaited. Premature traction on the baby, especially between contractions, must be avoided. This can lead to deflexion of the head and extension of the arms above or behind the head. It is important that the patient bear down with each contraction, and she must be encouraged to do so. Once the body has been born, the head is out of the upper contracting part of the uterus and in the lower segment, the cervix, or upper vagina. Since these organs do not have the power to expel the head, its descent and delivery must be effected by the voluntary action of the abdominal muscles, and the attendant's exerting suprapubic pressure. Fetal salvage will be increased by calmness and slowness rather than by agitation and speed.

Our experience has been that in normally progressing cases the best results are obtained by a policy of:

1. No interference (except episiotomy) until the body is born to the umbilicus. This permits the cervix to become not only fully dilated but also paralyzed, a factor which is important in minimizing dystocia with the aftercoming head.
2. Hard bearing down by the mother during contractions
3. The maintenance of suprapubic pressure during descent to aid delivery and to keep the head in flexion

The reasons for using this technic are:

1. It has proved to be successful.
2. It is safe. There is less trauma to the baby.
3. Flexion of the head is maintained.
4. The danger of extension of the arms above the head is reduced.
5. There is less chance of the cervix clamping down around the baby's head or neck.

Anesthesia: A combination of local and general anesthesia is employed. Pudendal block or perineal infiltration permits episiotomy without pain and facilitates delivery by relaxing the muscles. In addition, with each contraction the patient takes several breaths of an anesthetic vapor. This acts as an analgesic, eases the pain, and helps her to bear down more efficiently. Actual general anesthesia is not instituted until the baby is born to the umbilicus.

We have used epidural anesthesia with success. The drawback is that once the perineal dose takes effect, the reflex stimulation from pressure of the presenting part on the perineum may be reduced or removed, and the patient's desire to bear down with each contraction lost. This unwanted effect can be obviated by omitting the perineal dose, and using local anesthesia for the episiotomy. In this way the analgesic value of the epidural dose during labor is maintained without loss of the perineal reflex during the delivery.

Equipment Which Must Be at Hand:

1. A warm dry towel to be wrapped around the baby's body as soon as it is sufficiently born. The purposes of this are:
   a. To reduce the stimulating effect of cold air on the baby in the hope that

respiration will not begin while the head is in the pelvis, and aspiration of amniotic fluid or vaginal contents will not occur

b. To make it easier to hold the slippery baby

2. Piper forceps for the aftercoming head, if it does not deliver with assistance easily

3. Equipment for resuscitation of the infant must be in the delivery room and ready for immediate use.

Episiotomy: Since in many cases the breech dilates the perineum insufficiently to allow easy passage of the head, an adequate episiotomy is essential. It is safer to make a big episiotomy to avoid having to enlarge it while occupied with delivery of the head. The mediolateral incision is the better. The perineotomy must be done at the optimum time, that is, before the breech crowns or one is faced with the need for delivering the infant and making the incision simultaneously. On the other hand, if the incision is made too soon the blood loss can be excessive. Hence, the episiotomy should be performed just before the buttocks crown or when the attendant feels that their birth will occur with the next one or two contractions.

Delivery of the Breech:

1. The patient is encouraged to bear down with the contractions, but must rest between them.

2. When the buttocks are ready to crown, a wide mediolateral episiotomy is made and hemostasis secured.

3. As long as there is no fetal or maternal distress, spontaneous delivery to the umbilicus is awaited. Up to this point there is no urgency, and the operator should not interfere.

4. Once the umbilicus has been delivered, time becomes an important factor, and the remainder of the birth is expedited gently and skillfully. A free airway to the mouth should be available within 3 to 5 minutes to obviate anoxic brain damage.

5. The legs usually deliver spontaneously, or they are extracted easily.

6. The baby is covered with a warm towel and the body is supported.

7. A loop of umbilical cord is pulled down to minimize traction on it in case it is caught between the head and the pelvic wall. At the same time it is palpated for pulsations.

8. The anesthetist is asked to put the patient to sleep at this stage of the delivery.

Delivery of the Shoulders and Arms:

1. The assistant exerts suprapubic pressure on the head to maintain its flexion.

2. The operator depresses the buttocks and delivers the body to the anterior scapula so that the anterior shoulder comes under the symphysis.

3. To deliver the anterior arm the accoucheur passes his hand up the baby's back, over the shoulder, and down the chest, thus sweeping the arm and hand out under the pubis with his finger.

4. The baby is raised so that the posterior scapula and then the posterior arm are born over the perineum by the same maneuver.

5. Some obstetricians deliver the posterior arm first.

Fig. 20. Loop of umbilical cord being pulled down.

Fig. 21. Extraction of anterior arm.

Fig. 22. Extraction of posterior arm.

Delivery of the Head:

1. In almost every case the back will turn anteriorly spontaneously. This must be encouraged so that the head will rotate the occiput to the pubis and the face toward the sacrum. Rarely, there is a tendency for the back to turn posteriorly. The obstetrician must counteract this, and rotate the back anteriorly to prevent the head's rotating face to pubis, a serious and always avoidable complication.

2. Once the back has rotated anteriorly and the fetal head is in the anteroposterior diameter of the pelvis, the body is lowered so that the occiput appears under the symphysis, and the nape of the neck pivots there.

3. At the same time the assistant maintains suprapubic pressure to guide the head through the pelvis and to keep it flexed.

4. The body is then raised gently so that there is slight extension at the neck.

5. Then by further suprapubic pressure (Kristellar maneuver) the head is delivered in flexion, the chin, mouth, nose, forehead, bregma, and vertex being born in order over the perineum.

6. The speed of delivery of the aftercoming head must be considered. The rapid passage of the head through the pelvis causes sudden compression and decompression of the cranial contents. In the extreme, the ligaments of the brain will tear, leading to hemorrhage, cerebral damage, and death. On the other hand, too slow delivery of the head results in asphyxia, which may also be fatal. Experience teaches the middle road, slow enough to prevent injury to the brain and sufficiently rapid to avoid asphyxia.

Fig. 23. Body lowered so that nape of neck is in the subpubic angle. Assistant maintains flexion of the head.

Fig. 24. Kristellar maneuver: head born in flexion.

ARREST IN BREECH PRESENTATION

Most babies that present by the breech are born spontaneously, or with the help of, but not interference from, the attendant. The Kristellar maneuver (suprapubic pressure) is all that is needed to deliver the aftercoming head. However, progress may cease and active interference becomes mandatory. Arrest may take place at the head, neck, shoulders and arms, or the buttocks.

Arrest of the Head

When the head arrests the body, shoulders, and arms have been born, but the bearing-down efforts of the mother and the Kristellar maneuver are not successful in delivering the head. Several measures are available to extract the head.

Wigand-Martin Maneuver

The body of the baby is placed on the arm of the operator, the middle finger of the hand of that arm is placed in the baby's mouth, and the index and ring fingers on the malar bones. The purpose of the finger in the mouth is not for traction but to encourage and maintain flexion. With his other hand the obstetrician exerts suprapubic pressure on the head through the mother's abdomen.

Mauriceau-Smellie-Veit Maneuver

The position is the same as the Wigand-Martin, with one finger in the baby's mouth and two on the malar bones. The difference is that the accoucheur places his other hand astride the baby's shoulders and produces traction in this way. The efficiency of this procedure is increased by an assistant's applying suprapubic pressure on the fetal head while the operator is performing the Mauriceau maneuver.

Piper Forceps on the Aftercoming Head

1. The baby's feet are grasped by an assistant and the body is raised. Care must be taken not to elevate the body too much for fear of damage to the sternomastoid muscles. A good way to keep the arms out of the way is to use a folded towel as described by Savage.
2. The right hand is placed in the vagina, and the left forceps blade is guided into place over the parietal bone. Should there be a rim of cervix still present, the blade must be inserted inside of it.
3. The right blade is then applied using the left hand as a guide.
4. The forceps are locked. The blades fit along the occipitomental diameter, one over each ear.
5. With the exception of simple suprapubic pressure, the best method of delivering the aftercoming head is by the use of the Piper forceps. In contrast to those maneuvers where traction on the head is effected through the neck, the forceps exert traction directly on the head, and damage to structures in the baby's neck is avoided.

Fig. 25. Wigand–Martin maneuver.

Fig. 26. Mauriceau–Smellie–Veit maneuver.

Fig. 27. Management of fetal arms (Savage) as Piper forceps are applied.

6. Traction is made and the head extracted slowly (see Ch. 29). This operation should be performed only when the head is in the pelvis. Any type of forceps can be used to deliver the aftercoming head. The Piper forceps have a double curve in the blades and in the shanks, the shanks are long, and the handles are depressed below the arch of the shanks. This instrument should be employed whenever possible, since it is easier to use and more efficient than the regular forceps.

Airway

Where there is delay in delivery of the head and one is waiting for help or instruments, an ordinary vaginal retractor can be used temporarily to clear an airway in the vagina to the baby's mouth. The retractor is placed in the vagina, and pressure exerted posteriorly. The vaginal contents are sponged out, so that air can get to the baby should it breathe.

The Prague Maneuver

The Prague maneuver is used when the occiput is posterior. The fingers are placed over the shoulders, and outward and upward traction is made. The legs are grasped with the other hand, and the body is swung over the mother's abdomen. By this procedure the occiput is born over the perineum. This method carries with it the danger of overstretching or breaking the neck of the infant and is used rarely.

Embryotomy

When delivery of the head is not accomplished within reasonable time, the baby may die. If it does perish the mother's welfare alone should be considered. To save her from needless injury, reduction of the size of the child's head by perforation of the skull is preferable to its extraction by brute force.

Fig. 28.   Vaginal retractor providing airway to the baby's mouth and nose.

Fig. 29.   Prague maneuver.

Arrest of the Neck

Occasionally the cervix, which has opened sufficiently to allow the trunk and shoulders to be born, will clamp down around the baby's neck, trapping the head in the uterus. The possibility of this happening is greater in the premature baby, where the body has not yet developed its adipose tissue and is a poor dilating wedge. This dangerous situation calls for rapid action to break the spasm of the previously dilated cervix. This is accomplished by a single bold incision of the cervix with the scissors. The resultant relaxing of the spasm will permit the head to be born.

Arrest of the Shoulders and Arms

Extended Arms: The arms are simply extended over the baby's head.

Nuchal Arms: There is extension at the shoulder and flexion at the elbow so that the forearm is trapped behind the fetal head. One or both arms may be affected.

Prophylaxis

One method of reducing the incidence of this complication is to resist the temptation to pull on the baby's legs to speed the delivery, especially when the uterus is in a relaxed state.

Simple Extraction

When this problem does occur an attempt should be made first to deliver the arms by sweeping them over the chest in the usual way. This will succeed in most cases of simple extension and in some instances of nuchal arms when the upper limb is not jammed tightly behind the head.

Rotation of Body

If extraction fails in the case of a nuchal arm, the baby's body is rotated in the direction to which the hand is pointing. This will dislodge the arm from behind the head and its delivery is then usually possible as described above. If both arms are nuchal, the body is rotated in one direction to free the first arm, which is then extracted, and next in the opposite direction to free the other arm.

Fracture

In the rare instance where rotation fails, the humerus or clavicle must be fractured. This can be done directly, or it can be effected by simply pulling on the arm until it breaks. Once this occurs delivery can be accomplished. Since the fracture usually heals rapidly and well, and since the choice may be between a dead baby and a broken arm, extreme measures are justified.

Fig. 30. Arm extended above the head.

Fig. 31. Nuchal arm.

Fig. 32. Nuchal arm: rotation of the trunk of the child 90º in the direction to which the hand is pointing.

Fig. 33. Nuchal arm: hand introduced into the uterus to flex and bring down the nuchal arm.

Failure of Descent of the Breech

Etiology

In any situation the size of the passenger, the capacity of the pelvis, the dilatability of the maternal soft tissues, and the character of the uterine contractions all play a part in determining whether spontaneous delivery will take place.

In frank breech presentation there is an added factor. The splinting effect of the baby's legs across its abdomen can reduce the maneuverability of the fetus to an extent that progress is arrested.

Disproportion

In the presence of good uterine contractions, nondescent of the breech is an indication, not for hasty interference, but for the most careful reassessment. Keeping in mind the fact that one of the causes of breech presentation is a large head which cannot engage easily, the accoucheur must be assured, not of the general capacity of the pelvis, but of its adequacy with respect to that particular baby. More and more evidence is appearing in the literature that when, in spite of good contractions, a breech fails to descend, disproportion is present, and cesarean section must be considered seriously.

Decomposition

If there is good evidence that vaginal delivery is feasible, progress and descent can be expedited by reducing the bulk of the breech, an operation known as decomposition. This is done by bringing down the legs, both whenever possible. When there is complete flexion at the hips and the knees, the feet can be reached easily. The hand is placed in the uterus, the membranes are ruptured, a foot is grasped and brought down. Be sure it is not a hand. The same is done for the other foot. The position has been changed to a footling breech, and labor proceeds.

Pinard Maneuver

If the breech is frank (flexion at the hips and extension at the knees), it may be impossible to reach the feet, as they are high in the uterus near the baby's face. In such situations the Pinard maneuver is performed under anesthesia. With a hand in the uterus, pressure is made by the fingers against the popliteal fossa in a backward and outward direction. This will bring about flexion of the knee to a sufficient extent that the foot can be grasped with the other fingers and delivered. Where possible both feet should be delivered. Unless there are urgent indications for immediate delivery, labor is allowed to carry on as in a footling breech.

Footling

Sometimes a single footling breech is encountered which descends only to the midpelvis. Examination may show that either the other foot or flexed knee is impinged against the pubic symphysis, preventing further advance. Simple freeing of the foot or knee, and bringing down the leg will allow labor to proceed in many cases.

Cesarean Section

Sometimes breaking up a breech gives good results in multiparas. The belief is growing, on the other hand, that where this procedure is thought to be indicated in primigravidas cesarean section is the wiser and safer procedure.

Fig. 34. Decomposition of breech: bringing down a foot and leg.

Fig. 35. Pinard maneuver: first step.

Fig. 36. Pinard maneuver: second step.

TEST OF LABOR IN A BREECH PRESENTATION

In a vertex presentation a test of labor is based on the premise that if the relatively large fetal head will come through the pelvis, so will the rest of the baby. In a breech, however, by the time the head is entering the pelvis, the proportionately small body has been born, and it is too late to do anything but deliver per vaginam. To a degree every confinement in breech presentation is a test of labor. First the adequacy of the pelvis must be measured by manual and radiologic methods. Decisions with regard to the baby are based on clinical estimation of the size and clinical and radiologic determination of the presentation, configuration, and normalcy of the fetus.

In the presence of adequate pelvic and associated findings, the patient labors under careful observation. If the uterine contractions are efficient, if the fetal heart remains strong, regular, and normal in rate, if the cervix dilates well, and the presenting part descends steadily, labor is allowed to proceed. Experience has shown that in most cases where the buttocks are born spontaneously, the delivery of the rest of the baby will be successful and safe.

On the other hand, fetal distress, inefficient contractions, lack of descent or dilatation of the cervix for 2 or 3 hours in the presence of good labor, failure of advancement of the breech once complete dilatation of the cervix has been reached, labor which lasts over 12 hours, absence of good progress after spontaneous rupture of the membranes, are all ominous signs calling for reassessment of the entire situation and consideration of cesarean section. In those cases which ended with a dead or damaged baby there was a combination of these factors, and it was evident (on looking back) that in most instances things had been going badly for some time before the actual delivery.

The decision as to how long a test of labor should go on can be made only by the attendant obstetrician, preferably with consultation, and varies from one case to another.

BREECH EXTRACTION

This operation is the immediate vaginal extraction of the baby when signs of fetal distress demand delivery without delay.

Prerequisites: Conditions which must be present before this procedure may be performed include: 1. The pelvis must be ample, with no disproportion. 2. The cervix must be fully dilated. 3. The bladder and rectum should be empty. 4. Expert and deep anesthesia is essential. 5. Good assistance is mandatory. 6. The child must be alive.

Procedure: The patient is placed in the lithotomy position, the bladder is catheterized, and anesthesia is administered. As described in a previous section, the breech is decomposed, and the legs are brought down. The feet are pulled down if the breech is complete. The Pinard maneuver is used if the breech is frank. Instead of letting the patient go on to spontaneous delivery the baby is extracted rapidly. Traction from below is substituted for uterine contractions from above, but the maneuvers for delivery of the shoulders, arms, and head are those already set forth in the management of arrested cases.

While expert and experienced obstetricians have reported good results with routine breech extraction as soon as the cervix is fully dilated, we believe that, in the hands of the average doctor, this operation is hazardous for both mother and child. We feel that it should be carried out only in urgent situations where the danger of waiting for spontaneous delivery is greater than that of forceful extraction.

UTERINE INERTIA AND OXYTOCIN

A treacherous complication of labor in breech presentation is uterine inertia, primary (inefficient uterine action), or secondary (myometrial fatigue). Hall found that in inertic labors and in those lasting more than 30 hours, the perinatal loss rose to between 12 and 19 percent.

One of the major causes of fetal mortality during labor and delivery is unrecognized disproportion. Uterine inertia or failure of descent of the breech is so suggestive of disproportion, that this complication must be ruled out before treatment of the inertia is carried out.

The danger of stimulating labor by oxytocin is higher in breech than in cephalic presentations. It should not be used unless there is certainty that the pelvis is adequate for the baby. The employment of an oxytocin drip may be considered in selected cases of secondary inertia (especially in multiparas) where the pelvis is ample and when progress has been satisfactory up to the onset of inertia. In such cases a short trial of oxytocin stimulation is preferable to breech extraction, and may be indicated before a decision is made in favor of cesarean section.

Once the buttocks are pressing against the perineum and vaginal delivery is to be carried out, we have found an oxytocin drip to be valuable in ensuring that good contractions continue for the rest of the delivery.

BREECH PRESENTATION IN AN ELDERLY PRIMIGRAVIDA

This is a special case. If all conditions are favorable, a test of labor is permitted. If there is any doubt as to reasonably easy vaginal delivery, cesarean section should be elected.

BIBLIOGRAPHY

Foote, W. R. , and Sabin, M. The management of breech presentation in the primigravida. Amer. J. Obstet. Gynec. , 77:521, 1959.

Friedlander, D. External cephalic version in the management of breech presentation. Amer. J. Obstet. Gynec. , 95:906, 1966.

Hall, J. E. , Kohl, S. G. , O'Brien, F. , and Ginsberg, M. S. Breech presentation and perinatal mortality. Amer. J. Obstet. Gynec. , 91:665, 1965.

MacArthur, J. L. Reduction of the hazards of breech presentation by external cephalic version. Amer. J. Obstet. Gynec. , 88:302, 1964.

Neimand, K. M. , and Rosenthal, A. H. Oxytocin in breech presentation. Amer. J. Obstet. Gynec. , 93:230, 1965.

Savage, J. E. Management of fetal arms in breech extraction. Obstet. Gynec. , 3:55, 1954.

Todd, W. D. , and Steer, C. M. Term breech: Review of 1006 term breech deliveries. Obstet. Gynec. , 22:583, 1963.

19 Transverse Lie

Definition: When the long axes of mother and fetus are at right angles to one another, a transverse lie is present. Because the shoulder is placed so frequently in the brim of the inlet, this malposition is often referred to as "Shoulder presentation." The baby may lie directly across the maternal abdomen, or it may lie obliquely with the head or breech in the iliac fossa. Usually the breech is at a higher level than the head. The denominator is the scapula (Sc), the situation of the head determines whether the position is left or right, and that of the back indicates whether it is anterior or posterior. Thus LScP means that the lie is transverse, the head is on the mother's left side, and the baby's back is posterior. The part which actually lies over the pelvic brim may be the shoulder, the back, the abdomen, the ribs, or the flank.

Incidence: The incidence of transverse lie is around 1 in 500. This is a serious malposition whose management must not be left to nature.

Etiology: Anything that prevents engagement of the head or the breech may predispose to transverse lie. This abnormality is more common in multiparas than primigravidas because of the laxness of the uterine and abdominal muscles. Included are such factors as placenta previa; obstructing neoplasm; multiple pregnancies; fetal anomalies; polyhydramnios; prematurity; fetopelvic disproportion; uterine abnormalities such as uterus subseptus, uterus arcuatus, and uterus bicornis; and contracted pelvis. In many instances no etiologic factor can be determined, and we assume that the malposition is accidental. The head happens to be out of the lower uterine segment when labor starts, and the shoulder is pushed into the pelvic brim.

Fig. 1.   Transverse lie: L. Sc. P.

Fig. 2.   Oblique lie: breech in
iliac fossa.

Fig. 3.   Oblique lie: head in
iliac fossa.

Diagnosis of Position: Transverse Lie

Abdominal Examination

1. The appearance of the abdomen is asymmetrical.
2. The long axis of the fetus is across the mother's abdomen.
3. The uterine fundus is lower than expected for the period of gestation. It has been described as a "squat uterus." Its upper limit is near the umbilicus, and it is wider than usual.
4. Palpation of the upper and lower poles of the uterus reveals neither the head nor the breech.
5. The head can be felt in one maternal flank.
6. The buttocks are on the other side.

Fetal Heart

The fetal heart is heard best below the umbilicus, and has no diagnostic significance regarding position.

Vaginal Examination

The most important finding is a negative one; neither the head nor the breech can be felt by the examining finger. The presenting part is high. In some cases one may actually feel the shoulder, a hand, the rib cage, or the back. Because of the poor fit of the presenting part to the pelvis the bag of waters may hang into the vagina.

X-ray Examination

X-ray examination is valuable, both to confirm the diagnosis and to detect abnormalities in the fetus or the mother's pelvis.

Mechanism of Labor: Transverse Lie

A persistent transverse lie cannot deliver spontaneously, and if uncorrected, impaction takes place. The shoulder is jammed into the pelvis, the head and breech stay above the inlet, the neck becomes stretched, and progress is arrested. Transverse lies must never be left to nature.

Spontaneous Version

Spontaneous version takes place occasionally, more often with oblique than with transverse lies. Before, or shortly after, the onset of labor, the lie changes to a longitudinal one (cephalic or breech) and labor proceeds in the new position. Unfortunately, the chance of spontaneous version occurring is small, too small to warrant more than a very short delay in instituting corrective measures.

Fig. 4. Impacted shoulder.

Fig. 5. Prolapsed arm.

Fig. 6. Prolapsed umbilical cord.

Neglected Transverse Lie

Neglected transverse lie results from misdiagnosis or improper treatment. At first the contractions are of poor quality and the cervix dilates slowly. Because of the irregularity of the presenting part the membranes rupture early and the amniotic fluid escapes rapidly. As the labor pains become stronger the fetal shoulder is forced into the pelvis, the uterus molds itself around the baby, a state of impaction ensues, and progress is halted. From this impasse there is one of two outcomes:

1. Labor goes on, the upper part of the uterus becomes shorter and thicker, while the lower segment becomes more and more stretched and thinner and thinner, until it ruptures.
2. Uterine inertia sets in and the contractions cease. Intrauterine sepsis is followed by generalized sepsis.

In either event fetal death is certain and maternal mortality possible. Transverse lies must not be neglected!

Complications

Because the presenting part does not fill the inlet, the membranes tend to rupture early and may be followed by prolapse of a fetal arm or the umbilical cord. Both are serious complications necessitating immediate action.

Prognosis: Transverse Lie

Prognosis depends on the management. With early diagnosis and proper treatment the outcome is favorable. Neglect results in the death of all the infants and many mothers.

Management of Transverse Lie

Before Labor

1. Careful abdominal, pelvic, and radiologic examinations are performed to rule out fetal and pelvic abnormalities.
2. External version to a breech or preferably a cephalic presentation should be attempted. This may have to be repeated as there is a tendency for the transverse lie to recur.
3. Elective cesarean section is indicated where conditions exist which are incompatible with safe vaginal delivery. This includes such complications as placenta previa or fetopelvic disproportion.
4. In other cases the onset of labor is awaited, as there is a chance that the malposition will correct itself.

Early Labor

In early labor external version should be attempted, and, if successful, the new presentation is maintained by a tight abdominal binder until it is fixed in the pelvis.

Patient in Good Labor: Persistent Transverse Lie

Treatment is either cesarean section or internal podalic version and extraction. Before the decision as to management is made, five things are considered:

1. The cause of the transverse lie
2. The parity of the patient
3. The cervical dilatation
4. The state of the membranes
5. The condition of the child

Cesarean Section: Cesarean section should be performed in the following situations. The classical operation is preferred by many, as it may be difficult to extract the baby through a low transverse incision.
    a. When a condition is present which is incompatible with safe vaginal delivery
    b. In all primigravidas
    c. In a multipara with a bad obstetric history, such as a difficult delivery, a damaged baby, or a stillbirth
    d. In a multipara with a thick, closed cervix
    e. In a patient with a history of sterility

Internal Podalic Version and Extraction:* Because of the danger of prolapse of the umbilical cord, with the attendant high fetal mortality, most authorities no longer pursue the policy of allowing labor to go on in the hope that full dilatation of the cervix will be reached, at which time, version and extraction is performed. If the membranes have been ruptured for a long time and the amniotic fluid has drained away, version is dangerous, and cesarean section is preferred.

The use of podalic version and extraction (turning the baby to a footling breech and delivering it as such) is limited to the management of the following conditions:
    a. When the baby is premature, to the degree of nonviability, and the risk to the mother of cesarean section is not justified
    b. The delivery of the second twin
    c. When the patient is admitted to hospital with the membranes intact or ruptured a short time, the cervix fully or almost fully dilated, and prompt delivery is indicated and feasible

*See Chapter 30 for technic of internal podalic version.

Neglected Transverse Lie

The following conditions are present:

1. Prolonged labor
2. The membranes have been ruptured for a long time.
3. The lower uterine segment is stretched and thin.
4. Intrauterine infection is present.
5. Fetal impaction has taken place.
6. The cord, arm, or both have prolapsed.
7. The baby is dead.

Management under these circumstances is difficult.

1. Cesarean section, followed by hysterectomy if infection is present, is done in the interest of the mother even if the baby is dead.
2. Version and extraction may be considered. This carries a grave risk of rupturing the uterus and killing the mother.
3. In desperate situations a destructive operation on the child can be performed. Decapitation is carried out, the trunk is delivered, and then the head is extracted by forceps.

Conclusions

1. Transverse lies at term, after failure of external version, are treated best by cesarean section.
2. Transverse lies must never be neglected or left to nature.

BIBLIOGRAPHY

Hall, J. E., Kohl, S. G., and Kavaler, F. Transverse lie and perinatal mortality. N. Y. State J. Med., 62:2186, 1962.

Harris, B. A., and Epperson, J. W. W. An analysis of 131 cases of transverse presentation. Amer. J. Obstet. Gynec., 59:1105, 1950.

Johnson, C. E. Transverse presentation of fetus. J.A.M.A., 187:642, 1964.

MacGregor, W. G. Aetiology and treatment of the oblique, transverse, and unstable lie of the foetus with particular reference to antenatal care. J. Obstet. Gynaec. Brit. Comm., 71:237, 1964.

Posner, L. B., Tychowsky, E., and Posner, A. C. The transverse lie. Amer. J. Obstet. Gynec., 88:225, 1962.

20   Compound Presentations

PROLAPSE OF HAND AND ARM OR FOOT AND LEG

Definition: A presentation is compound when there is prolapse of one or more of the limbs along with the head or the breech, both entering the pelvis at the same time. Footling breech or shoulder presentations are not included in this group. Associated prolapse of the umbilical cord occurs in 15 to 20 percent.

Incidence: Easily detectable compound presentations occur probably once in 500 to 1,000 confinements. It is impossible to establish the exact incidence because:

1. Spontaneous correction occurs frequently, and examination late in labor will not make the diagnosis.
2. Minor degrees of prolapse will be detected only by early and careful vaginal examination.

Classification of Compound Presentation:

1. Cephalic presentation with prolapse of:
   a. Upper limb (arm-hand), one or both
   b. Lower limb (leg-foot), one or both
   c. Arm and leg together
2. Breech presentation with prolapse of the hand or arm

By far the most frequent combination is that of the head with the hand or arm. In contrast the head-foot and breech-arm groups are uncommon, about equally so. Prolapse of both hand and foot alongside the head is rare. All combinations may be complicated by prolapse of the umbilical cord, which then becomes the major problem.

Etiology: The etiology of compound presentation includes all conditions which prevent complete filling and occlusion of the pelvic inlet by the presenting part. The most common causal factor is prematurity. Others include high presenting part with ruptured membranes, multiparity, contracted pelvis, and twins.

Fig. 1. Compound presentation: head and hand.

Diagnosis

Diagnosis is made by vaginal or rectal examination. In many cases the condition is not noted until labor is well advanced and the cervix fully dilated.

Prognosis

The older authors suggested a poor prognosis for the child. However, the increased incidence of prematurity and associated prolapse of the cord make it difficult to evaluate accurately the danger to the fetus of uncomplicated prolapse of the hand or foot.

Because of the historically high fetal mortality associated with compound presentations, active therapy, repositioning of the prolapsed part or version and extraction, has been the most popular method of management. Recent studies have shown that the high fetal and maternal death rates have resulted from the overzealous treatment, and not from the compound presentation itself. With conservative management the results should be no worse than with other presentations.

Mechanism of Labor

The mechanism of labor is that of the main presenting part. Because the diameter is increased, the chance of arrested progress is greater. In many cases labor is not obstructed, and the leading part is brought down to the outlet. If dystocia occurs the baby will remain high, and operative treatment will be needed.

MANAGEMENT OF COMPOUND PRESENTATIONS

In choosing the therapeutic procedure, these factors are considered:

1. The presentation
2. The presence or absence of prolapse of the cord
3. The state of the cervix
4. The condition of the membranes
5. The condition and size of the baby
6. The presence of twins

The Progressing Case

The best treatment for compound presentations (in the absence of complications such as prolapse of the cord) is masterful inactivity. In most cases, as the cervix becomes fully dilated and the presenting part descends, the prolapsed arm or leg will rise out of the pelvis, allowing labor to proceed normally. Hence, as long as progress is being made there should be no interference.

Arrest of Progress

1. Reposition of the prolapsed part: In a normal pelvis if progress is arrested the arm or leg should be replaced, under anesthesia, and the head pushed into the pelvis. If the head is low in the pelvis and the cervix is fully dilated, it is extracted with forceps. High forceps must never be used.
2. Cesarean section: If there is cephalopelvic disproportion, if reposition is not feasible or is unsuccessful, or if there is some other condition which militates against vaginal delivery, cesarean section should be performed.
3. Internal podalic version and extraction: This procedure carries with it the danger of uterine rupture and fetal death. Hence, it should not be used in the management of uncomplicated compound presentations. An exception is made in the case of a second twin.

Prolapse of the Cord

In 13 to 23 percent the compound presentation is complicated by prolapse of the umbilical cord. This then becomes the major and urgent problem, and the treatment is directed primarily to it (see Ch. 21).

BIBLIOGRAPHY

Goplerud, J., and Eastman, N. J. Compound presentation. Obstet. Gynec., 1:59, 1953.
Quinlivan, W. L. G. Compound presentation. Can. Med. Ass. J., 76:633, 1957.
Sweeney, W. J., and Knapp, R. C. Compound presentation. Obstet. Gynec., 17:333, 1961.

21 Prolapse of the Umbilical Cord

This is the situation where the umbilical cord lies beside or below the presenting part. Although an infrequent complication—less than 1 percent (0.3 to 0.6 percent)—its significance is disproportionately great because of the high fetal mortality rate, and the increased maternal hazard from the operative procedures used in treatment.

Compression of the umbilical cord between the presenting part and the maternal pelvis reduces or cuts off the blood supply to the fetus, and, if uncorrected, leads to the death of the baby.

Classification of Prolapsed Cord

Umbilical Cord Presentation

The membranes are intact.

Umbilical Cord Prolapse

The membranes are ruptured. The cord may occupy three positions:

1. It may lie beside the presenting part at the inlet. Such an occult prolapse of the cord may be more common than generally accepted. It could kill a baby during labor without leaving a trace of evidence at vaginal delivery.
2. It may descend into the vagina.
3. It may pass through the introitus and out of the vagina.

Etiology

Whenever the presenting part does not fit closely and fails to fill the inlet of the pelvis, the danger of prolapse of the umbilical cord exists. Compound presentation and rupture of the bag of waters increases the risk.

Fetal

1. Abnormal presentation: Abnormal presentation is present in almost half the cases of prolapse of the cord. Since 95 percent of all presentations are cephalic, the greatest number of prolapsed cords occur when the head leads the way. The highest relative incidence, however, is in the following order: 1, transverse lie; 2, breech presentation, especially the footling variety; and 3, cephalic presentation.

238

Fig. 1.   Cord prolapsed at the
inlet.

Fig. 2.   Cord prolapsed into the
vagina.

Fig. 3.   Cord prolapsed through
the introitus.

2. Prematurity: Two factors play a part in the failure to fill the inlet: 1, the smallness of the presenting part; and 2, the frequency of abnormal positions in premature labors. The fetal mortality is high. One reason for this is that small babies withstand trauma and anoxia badly. The second is the reluctance to submit the mother to a major operation when the chance of saving the baby is almost nil.
3. Multiple pregnancy: The factors involved here include interference with good adaptation, greater frequency of abnormal presentation, high incidence of polyhydramnios, and rupture of the membranes of the second twin while it is still high.
4. Polyhydramnios: When the membranes rupture, the large amount of fluid pours out and the cord may be washed down.

Maternal and Obstetric

1. Cephalopelvic disproportion: Disproportion between pelvis and baby causes failure of engagement, and rupture of the membranes may be attended by prolapse of the cord.
2. High presenting part: Temporary delay of engagement may occur even in the normal pelvis, especially in multiparas. Should the membranes rupture during this period, the cord may come down.

Cord and Placenta

1. Long cord: The longer the umbilical cord the easier it is for it to prolapse.
2. Low lying placenta: When the placenta is located near the cervix it hinders engagement. In addition the insertion of the cord is nearer the cervix.

Iatrogenic

One third of prolapses of the cord are produced during obstetric procedures.

1. Artificial rupture of the membranes: When the head is high, or when there is an abnormal presentation, rupture of the membranes may be attended by prolapse of the cord.
2. Disengaging the head: Elevation of the head out of the pelvis to facilitate rotation
3. Flexion of an extended head
4. Version and extraction
5. Insertion of a bag (rarely used today)

Diagnosis: Prolapse of the Cord

The diagnosis of prolapse of the cord is made in two ways: 1, seeing the cord outside the vulva; and 2, feeling the cord on vaginal examination.

Since the fetal mortality is high once the cord has protruded through the introitus, means of earlier diagnosis must be sought.

Vaginal Examination

Vaginal examination should be made:

1. When there is unexplained fetal distress, and especially if the presenting part is not well engaged. Unfortunately fetal distress may be a late sign.
2. When the membranes rupture with a high presenting part
3. In all cases of malpresentation when the membranes rupture
4. When the baby is markedly premature
5. In cases of twins

Prognosis: Prolapse of the Cord

Labor: Labor is not affected by the prolapsed cord.

Maternal: Maternal danger is caused only by traumatic attempts to save the child.

Fetal: The uncorrected perinatal mortality is around 35 percent. The baby's chances depend on the degree and duration of the compression of the cord and the interval between diagnosis and delivery. The fetal results depend upon the following factors:

1. The better the condition of the baby at the time of diagnosis, the greater its chance of survival. A strong pulsating cord is a sign of hope, while a cord with a weak pulse is an ill omen.
2. The sooner the baby is delivered after the cord comes down, the better are the results.
3. The more mature the fetus, the greater is its ability to withstand traumatic processes.
4. The less traumatic the actual delivery of the child, the better is the prognosis for mother and baby.
5. Cervical dilatation is probably the most important point. If the cervix is fully dilated when the diagnosis is made, many babies can be saved. The less the dilatation the worse the prognosis. The exception to this situation is when rapid cesarean section can be done, in which case the prognosis is equally good or better when the cervix is dilated only to a small degree.
6. The fetal mortality increases as the interval between rupture of the membranes and delivery increases.

Management of Prolapsed Cord

1. The prolapsed cord is ignored and labor allowed to proceed under the following conditions:
   a. When the baby is dead
   b. When the baby is known to be abnormal, e.g., anencephaly
   c. When the fetus is so premature that it has no chance of survival. There is no point in subjecting the mother to needless risk.

2. Measures to lessen cord compression and improve the condition of the infant include:
   a. The attendant places a hand in the vagina and pushes the presenting part up and away from the cord. At the same time preparations are made for delivery.
   b. The patient is placed in the knee-chest or Trendelenburg position, with the hips elevated and the head low.
   c. The woman is given oxygen by mask.
   d. The fetal heart is checked carefully and often.
   e. Vaginal examination is made to ascertain the presentation, cervical dilatation, station of the presenting part, and condition of the cord.
3. The cervix is fully dilated:
   a. Cephalic presentation, head low in the pelvis: Extraction by forceps
   b. Cephalic presentation, head high: Internal podalic version and extraction as a breech. This procedure carries with it the danger of rupture of the uterus, but since this is a desperate attempt to save the child, the chance must be taken.
   c. Breech presentation: Both feet should be brought down and the baby extracted as a footling breech as soon as possible.
   d. Transverse lie: Internal podalic version to a footling and extraction are done immediately.
4. The cervix is incompletely dilated:
   a. Cesarean section is the treatment of choice as long as the child is mature and in good condition. The fetal results with cesarean section are far superior to other methods of delivery. The danger to the mother is considerably less than forceful delivery through an undilated cervix. While preparations for surgery are being made, the measures previously described for reducing compression of the cord are carried out. Spinal anesthesia can be given to stop uterine contractions.
   b. Reposition of the cord may be attempted if cesarean section cannot be performed. The cord is carried up into the uterus, and the presenting part is pushed down into the pelvis and held there. Reposition of the cord is successful occasionally, but in most cases valuable time is lost in attempting it.
   c. These measures failing, the patient is kept in the Trendelenburg position in the hope that pressure will be kept off the cord so that the child survives until the cervix is dilated enough to enable delivery to be effected.
   d. Manual dilatation of the cervix, cervical incisions, and other forceful methods of opening the cervix are almost never justified. Their success is small, and the risk to the mother is great.
5. Prophylaxis: Obstetric manipulations which encourage premature rupture of the membranes, such as artificial rupture of the membranes when the leading part is unengaged or where there is a malpresentation, and which increase the incidence of prolapse of the umbilical cord should be avoided. Patients whose membranes rupture at home, either before or during labor, should be admitted to hospital.

CORD ENTANGLEMENTS

The most common variety is the umbilical cord around the fetal neck.
Four coils have been seen from time to time and as many as nine coils have
been reported. The cord may be looped around the trunk, shoulders, and upper
or lower limbs. This condition is associated with excessive amounts of amniotic fluid, long cords, and small infants.

During pregnancy trouble is unusual. Sometimes, as the fetus descends
during labor, the coils tighten sufficiently to reduce the flow of blood through
the cord, and thus fetal anoxia is caused.

Only rarely are cord entanglements responsible for fetal or neonatal death.
However, abnormalities of the fetal heart, meconium stained amniotic fluid,
and babies requiring resuscitation are seen more often when there is an entan-
glement of the cord. Significantly lower Apgar scores have been reported.
Radical or hasty delivery is almost never indicated for cord abnormalities other than prolapse.

TRUE KNOT

Occasionally a true knot of the umbilical cord is noted after delivery. This
complication can occur where there is a long cord, large amounts of amniotic
fluid, a small infant, monoamniotic twins, an overactive fetus, or as a result
of external version. In many instances the knot is formed when a loop of cord
is slipped over the infant's head or shoulders during delivery. Rarely is there
serious trouble, although when pulled tight, the knot may produce fetal asphyxia.

LONG AND SHORT CORDS

A long cord is more likely to prolapse and to become entangled about various parts of the fetus. The average cord is 50 cm long. An otherwise normal
cord measuring 115 cm has been reported.

A short cord (e.g., 25 cm) may cause delay in descent of the fetus, abnormal position, and fetal distress, but seldom is operative interference needed.

BIBLIOGRAPHY

Cushner, I. M. Prolapse of the umbilical cord, including a late follow-up of
    fetal survivors. Amer. J. Obstet. Gynec., 81:666, 1961.

Dippel, A. L. Maligned umbilical cord entanglements. Amer. J. Obstet.
    Gynec., 88:1012, 1964.

Donaldson, I. A. Abnormal positions of the umbilical cord. Postgrad, Med.
    J., 42:20, 1966.

Nelson, H. B., and Burns, D. R. Prolapse of the umbilical cord. West. J.
    Surg. Gynec. Obstet., 71:205, 1963.

Spellacy, W. N., Gravem, H., and Fisch, R. O. The umbilical cord complica-
    tions of true knots, nuchal coils, and coils around the body. Amer. J. Ob-
    stet. Gynec., 94:1136, 1966.

Winch, G. C., and Claman, A. D. Prolapse of the cord. Can. M.A.J.,
    84:1369, 1961.

22 Shoulder Dystocia

Definition: True shoulder dystocia refers to the following situation: the presentation is cephalic, the head has been born, but the shoulders cannot be delivered by the usual methods. There is no other cause for the difficulty.

Incidence: The general incidence is less than 1 percent (0.15 to 0.2 percent). In babies weighing over 4,000 g the incidence is 1.6 percent.

Etiology: Shoulder dystocia is associated with: 1, maternal obesity; 2, excessive weight gain; 3, oversized infants; 4, history of large siblings; and 5, maternal diabetes.

Mechanism of the Shoulders

Normal Mechanism

In most cases the shoulders enter the pelvis in an oblique diameter. As labor progresses the shoulders descend, and, under the rifling effect of the birth canal, rotate the bisacromial diameter toward the anteroposterior diameter of the pelvis. By this mechanism the anterior shoulder comes under the pubic symphysis a little to the side of the midline, and is then delivered.

Mechanism in Shoulder Dystocia

Impaction of the shoulders is favored when they attempt to enter the pelvis with the bisacromial diameter in the anteroposterior diameter of the inlet, instead of utilizing one of the oblique diameters. Rarely do both shoulders impact above the pelvic brim. Usually the posterior shoulder can negotiate its way past the sacral promontory, but the anterior one becomes arrested against the pubic symphysis. Some authors restrict the definition of shoulder dystocia to cases where the shoulders try to enter the pelvis with their bisacromial diameter in the anteroposterior diameter of the inlet.

244

Fig. 1. Shoulder dystocia: bisacromial diameter in the antero-posterior diameter of the pelvis.

Causes of Dystocia after Birth of the Head

1. Short umbilical cord
2. Abdominal or thoracic enlargement of the infant (anasarca, monsters, neoplasms)
3. Locked or conjoined twins
4. Uterine constriction ring
5. True shoulder dystocia

Effects of Shoulder Dystocia

Effects on the Fetus

With each uterine contraction large amounts of blood are transferred from the baby's trunk to its head. The angulation of the neck and the compression of chest, which interfere with cardiac function, impair the venous return. The intracraniel vascular system of the fetus cannot compensate for the excessive intravascular pressure. Under these conditions anoxia develops and may be accompanied by hemorrhagic effusions. If this condition persists too long the baby suffers irreparable brain damage. It may die during the attempts at delivery or in the neonatal period.

Complications

1. Fetal:
   a. Death, intrapartum and neonatal
   b. Brachial plexus palsy (Erb's)
   c. Fractures of the clavicle
2. Maternal: Extensive lacerations of the perineum and vagina

<u>The Clinical Picture</u>

The clinical picture has been described by Morris:

    The delivery of the head with or without forceps may have been quite easy, but more commonly there has been a little difficulty in completing the extension of the head. The hairy scalp slides out with reluctance. When the forehead has appeared it is necessary to press back the perineum to deliver the face. Fat cheeks eventually emerge. A double chin has to be hooked over the posterior vulval commissure, to which it remains tightly opposed. Restitution seldom occurs spontaneously, for the head seems incapable of movement as a result of friction with the girdle of contact of the vulva. On the other hand, gentle manipulation of the head sometimes results in a sudden 90 degree restitution as the head adjusts itself without descent to the anteroposterior position of the shoulders.

    Time passes. The child's head becomes suffused. It endeavors unsuccessfully to breathe. Abdominal efforts by the mother or by her attendants produce no advance, gentle head traction is equally unavailing.

    Usually equanimity forsakes the attendants. They push, they pull. Alarm increases. Eventually
<blockquote>
By greater strength of muscle
Or by some infernal juggle
</blockquote>
the difficulty appears to be overcome, and the shoulders and trunk of a goodly child are delivered. The pallor of its body contrasts with the plum-colored cyanosis of the face, and the small quantity of freshly expelled meconium about the buttocks. It dawns upon the attendants that their anxiety was not ill-founded, the baby lies limp and voiceless, and too often remains so despite all efforts at resuscitation.

Diagnosis

Diagnosis can be made only once the head has been delivered.   Certain signs then appear:

1. There is a definite recoil of the head back against the perineum.
2. Restitution rarely takes place spontaneously.   Because of the friction with the vulva, the head seems incapable of movement.
3. The problem is usually recognized when traction from below and pressure from above fail to deliver the child.
4. Vaginal examination is made to rule out other causes of difficulty, as listed above (p. 245).

Management of Shoulder Dystocia

Prophylaxis

While this complication cannot be prevented, the results can be improved by recognizing the situations in which it occurs and by insisting on expert obstetric care for these patients.

Accessory Measures

1. Anesthesia is administered, or if already in progress, it should be deepened, as complete muscle relaxation is of great value.   Time is precious, and while the anesthesia is being given, the operator must act.
2. The respiratory tract is cleared of mucus and debris to provide a clear airway.
3. Vaginal examination of the infant and the pelvis is made to rule out the other complications which prevent descent of the body.   These include short umbilical cord, locked or conjoined twins, enlargement of abdomen or thorax, and uterine constriction ring.
4. An episiotomy, preferably mediolateral and large, is made to make more room and to prevent tears into the rectum.

Basic Method of Delivery of Shoulders

Gentle backward traction is made on the delivered head, without forced rotation and without excessive angulation. At the same time the patient is told to
bear down, if she is awake; if the patient is asleep, pressure on the fundus is
made by an assistant at the same time that traction is being exerted on the head.
The traction must be smooth and continuous and sudden jerks avoided.   The duration of these efforts should rarely exceed 4 or 5 seconds. If the cause of the
difficulty is merely the friction of large shoulders in the oblique or transverse
diameters, these simple measures will almost always produce advancement.
One or two efforts, however, are sufficient. If they fail this method of delivery
should be abandoned.

Operative Methods of Treating Shoulder Dystocia

Delivery of the Anterior Shoulder

1. The hand is placed deeply in the vagina behind the anterior shoulder.
2. With the next contraction the axis of the shoulders is rotated into an oblique
   diameter of the pelvis.
3. Firm traction is made on the head, deflecting it toward the floor.
4. Suprapubic pressure is exerted, and this will usually succeed in bringing
   the anterior shoulder into and through the pelvis.
5. Sometimes the extraction may be furthered by the operator's hooking a
   forefinger under the axilla.

Fig. 2. Basic method of delivery of shoulders.

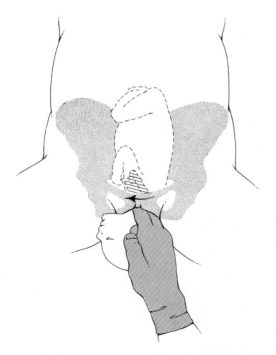

Fig. 3. Shoulder dystocia: rotation of bisacromial diameter from antero-posterior diameter of the pelvis into the oblique.

Extraction of the Posterior Shoulder and Arm

1. The hand is placed deeply into the vagina behind the posterior shoulder.
2. The arm is grasped and carried up over the front of the baby's abdomen. The hand is then seized and extracted with the arm.
3. Once this is accomplished the anterior shoulder will deliver. If it does not, the body is rotated 180 degrees so that the anterior shoulder is now posterior. It is then delivered in the same way as the first one.

Fig. 4. Extraction of posterior shoulder and arm: first step.

Fig. 5. Extraction of posterior shoulder and arm: second step.

The Screw Principle of Woods

1. The position of the head is LOT. This technic is not possible until the posterior shoulder has passed the spines.
2. Downward pressure is made on the baby's buttocks through the mother's abdomen by the operator's hand.
3. Two fingers of the left hand are placed on the anterior aspect of the posterior shoulder. Pressure is made against the shoulder so that it moves counter clockwise, the posterior aspect leading the way. It is turned 180 degrees, past 12 o'clock. In this way the posterior shoulder is delivered under the pubic arc. The head has turned from LOT to ROT.
4. The posterior shoulder has been delivered. The anterior shoulder is now posterior.
5. Pressure is again made on the buttocks in a downward direction.
6. At the same time two fingers are placed against the anterior aspect of the newly posterior shoulder. By pressure against the shoulder, it is moved in a clockwise direction, the posterior aspect leading the way. It is turned 180 degrees, past 12 o'clock, and the posterior shoulder is again delivered. The head rotates from ROT to LOT.

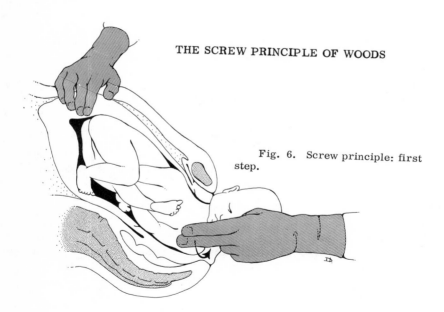

THE SCREW PRINCIPLE OF WOODS

Fig. 6.   Screw principle: first step.

Fig. 7.   Screw principle: second step.

Fig. 8.   Screw principle: third
step.

Fig. 9.   Screw principle: fourth
step.

BIBLIOGRAPHY

Barnum, G.   Dystocia due to the shoulders.   Amer. J. Obstet. Gynec., 50:439, 1945.

Mazzanti, G. A.   Delivery of the anterior shoulder.   Obstet. Gynec., 13:1603, 1959.

Morris, W. I. C.   Shoulder dystocia.   J. Obstet. Gynec. Brit. Emp., 62:302, 1955.

Schwartz, B. C., and Dixon, D. M.   Shoulder dystocia.   Obstet. Gynec., 11:468, 1958.

Swartz, D. P.   Shoulder girdle dystocia in vertex delivery.   Obstet. Gynec., 15:194, 1960.

Woods, C. E.   A principle of physics as applicable to shoulder delivery.   Amer. J. Obstet. Gynec., 45:796, 1943.

23 Multiple Pregnancy

Incidence: Hellin's law propounds the following rates of multiple pregnancy:

Twins (two children)	$1/89$
Triplets (three)	$1/89^2$
Quadruplets (four)	$1/89^3$
Quintuplets (five)	$1/89^4$

Another way of expressing the approximate incidence is:

Twins	$1/100$
Triplets	$1/10,000$
Quadruplets	$1/750,000$

A tendency to plural births runs in families, more often on the maternal side. The incidence is higher in multiparas, and in colored races.

TWIN PREGNANCY

Double Ovum

About 75 percent of twins are binovular. Two fetuses develop from the fertilization of two ova liberated during the same menstrual cycle. The incidence of double ovum twins is influenced by heredity, race, maternal age, and parity. Each twin has its own placenta, chorion, and amniotic sac. When the ova are implanted near each other the two placentas may seem to fuse. The circulations, however, remain completely separate. These children are fraternal twins. They resemble each other only to the extent that siblings of the same age would. They may be of different sex and sometimes look entirely dissimilar. Weinberg's rule states that the number of dizygous twins in any population is twice the number of twins of different sex; the remainder are monozygous.

Single Ovum

Some 25 percent of twins are uniovular—identical, or true twins. They represent complete cleavage of the blastodermic vesicle. There is one egg fertilized by a single sperm, and, therefore, the offspring arise from the same germ plasm. The frequency of single ovum twinning is independent of heredity, race, maternal age, and parity. These children are always of the same sex and look alike. Incomplete division results in anything from conjoined twins to double monsters. There is one placenta, one chorion, and two amniotic sacs. The blood circulations of the twins intercommunicate in the common placenta. In some cases a stronger twin will monopolize the circulation, which results in poor development of the other fetus.

Monoamniotic Twins

Monoamniotic twins, where both babies lie in one amniotic cavity, are rare. The exact incidence is not known. There are two etiologic theories:

1. At first there are two amnions. Early in the pregnancy the partition between them breaks down, and a single amniotic sac results.
2. A single ovum gives rise to two blastodermic vesicles which split after formation of the amnion. Thus, there is only one original sac.

Because the fetuses are not separated by membrane there is a great likelihood of knotting, tangling, and strangulation of the cords, resulting in fetal death. Therefore the prognosis for monoamniotic twins is poor. If after the birth of the first baby, the umbilical cord is observed to be twisted or knotted, or if there is no second bag of waters, the other twin should be delivered immediately.

Superfetation

Superfetation is the fertilization of a second ovum at a later ovulation. In theory, this is possible up to the fourth month of pregnancy. After the fourteenth week the uterine cavity is sealed off by the enlarging fetal sac. In practice, there is doubt that superfetation takes place.

Superfecundation

Superfecundation is the fertilization of two ova expelled at the same ovulation but fertilized at different copulations. This can be proved only if the resulting children are of identifiably different races.

DIAGNOSIS OF MULTIPLE PREGNANCY

1. Suggestive findings
   a. Familial history
   b. The uterus and abdomen seem larger than expected for the period of amenorrhea.
   c. Uterine growth is more rapid than normal.
   d. Unexplainably excessive weight gain
2. Positive signs
   a. Palpation of two heads or two breeches
   b. Two fetal hearts auscultated at the same time by two observers and differing in rate by at least 10 beats per minute
   c. X-ray of the abdomen shows two skeletons. These may appear by the eighteenth week or sooner, but a second skeleton cannot be ruled out until the twenty-fifth week.
   d. At birth, the delivery of more than one child is positive evidence.
3. The diagnosis of twins is not easy unless there is a high index of suspicion. The frequency of premature labor makes the diagnosis even more difficult.

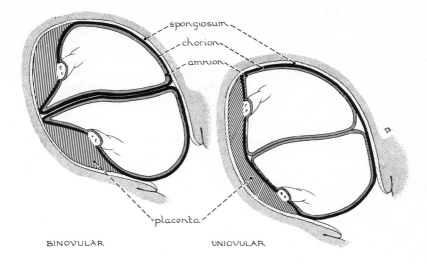

Fig. 1. Placenta and membranes in twin pregnancy.

EFFECTS OF MULTIPLE PREGNANCY

Maternal

1. Because the volume of the intrauterine contents is large, symptoms rang-
    ing from discomfort to actual abdominal pain are frequent. Pressure
    against the diaphragm leads to dyspnea.
2. The mechanical and metabolic loads increase with the multiplicity of the
    pregnancy.
3. Polyhydramnios, an excessive amount of amniotic fluid, is more common
    than in single pregnancies.
4. Twins increase the incidence of preeclampsia fivefold.
5. Anemia is prevalent.
6. Excessive gain of weight occurs for several reasons, including overeating,
    water retention, more than one fetus, and polyhydramnios.
7. Complaints of fetal overactivity are made frequently.

Fetal

1. While the individual child is smaller than average, the combined weight of
    the babies is larger than a single child. One twin may be 50 to 1,000 g
    heavier than the other. In half the cases the children are of term size. In
    one eighth of pregnancies both babies are under 1,500 g. The remaining
    three eighths are between 1,500 and 2,500 g.
2. The combination of small babies and large amounts of amniotic fluid leads
    to an increased incidence of malpresentations.

3. Fetal mortality is increased in twin pregnancy to four times that of single-tons. The gross mortality varies from 9 to 14 percent. While malpresen-tations and congenital abnormalities play a part, the major cause of death is prematurity. Birthweight is an important factor; 2,000 g seems to be a critical point. The survival rate of twins born after 36 weeks gestation is several times higher than that of twins born before this period.

4. The risk to the second twin is almost twice that of the first. Reasons for this include:
   a. The greater incidence of operative deliveries
   b. Too long an interval between the birth of the first and second twins
   c. The reduction of the uterine capacity after the birth of the first baby: This may alter the placental hemodynamics, and result in fetal anoxia.
   d. The second twin occupies a less favorable position in the actively con-tracting upper uterine segment.
   e. There is an increased incidence of malpresentation in the second twin.

   The least possible delay should be permitted between the delivery of the children. After the first is born it may be wise to give the mother oxygen to breathe in an effort to prevent anoxia of the second twin.

5. Congenital malformations are more common in twins than in singletons.
6. Kurtz found that in no set of triplets did the combined weights reach 7,500 g, indicating that triplets average under 2,500 g. The second and third ba-bies have a higher mortality than the first.

Labor

1. The overstretching of the uterus by the large combined weights of the ba-bies, the two placentas, and the copious amniotic fluid, lead to the follow-ing:
   a. Premature labor occurs, on the average, three weeks before term.
   b. Early rupture of the membranes is frequent and is one cause of prema-ture labor.
   c. Most twin labors are satisfactory. Sometimes the overlengthened uter-ine muscles produce weak and inefficient contractions, resulting in slow progress.
   d. The increased incidence and danger of postpartum hemorrhage must be kept in mind.
   e. Malpresentations are common.
   f. Umbilical cord prolapse is caused by rupture of the membranes with the gushing out of large amounts of fluid, especially with the second twin.
2. In 80 percent of cases the second twin is born within 30 minutes of the first.
3. The two babies are born first and then the two placentas.
4. The combinations of presentations are, in descending order of frequency:
   a. Two vertexes: This is the most common and most favorable presentation.
   b. Vertex and breech
   c. Two breeches
   d. Vertex and transverse lie
   e. Breech and transverse lie
   f. Both in the transverse

TWIN PRESENTATIONS

Fig. 2. Two vertices.

Fig. 5. Vertex and transverse lie.

Fig. 3. Vertex and breech.

Fig. 6. Breech and transverse lie.

Fig. 4. Two breeches.

Fig. 7. Two transverse lies.

MANAGEMENT OF MULTIPLE PREGNANCY

Management During Pregnancy

Early diagnosis enables the parents to make preparations for more than one child, and alerts the doctor to the problems of multiple pregnancy. The two main complications, premature labor and preeclampsia, call for special care during the prenatal period.

1. The patient should cease outside work by 24 weeks. She needs frequent rest periods.
2. Travel is restricted, since the probability of early labor is strong.
3. Coitus is forbidden during the last three months.
4. It is believed that one reason for premature labor is the inability of the cervix to contain the enlarging products of conception. If, at any time, the cervix becomes effaced and open, the patient should be put to bed.
5. A sodium poor diet is prescribed as soon as the diagnosis of twins is made.
6. Prenatal visits are made more often so that the presence of toxemia can be noted as soon as possible.
7. The anemia that occurs in many of these patients must be treated vigorously.
8. Since the greatest cause of fetal mortality is prematurity, the maintenance of the pregnancy to at least 36 or 37 weeks is desirable. Many obstetricians believe that bed rest, at home or in hospital, helps to achieve this goal. The period of confinement to bed (with bathroom privileges) recommended by different authors varies between 30 to 36 weeks and 28 to 38 weeks. Once the babies have attained a good size, the patient is permitted to resume her activities.

Management During Labor

1. Accurate diagnosis of the presentations is essential. The x-ray is used when needed.
2. Sedatives and analgesics are administered with care since the small babies are more susceptible to drugs which depress the vital centers.
3. The higher incidence of postpartum hemorrhage calls for precautionary measures, even to the extent of having cross-matched blood available, especially if the patient is anemic.
4. Watchful expectancy is the procedure of choice during labor. The best results are obtained when the least interference is employed.
5. When delivery is near, the patient is placed on the delivery table, and an intravenous infusion of 5 percent glucose in water is started. This precautionary measure has two uses: 1, should uterine atony occur, either before or after the birth of the baby, oxytocin can be added to the solution to stimulate the myometrium; 2, if postpartum hemorrhage does take place, the route for the administration of fluids or blood is available immediately.
6. The first baby is delivered in the usual way, as if it were a single pregnancy.

7. The umbilical cord must be clamped doubly. This is to prevent the second baby's bleeding through the cord of the first in uniovular twins, where the placental circulations communicate.

8. Intravenous egometrine should not be given before the birth of the second twin is complete. The strong contraction which results may be dangerous to the baby still in utero, especially if it is placed badly.

9. Careful examination is made to determine the position and station of the second baby. If the vertex or breech is in or over the inlet, and the uterus is contracting, the membranes should be ruptured artificially, care being taken that the cord does not prolapse. If uterine inertia has set in, an oxytocin drip may be given to reestablish uterine contractions, and when this has been achieved, amniotomy is performed. The presenting part is guided into the pelvis by the vaginal hand. If necessary, pressure is made on the fundus with the other hand. Since the first baby has already dilated the birth canal, the second one descends rapidly to the pelvic floor.

10. Once the presenting part is on the perineum it is delivered spontaneously or by simple operative measures.

11. If the presentation is abnormal, if fetal or maternal distress supervenes, or if spontaneous delivery of the second twin has not taken place within 15 minutes, operative interference is considered, since the risk to the second baby increases with time. The second baby should be extracted as a breech if it so presents, and by version and extraction if it is a cephalic presentation or transverse lie. We do not believe in routine version and extraction for normal positions.

12. The sudden reduction of the intrauterine contents by delivery of the first twin may lead to premature separation of the placenta, endangering the second baby.

13. The placentas are delivered after both twins have been born.

14. Cesarean section is never performed when the presence of twins is the sole indication. The reason for operative delivery is some accompanying complication, such as: 1, toxemia of pregnancy; 2, antepartum hemorrhage (placenta previa and abruptio placentae); 3, transverse lie; or 4, prolapse of the umbilical cord. Twin pregnancy does not impose a special threat to the integrity of a preexisting low transverse cesarean scar. It is not necessary to schedule a repeat cesarean any earlier for a twin pregnancy than for a singleton.

LOCKING OF TWINS

Locking of twins is the situation where one baby impedes the descent and delivery of the other. This complication is so rare that most obstetricians never see a case. There are three varieties:

Crowding

Crowding or wedging is the attempted entry of both children into the pelvis at the same time.

Blocking

Both babies present by the vertex. The head of the second is jammed against the throat of the first, between the chin and the thorax.

Interlocking

Interlocking is a rare condition; the incidence is approximately 1/1,000 twin births. The first infant presents as a breech and the second as a vertex. Interlocking takes place between the chins. The first child delivers uneventfully until the scapula is born. The interlocking makes further descent impossible. Unless the condition is relieved rapidly, the first child will die of asphyxia, and only the second one can be saved.

Management

Management of Crowding and Blocking

1. Under deep anesthesia attempts are made to push the second twin out of the pelvis, so that the first one can be born. The second twin is delivered in the usual way.
2. If this method fails, cesarean section is performed.

Management of Interlocking

1. Under anesthesia an attempt is made to unlock the chins, so that the second twin can be pushed out of the way, enabling the first to be born. Traction on the first twin must be avoided as this aggravates the problem.
2. If this does not succeed within a short time, the first baby will die from asphyxia and trauma in the attempted delivery. The following treatment is carried out:
    a. The first twin is decapitated.
    b. The second is delivered.
    c. The head of the first is extracted by forceps.
    d. A couple of strong sutures should be placed in the head of the first twin above the line of decapitation. Later, by traction on these sutures, the head can be fixed, making it easier to apply the forceps.
3. Cesarean section is contraindicated. It would entail pulling the body of the first twin, which is outside of the vulva, back through the vagina, uterus, and peritoneal cavity. This would carry with it grave danger to the mother of peritonitis and general sepsis when there is nothing to gain by this procedure.
4. In the rare case where the fetuses are viable, and the diagnosis of interlocking is made by x-ray before or during labor, but before the actual delivery has begun, cesarean section can be performed.

Fig. 8. Crowding.

Fig. 9. Blocking

Fig. 10. Interlocking.

Siamese Twins

Siamese twins are a variety of conjoined fetuses. The incidence of conjoined twins is one in 50,000 to 100,000 births. They are uniovular twins whose misfortune it is that the embryonic area failed to split completely, and the two individuals remain attached. They are predominantly female. In the most common variety the point of juncture is at the sacrum. Delivery is effected best by cesarean section. Many of these pregnancies do not go to term, and if the fetuses are small, delivery may be per vaginam.

BIBLIOGRAPHY

Barter, R. H., Hsu, I., Erkenbeck, R. V., and Pugsley, L. Q. The prevention of prematurity in multiple pregnancy. Amer. J. Obstet. Gynec., 91:787, 1965.

Cohen, M., Kohl, S. G., and Rosenthal, A. H. Fetal interlocking complicating twin gestation. Amer. J. Obstet. Gynec., 91:407, 1965.

Guttmacher, A. F. Multiple pregnancy; biologic aspects. G. P., 13[No. 4]: 105, 1956.

_____ Multiple pregnancy; clinical aspects. G. P., 13[No. 5]:97, 1956.

_____ and Kohl, S. G. The fetus of multiple gestations. Obstet. Gynec., 12:528, 1958.

_____ and Kohl, S. G. Cesarean section in twin pregnancy. Amer. J. Obstet. Gynec., 83:866, 1962.

Kurtz, G. R., Davis, L. L., and Loftus, J. B. Factors influencing the survival of triplets. Obstet. Gynec., 12:504, 1958.

Spurway, J. H. The fate and management of the second twin. Amer. J. Obstet. Gynec., 83:1377, 1962.

Timmons, J. D., and DeAlvarez, R. R. Monoamniotic twin pregnancy. Amer. J. Obstet. Gynec., 86:875, 1963.

Wood, W. R., and Perry, H. B. Intravenous oxytocin stimulation in the second stage of labor in twin pregnancies. Amer. J. Obstet. Gynec., 87:337, 1963.

24   Obstetric Forceps

The obstetric forceps, invented by Peter Chamberlen in the beginning of the seventeeenth century, is an instrument designed for the extraction of the fetal head. While many varieties of forceps have been described the basic design and purpose have remained unchanged.

PARTS OF THE FORCEPS

1. Handles
2. The lock holds the forceps together. It is so constructed that the right one fits on over the left. For this reason, unless the particular situation necessitates doing otherwise, the left blade should be applied first. The main types of lock are:
   a. The English lock (e.g., Simpson forceps) has a shoulder and flange in each shank which fit into each other. Articulation is fixed at a given point.
   b. The French lock (e.g., Tarnier and De Wees) has a pinion and screw. The left shank bears a pivot fitting into a notch on the right shank. After articulation the pivot is tightened by screwing it home.
   c. The sliding lock (e.g., Kjelland) is built in the left blade only. The right blade fits into the lock, but articulation is not fixed. This type of lock is useful when application is not perfect, as when the head is asynclitic.
3. The shank connects the handle and the blade. A short-shanked instrument is satisfactory when the fetal head is low in the pelvis. Where the head has not reached the perineum a longer shank is needed.
4. The blades, which enclose the head, may be solid or fenestrated. They are designed to grasp the head firmly, but without excessive compression. The solid blades may cause less trauma, but the fenestrated blades are lighter, grip the fetal head better, and are less likely to slip. The edges are smooth to reduce damage to the soft tissues.
5. Forceps are right or left depending on the side of the maternal pelvis to which they are applied. Since most forceps cross at the lock, the handle of the right forceps is held in the operator's right hand, and fits the right side of the pelvis. The left blade fits the left side of the maternal pelvis, and its handle is held in the left hand of the operator.

6. The front of the forceps is the concave side.
7. The apex is the tips of the blades.
8. The diameter is the widest distance between the blades. It measures about 7.5 cm.
9. The forceps have two curves:
   a. The cephalic curve fits the shape of the baby's head, and reduces the danger of compression.
   b. The pelvic curve follows the direction of the birth canal. It makes application and extraction easier, and decreases damage to the maternal tissues.

TYPES OF FORCEPS

There are many general duty forceps, and several with specialized functions. We believe that the new obstetrician should learn to use one instrument well, so that he becomes thoroughly at home with it. Once he has achieved this experience he must try other instruments, so that he has several familiar types at his command.

1. Simpson: This is the common parent forceps. It has a cephalic and a pelvic curve. The shank is straight. The lock is of the English variety. This is a good general duty forceps, and is used widely and successfully for all obstetric forceps operations.
2. DeLee: This is the Simpson forceps with a few minor modifications. The shank is a little longer to keep the handle away from the anus. The handle is changed to secure lightness, a better grip, and ease of cleaning.
3. Tucker-McLane: The blades are solid.
4. Kjelland: This forceps has a very slight pelvic curve, and a sliding lock which makes easier the locking of the blades. It is useful in rotating transverse positions of the occiput.
5. Barton: The anterior blade is attached to the shank by a hinge. This feature, plus the sliding lock, allows the blades to be locked even when there is marked asynclitism.
6. Piper: The blade of this forceps is similar to that of the Simpson forceps. The shank has been lengthened and curved downward so that the handles are lower than the blades. Thus the forceps has a double pelvic curve which facilitates application to the aftercoming head in breech presentations.
7. DeWees: The blades are standard. The handles are modified so that an axis-traction bar can be attached.
8. Axis-traction forceps: These are forceps specially designed so that a traction apparatus can be attached either to the blades at the bases of the fenestra (Tarnier and Milne-Murray) or to the handles (DeWees). The traction bar is attached to the forceps by a series of joints, which has the effect of a universal joint. The forceps are applied to the head in the usual way, and the traction apparatus is attached. The baby's head is then extracted by pulling only on the traction bar. The advantages of this technic are:
   a. The line of traction is in the axis of the birth canal.
   b. The universal joint permits the blades to rotate with the head, and thus to follow the natural rotation of the head as it accommodates itself to the maternal pelvis in its descent.
   c. Axis traction was of value in difficult high and midforceps deliveries. Since in modern obstetrics we try to eliminate these traumatic operations, axis traction is needed rarely today.

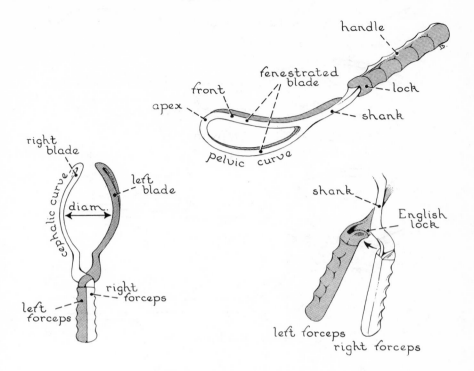

Fig. 1. Simpson forceps showing the various parts.

Fig. 2. French lock.

Fig. 3. Sliding lock.

Fig. 4. Front view of some commonly used forceps. (From Douglas and Stromme. <u>Operative Obstetrics</u>, Appleton-Century-Crofts, 1957.)

Tucker-McLane

Simpson

Elliot

Kjelland

Barton

Piper

Bailey-Williamson

Fig. 5. Lateral view of some commonly used forceps. (From Douglas and Stromme. <u>Operative Obstetrics</u>, Appleton-Century-Crofts, 1957.)

APPLICATION OF FORCEPS

Cephalic Application

A cephalic application is made to fit the baby's head. An ideal cephalic application in occipitoanterior positions is:

1. Biparietal, along the occipitomental diameter, with the fenestra including the parietal bosses, and the tips lying over the cheeks.
2. The concave edges point to the denominator.
3. The convex edges point toward the face.

With this application, pressure on the head will cause the least damage. If the forceps are applied so that one blade lies over the face and the other over the occiput, a relatively small degree of compression may cause tentorial tears and intracranial hemorrhage.

Pelvic Application

A pelvic application is made to fit the maternal pelvis regardless of how the forceps grip the fetal head. The best pelvic application is achieved when:

1. The left blade is next to the left side of the pelvis.
2. The right blade is on the right side of the pelvis.
3. The concave margin is near the symphysis pubis.
4. The convex margin is in the hollow of the sacrum.
5. The diameter of the forceps is in the transverse diameter of the pelvis.

Perfect Application

A perfect application is achieved when both the cephalic and pelvic requirements have been fulfilled. When the occiput has rotated under the symphysis pubis, and the sagittal suture is in the anteroposterior diameter, an ideal application is possible.

Fig. 6.   Cephalic application.

Fig. 7.   Pelvic application.

Fig. 8.   Perfect application.

FUNCTIONS OF OBSTETRIC FORCEPS

Of the six original uses of forceps—traction, rotation, compression, dilation, leverage, irritation—only traction and rotation are acceptable today. Compression of the head may be an unavoidable accompaniment, but is never a function, of forceps.

Traction

In other than expert hands the use of forceps should be restricted to that of traction. The direction of traction must be along the pelvic curvature, and as the station changes during descent, so does the line of traction. The direction of pull should be perpendicular to the plane of the level at which it is being applied. The higher the level, the more posterior is the line of traction.

Rotation of the Head from Posterior or Transverse Positions

An important principle must be remembered when using the forceps for rotation. The handles should be swung through a wide arc in order to reduce the arc of the blades. This lowers the incidence and extent of vaginal lacerations, and, at the same time, makes the operation easier. Rotation is carried out best in the midpelvis.

CLASSIFICATION OF FORCEPS OPERATIONS

Low Forceps

Low forceps is the application of forceps after the head has become visible, the skull (not the caput) has reached the perineal floor, and the sagittal suture is in or near the anteroposterior diameter of the pelvis. The station is +3.

Mid Forceps

Mid forceps is the application of forceps before the criteria of low forceps have been met, but after engagement has taken place. The biparietal diameter has passed through the inlet and the lowest part of the skull has reached the level of the ischial spines. The station is 0 to +2. Frequently rotation is not complete. This can be a difficult operation, even for the experienced obstetrician. Dennen has suggested the following subdivisions:

1. Midforceps delivery is one where the leading bony part of the head is at or just below the plane of the ischial spines with the biparietal diameter below the superior strait (inlet). The head nearly fills the hollow of the sacrum.
2. A low midforceps delivery is one in which the biparietal diameter is at or below the plane of the ischial spines with the leading point within a finger breadth of the perineum between contractions. The head fills the hollow of the sacrum completely.

Fig. 9. Traction with forceps. (From Douglas and Stromme. Operative Obstetrics, Appleton–Century–Crofts, 1957.)

Fig. 10. Rotation with forceps, incorrect technic. (From Douglas and Stromme. Operative Obstetrics, Appleton–Century–Crofts, 1957.)

Fig. 11. Rotation with forceps, correct technic. (From Douglas and Stromme. Operative Obstetrics, Appleton–Century–Crofts, 1957.)

High Forceps

The head has entered the pelvis, but is not engaged. The widest diameter has not passed through the inlet, and the bony presenting part has not reached the level of the ischial spines. The danger of damage to the baby and the mother is great, and this operation is carried out rarely.

Floating Forceps

The whole fetal head is above the pelvic brim. This procedure is not performed today, and has been superseded by cesarean section.

The average case fits nicely into these categories. However, where there is extreme molding, marked asynclitism, large caput succedaneum, attitude of extension, or abnormal pelvis, errors are often made in thinking that the station is lower than it really is. The operator believes he is about to perform a midforceps operation and finds himself doing a high forceps.

A. C. O. G. Classification

In 1964 the Executive Board of the American College of Obstetricians and Gynecologists adopted the following classification of forceps deliveries.

1. Outlet forceps: The application of forceps when the scalp is or has been visible at the introitus without separating the labia, the skull has reached the pelvic floor, and the sagittal suture is in the anteroposterior diameter of the pelvis.

2. Midforceps: The application of forceps when the head is engaged, but the conditions for outlet forceps have not been met. In the context of this term, any forceps delivery requiring artificial rotation, regardless of the station from which extraction is begun, shall be designated a "midforceps delivery." The term "low midforceps" is disapproved. A record shall be made of the position and station of the head when the delivery is begun. In addition, a description of the various maneuvers and of any difficulties encountered in the application of the forceps and in the extraction of the infant shall be recorded.

3. High forceps: The application of forceps at any time prior to full engagement of the head. High forceps delivery is almost never justified.

CONDITIONS AND PREREQUISITES

Before obstetric forceps may be used safely certain conditions, requirements, or prerequisites must be present.

1. An adequate pelvis with no disproportion is an absolute condition. Failure to observe this rule may lead to disaster for fetus and mother.
2. There must be no serious bony or soft tissue obstruction, such as presenting ovarian cysts or uterine fibromyomata.
3. The fetal head must be engaged so that the bony skull (not the caput succedaneum) is at least at the level of the ischial spines.

4. The cervix must be completely dilated and retracted. Disregard for this rule will lead to tears of the cervix, hemorrhage, and may result in "failed forceps."

5. Accurate diagnosis of position and station is essential.

6. The membranes should be ruptured. If they are not there is increased chance of the blades slipping, and there is danger of pulling the placenta away from the uterine wall. If the bag of waters is intact it should be broken. Frequently this results in better labor and progress, so that the need for forceps is obviated.

7. The patient is placed on a good delivery table, with the legs in stirrups, and the buttocks well down and a little past the end of the table.

8. Some form of anesthesia, general, conduction, or local, should be used. This achieves both relaxation and relief of pain.

9. The bladder must be emptied by using a rubber catheter before the forceps are applied. An empty bladder occupies less space than a full one, and is less liable to injury.

10. The rectum should be empty. This has usually been accomplished by an enema earlier in labor.

11. The operation is performed under strictly aseptic conditions.

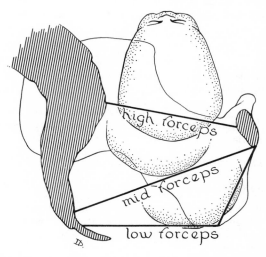

Fig. 12. Classification of forceps operations according to station.

INDICATIONS FOR THE USE OF FORCEPS

Fetal Distress

Signs which suggest that the baby is suffering from lack of oxygen include:

1. An irregular fetal heart
2. Bradycardia, under 100 beats per minute, between uterine contractions
3. A rapid fetal heart—more than 160 beats per minute
4. The passage of meconium in cephalic presentations

Once fetal distress has developed the baby must be delivered immediately, providing the prerequisites have been met.

The more serious signs are irregularity and slowness of the fetal heart. Prolapse of the umbilical cord may be in the background. Occasionally a loop of cord around the baby's neck tightens as the fetus descends, the flow of blood through the cord is reduced, hypoxia or anoxia results, with bradycardia as a clinical sign. Often babies who demonstrated intrauterine bradycardia, or passed meconium, are born in good condition and remain so. Thus, when signs of distress are present and delivery can be expedited by an easy low forceps delivery, this should be done immediately. On the other hand, in the panicky attempt to save a baby with possible anoxia, one should beware of damaging it or even killing it by a difficult, traumatic, and sometimes needless forceps extraction.

Maternal Conditions

An extraction of the baby for maternal reasons is justified if the risk to mother and child is less than that of waiting for spontaneous delivery.

Maternal Distress or Exhaustion: This is shown by dehydration, concentrated urine, pulse and temperature above 100. These patients are not in shock; they are simply becoming exhausted.

Maternal Disease: When the mother has cardiac disease, tuberculosis, toxemia, or any debilitating condition, forceps can be used to shorten the second stage and obviate the need for prolonged bearing-down efforts by the patient.

It is essential in these situations that the forceps delivery be easy. The patient will not be helped by a difficult forceps extraction with attendant lacerations and hemorrhage. If the latter is likely, it is better to leave the case to nature.

Failure of Progress in the Second State

1. Failure of descent
2. Failure of internal rotation

Providing the conditions for the use of forceps have been met, lack of advancement in the presence of good uterine contractions for one hour in a multipara, or two hours in a primigravida, is an indication for assessment of the situation, and probable delivery of the baby by forceps. A delay of only two hours in the second stage is permitted, because experience has shown that the incidence of fetal and maternal damage rises definitely after this period.

Situations which predispose to arrest of progress include:

1. Poor uterine contractions
2. Minor degrees of relative disproportion caused by such conditions as a large baby or prominent ischial spines
3. Abnormal fetal position such as posterior position of the occiput or attitudes of extension
4. A rigid perineum which the advancing head cannot thin out
5. Diastasis of the rectus abdominis muscle
6. A lax pelvic floor which inhibits proper rotation of the head

Elective Outlet Forceps: Prophylactic Forceps

This procedure is prophylactic in that it is designed to prevent fetal asphyxia and death and to reduce injury and needless suffering of the mother. It is done in conjunction with early episiotomy. The reasoning is:

1. It is better to do the episiotomy before the tissues are overstretched. This may reduce the incidence of relaxation of the perineum and pelvic floor and of prolapse of the uterus in later life.
2. It saves the mother a certain period of bearing down, and may prevent painful hemorrhoids.
3. The extraction of the baby with outlet forceps is less damaging than prolonged pounding of the head on the perineum.

The Optimum Time to Use Forceps

The indications, conditions, and time limits, as detailed previously, cannot be considered as rigid and unchangeable. The attendant must, at all times, exercise his prerogative to modify the indications to suit the situation at hand. Sometimes interference is carried out sooner than usual, while in other instances more time is allowed before operative measures are instituted.

Once fetal distress is present, interference is mandatory. However, rather than waiting for marked bradycardia with subsequent desperate activity by the obstetrician, it is better to extract the infant while it is still in good condition and able to stand better the trauma of the operation and anesthesia. In cases of prolonged labor with slow advance, for example, the possibility of fetal distress should be anticipated.

Maternal distress is a definite indication for operative delivery. One should not permit the patient to become completely exhausted before offering assistance. Once the second stage has been reached the patient must be observed carefully for signs of fatigue. When they appear, extraction should be carried out without waiting for the usual time limit to expire.

The rule to wait until progress in the second stage has ceased for one hour in a multipara and two hours in a primipara is not absolute. Often the attendant can decide much sooner whether there is hope of advancement.   For instance, when the head is on the perineum there is no justification in running out the clock, when an episiotomy or low forceps would be of assistance to the fetus, the mother, and the perineum.

The best time to use forceps is a matter of judgment.   One should not resort to operative delivery needlessly or too quickly.   On the other hand, one must not wait so long that the life of the baby and the health of the mother have been jeopardized.

CONTRAINDICATIONS TO THE USE OF FORCEPS

1. Absence of a proper indication.
2. Incompletely dilated cervix.
3. Marked cephalo-pelvic disproportion.
4. Unengaged fetal head.
5. Lack of experience on the part of the operator.

DANGER OF FORCEPS

Maternal

1. Lacerations of the vagina and cervix.
2. Rupture of the uterus.
3. Injury to bladder and/or rectum.
4. Hemorrhage.
5. Infection.

Fetal

1. Cephalhematoma (subperiosteal hemorrhage).
2. Brain damage and intracranial hemorrhage.
3. Skull fracture.
4. Facial paralysis.
5. Bruising.
6. Cord compression.

TRIAL FORCEPS AND FAILED FORCEPS

Trial Forceps

The theory of trial forceps postulates that after successful application and locking is achieved, a few tractions of moderate strength are made.   Should the head come down easily the operation is continued and the head delivered.   If, on the other hand, the operator decides that the amount of force needed to extract the child would damage it and the mother, the forceps are removed and delivery effected by cesarean section.

Failed Forceps

There are two situations in which failed forceps occur:

1. A proper application cannot be achieved.
2. The forceps are applied correctly, but, even though an all out effort has been made, delivery cannot be accomplished.

The three main causes of failed forceps are:

1. Incomplete dilatation of the cervix
2. Malpositions of the head
3. Unrecognized cephalopelvic disproportion

In most instances the obstetrician is able to decide beforehand which patients can be delivered safely with forceps. Sometimes, however, the evidence of trouble is found only after the forceps are applied and rotation and/or traction have been attempted. When this happens the forceps should be removed and the whole situation reevaluated. Then if the operator feels that vaginal delivery is feasible, he may apply the forceps again. Should the difficulty persist at the second attempt, or should examination reveal an unrecognized disproportion or undilated cervix, the wise accoucheur will abandon the forceps and turn to cesarean section.

Many authorities emphasize the difference between trial and failed forceps, describing the first as an exercise of skill and judgment and the second as an example of poor obstetrics and mismanagement. In many instances, it seems to us, these two entities lose their distinguishing characteristics, and the nomenclature becomes a matter of semantics or self-deception.

THE VACUUM EXTRACTOR

Attempts to use suction on the fetal scalp as a means of exerting traction on the skull have been carried on since 1706. The first successful apparatus was made by Malmström in 1954, and the presently used modification in 1957.

The modern instrument consists of an all metal cup of four sizes—30, 40, 50, and 60 mm in diameter. The largest diameter is in the interior of the cup. A rubber tube extends from the cup to a pump which creates the suction. Attached to the cup and inside the tubing is a chain by which traction on the cup is effected. The scalp is drawn into the cup, and an artificial caput succedaneum is formed. A dusky ring remains after the cup is removed; this is gone by the time the baby leaves the hospital.

Indications: These are much the same as those for forceps. The vacuum extractor cannot be used for face presentations, or on the aftercoming head in breeches.

Advantages: The instrument can be used before the cervix is completely dilated. It can be applied at any station but is safest after engagement. The vacuum extractor does not encroach on the space in the pelvis. The head is not fixed in a certain position, so it can perform spontaneously the rotations which its shape and the configuration of the birth canal make necessary.

Application: The cervix should be at least 4 cm dilated. The patient is positioned and prepared just as for a forceps delivery. The lubricated suction cup is placed on the fetal head, over the posterior fontanelle whenever possible. Slowly the negative pressure is pumped up until it reaches 0.7 to 0.8 kg per cm. This takes 8 to 10 minutes. The apparatus is now ready for traction.

Delivery: If the uterine contractions are weak an oxytocin drip can be used. A series of tractions synchronized with the labor pains are applied, the right hand pulling the chain-tube, while the left hand presses the traction cup and the fetal head posteriorly against the sacrum. This produces a force in the direction of the birth canal. The total extraction time takes about 15 minutes, or 5 to 10 tractions during uterine contractions. If the cervix is not fully dilated it may take longer. The upper time limit is 30 minutes (rarely 45) to prevent damage to the baby. If delivery is not accomplished during this time, the case is considered unsuitable for vaginal delivery, and cesarean section is performed. After delivery the vacuum is released and the cup removed. The large artificial caput disappears in about 10 minutes, and by the end of a week only a slight circular area of redness is seen.

Maternal complications: These are rarely severe, consisting of small cervical and vaginal tears.

Fetal complications: Most of the ill effects are similar in type and in incidence to those associated with forceps deliveries. In properly selected cases the results are good. Included here are:

1. Large caput, which disappears by the fourth day
2. Necrosis and ulceration at the site of the application of the cup are rare, and are caused, probably, by the instrument's being left on too long.
3. Cephalhematomas
4. Occasionally there is bleeding from the sagittal sinus into the subgaleal space.
5. Postnatal asphyxia
6. Cerebral irritation is related to the number of pulls, and seems to increase after 5 or 6 tractions.

BIBLIOGRAPHY

Barth, W. H., and Newton, M. The use of the vacuum extractor. Amer. J. Obstet. Gynec., 91:403, 1965.

Dennen, E. H. A classification of forceps operations according to station of head in pelvis. Amer. J. Obstet. Gynec., 63:272, 1952.

_____ Forceps Deliveries. Philadelphia, F. A. Davis Co., 1955.

Douglas, R. G., and Stromme, W. B. Operative Obstetrics, 2nd ed. New York, Appleton-Century-Crofts, 1960.

Schroeder, H. J. Trial and failed forceps. Amer. J. Obstet. Gynec., 83:1491, 1962.

25 Anterior Positions of the Occiput: Delivery by Forceps

LOW FORCEPS DELIVERY: OCCIPUT ANTERIOR

In order to prevent the omission of essential steps, the obstetrician should train himself to perform forceps operations with a definite routine in mind. After a time these procedures become automatic. The exact details of application will be described here and will not be repeated in succeeding sections.

Preparations

1. The conditions and indications are rechecked to be certain that the correct procedure is being carried out.
2. The patient is placed on the delivery table with the legs in stirrups and the buttocks a little past the lower end of the table (Ch. 11, Fig. 20, p. 111).
3. Vulvar preparation is performed with green soap and water. This wash includes the upper thighs and lower abdomen. The bladder is catheterized.
4. If spinal or epidural anesthesia is to be used, it will have been administered by this time. If local anesthesia has been chosen, the injection is made. If general anesthesia is to be employed, the patient is put to sleep at this point.

Orientation

Vaginal Examination (Fig. 1)

Vaginal examination is made to diagnose accurately the position and station of the head, whether there is flexion or extension, and the presence of synclitism or asynclitism.   Since this is a low forceps procedure for occipitoanterior position, the following conditions will be present:

1. The presentation is cephalic.
2. The sagittal suture is in the anteroposterior diameter of the pelvis.
3. The occiput and posterior fontanelle are next to the pubis.
4. The face and bregma are in the hollow of the sacrum.
5. The station is at least +3.

Orientation and Desired Application

The locked forceps are positioned outside the vagina, in front of the perineum, in the way they are to be when they are applied to the fetal head in the pelvis.   By this simple procedure the operator fixes in his mind exactly how and where each blade should fit.   In the occipitoanterior position both a perfect cephalic and an ideal pelvic application are possible (see Figs. 2A and 2B, p. 283).

1. Cephalic application
   a. The blades are over the parietal bones in an occipitomental application.
   b. The front of the forceps (concave edges) point to the denominator (occiput).
   c. The convex edges point to the face.
2. Pelvic application
   a. The left blade is next to the left sidewall of the pelvis and the right blade near the right sidewall.
   b. The concave edges point to the pubis.
   c. The convex edges point to the sacrum.
   d. The diameter of the forceps is in the transverse diameter of the pelvis.

Fig. 1. Occiput Anterior.

Fig. 2A. O. A. Orientation. Low forceps, Simpson.

Fib. 2B. O. A. Orientation. Low forceps, Simpson.

Application of the Left Forceps

1. The left blade is inserted first. The handle is held by the thumb and the first two fingers of the left hand. At first the forceps is in an almost vertical position, with the handle near the mother's right groin (Fig. 3).
2. The fingers of the right hand are placed in the vagina between the fetal head and the left vaginal wall.
3. The left blade is inserted gently into the vagina at about 5 o'clock, between the fingers and the fetal head.
4. The handle is lowered slowly to the horizontal, and toward the midline, and at the same time the blade is moved up by the vaginal fingers over the left side of the head giving an occipitomental application. The blade lies between the left parietal bone and the left pelvic wall (Fig. 4).
5. The fingers are removed and the handle is supported by an assistant, if one is available.

Application of the Right Forceps

1. The right forceps is grasped in the right hand, and is held in an almost vertical position, with the handle near the mother's left groin.
2. The fingers of the left hand are inserted in the right side of the vagina between the fetal head and the vaginal wall.
3. The right blade is inserted over the left forceps, between the fingers and the fetal head, at about 7 o'clock (Fig. 5).
4. The handle is lowered to the horizontal and toward the midline. At the same time the blade is moved by the vaginal fingers up over the right side of the head to the occipitomental position. The blade fits between the right parietal bone and the right pelvic wall (Fig. 6).
5. The fingers of the left hand are removed from the vagina and the forceps are ready for locking.

Fig. 3. O. A. Insertion of left blade between the fetal head and the left side of pelvis.

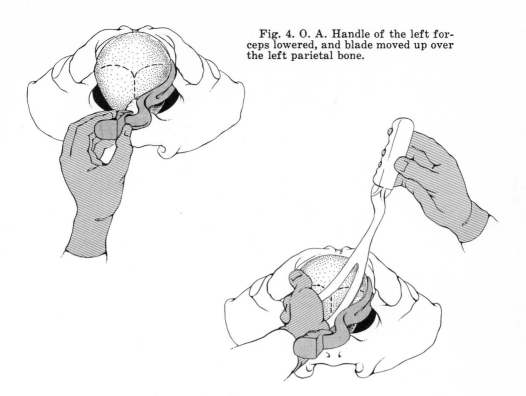

Fig. 4. O. A. Handle of the left forceps lowered, and blade moved up over the left parietal bone.

Fig. 5. O. A. Insertion of the right blade between fetal head and the right side of the pelvis.

Fig. 6. O. A. Handle of the right forceps is lowered, and the blade is moved up over the right parietal bone.

Locking

When both blades have been applied correctly locking is easy. There should be no difficulty, and the handles must never be forced together (Figs. 7A and 7B).

Extraction of the Head

Preextraction Reexamination

1. Auscultation of the fetal heart
2. Vaginal examination is made to be sure that there is nothing between the forceps and the fetal head. This includes umbilical cord, cervix, and membranes.
3. Vaginal examination is performed to check the application. The blades of the forceps must be over the sides of the fetal head in a biparietal application. The left blade should be next to the left side of the pelvis and the right blade on the right side. The concave edges of the forceps should be under the pubis and the convex edges near the sacrum. The diameter of the blades should be in the transverse diameter of the pelvis. Sometimes the blades may be a little off center, with one blade nearer the occiput and the other closer to the face. In such cases the forceps must be unlocked and the blades moved so that the application becomes symmetrical.

Trial Traction

A gentle pull on the forceps ought to bring about a small advancement of the head.

Indications for Complete Reassessment

1. When locking is difficult or impossible
2. When trial traction fails to advance the head
3. When vaginal examination reveals an incorrect application. The forceps should be removed and the whole situation reassessed. Reasons for the failure include:
   a. Wrong diagnosis of position
   b. Incorrect application of the forceps
   c. Cephalopelvic disproportion
   d. Cervix between the blades and the head
   e. Uterine constriction ring

Fig. 7A.   O. A.   Forceps locked in cephalic and pelvic application.

Fig. 7B.   O. A.   Forceps locked in cephalic and pelvic application.

Extraction of the Head

1. The operator sits on a stool and grasps the forceps with both hands, one hand on the handles and the other on the shanks (Ch. 24, Fig. 9, p. 273).

2. The traction must be intermittent, every 1 to 2 minutes, and lasting 30 to 40 seconds.

3. Between periods of traction the forceps should be unlocked to relieve the compression of the baby's head. The fetal heart must be checked often.

4. If the patient is under general or spinal anesthesia the uterine contractions are of little help, and since the patient cannot bear down, the baby is delivered by traction alone, or with the help of pressure on the uterus exerted by the assistant. On the other hand, if the patient has been given a local or epidural anesthetic, traction should be made during the uterine contractions and with the patient bearing down. The combined effort makes the delivery much easier.

5. The direction of traction must follow the birth canal. First the pull should be outward and posteriorly until the occiput comes under the symphysis of the pubis and the nape of the neck pivots in the subpubic angle (Fig. 8). In performing Pajot's maneuver, the hand on the handles makes traction in an outward direction, while the hand on the shanks pulls the head posteriorly.

6. Then the direction is changed to outward and anterior to promote extension of the head. This mimics the course of events in spontaneous birth (Fig. 9).

7. In all primigravidas and in most multiparas an episiotomy should be made before the baby is extracted and before the perineum is overstretched.

Fig. 8. O. A. Traction is made outward and posteriorly until the nape of the neck is under the pubic symphysis.

Fig. 9. O. A. The direction of traction is changed to outward and anteriorly to promote extension of the head.

Birth of the Head and Removal of Forceps

Birth of the head and removal of the forceps can be accomplished in two ways:

1. Traction with the forceps is continued, and by a process of extension the forehead, face, and chin are born over the perineum. The forceps are now out of the vagina, and slip off the head easily.
2. When the head is crowning, the forceps are removed by a process which is the reverse of their application. First the handle of the right blade is raised toward the mother's left groin and the blade slides around the head and out of the pelvis (Fig. 10). Then the same is done with the left forceps by raising the handle toward the right groin (Fig. 11). Once this has been accomplished the head is delivered by the modified Ritgen maneuver. Removing the forceps has the advantage of reducing the circumference of the part passing through the introitus by 0.5 cm to 0.75 cm.

Lacerations of the vagina, cervix, and uterus must be ruled out by careful examination after all forceps deliveries. If tears are found they are repaired.

Fig. 10. O. A. Removal of right forceps.

Fig. 11. O. A. Removal of left forceps.

FORCEPS DELIVERY: LOA

Orientation

Vaginal Examination

1. The presentation is cephalic.
2. The sagittal suture is in the right oblique diameter of the pelvis.
3. The posterior fontanelle is in the left anterior quadrant of the pelvis (Fig. 12).
4. The bregma is in the right posterior quadrant.
5. The station is 0 to +3 in most cases.

Orientation and Desired Application

1. The aim is for a perfect cephalic application.
   a. The blades are over the parietal bones in an occipitomental application.
   b. The concave edges point to the occiput.
   c. The convex edges point to the face.
2. The pelvic application is not perfect.
   a. The diameter of the forceps is in the left oblique diameter of the pelvis.
   b. The left blade is in the left posterior quadrant.
   c. The right blade is in the right anterior quadrant.
   d. The concave edges point anteriorly and to the left.
   e. The convex edges point posteriorly and to the right.
   f. This can be a low to mid forceps, depending on the exact station of the head (Fig. 13).

Fig. 12. Left Occiput Anterior.

Fig. 13. L. O. A. Orientation. Low forceps, Simpson.

Application of the Forceps

1. The left forceps is inserted into the vagina at 5 o'clock so that it lies over the left parietal bone in an occipitomental application and in the left posterolateral quadrant of the pelvis (Fig. 14).
2. The right blade is inserted into the vagina at 7 o'clock (Fig. 15).
3. It is then moved anteriorly around the fetal head so that it lies over the right parietal bone in an occipitomental application, and in the right anterior quadrant of the pelvis.
4. The forceps are now locked, and vaginal examination is made to be sure that the application is correct. If not, the forceps are unlocked and the necessary adjustments made (Fig. 16).
5. The cephalic application is ideal, but not the pelvic, for the diameter of the blades is in the oblique diameter of the pelvis.

Rotation and Extraction

1. Traction is made in an outward and posterior direction until the occiput comes under the symphysis and the nape of the neck pivots in the subpubic angle.
2. In many cases as traction is being made the head will rotate spontaneously from the LOA to the OA position. If this does not occur the operator must rotate the occiput 45 degrees to the anterior at the same time that he is exerting traction (Fig. 17).
3. Once the name of the neck pivots in the subpubic angle the direction is changed from outward and posterior to outward and anterior so that the head is born over the perineum by extension (Fig. 9).

BIBLIOGRAPHY

Douglas, R. G., and Stromme, W. B. Operative Obstetrics, 2nd ed. New York, Appleton-Century-Crofts, 1960.
Wilson, J. R. Atlas of Obstetric Technic. St. Louis, C. V. Mosby Co., 1961.

Fig. 14. L. O. A. Insertion of the left blade between the fetal head and the left postero-lateral quadrant of the pelvis.

Fig. 15. L. O. A. Insertion of the right blade between the fetal head and the right postero-lateral quadrant of the pelvis; followed by upward movement of the blade to the right antero-lateral quadrant of the pelvis.

Fig. 16. L. O. A. Locking of forceps in cephalic application.

Fig. 17. L. O. A Head is rotated from L O. A. to O. A. It is now ready for extraction.

BIBLIOGRAPHY

Douglas, R. G., and Stromme, W. B. Operative Obstetrics, 2nd ed. New
    York, Appleton-Century-Crofts, 1960.
Wilson, J. R. Atlas of Obstetric Technic. St. Louis, C. V. Mosby Co., 1961.

26 Transverse Positions of the Occiput: Deep Transverse Arrest

The problem of deep transverse arrest can be treated in two ways:

1. Application of forceps in the LOT position, rotation with forceps to OA, followed by extraction. This is always a midforceps operation.
2. Manual rotation of the head 90 degrees to the occipitoanterior position, LOT to LOA to OA. The head is then extracted with forceps as an occiput anterior. Sometimes the rotation can be carried out only 45 degrees, LOT to LOA. The forceps are applied to the LOA, and rotation and extraction are completed.

FORCEPS ROTATION AND EXTRACTION: LOT

Orientation

Vaginal Examination

1. The presentation is cephalic.
2. The sagittal suture is in the transverse diameter of the pelvis.
3. The posterior fontanelle and occiput are on the left side at 3 o'clock (LOT) (Fig. 1).
4. The bregma and face are on the right side at 9 o'clock.
5. This situation is associated frequently with the military attitude, so the bregma and the posterior fontanelle may be at almost the same level in the pelvis (neither flexion nor extension).
6. The baby's right ear is next to the bladder, and the left one is near the rectum.
7. Asynclitism is common, and the sagittal suture may be nearer the pubis (posterior asynclitism) or closer to the sacral promontory (anterior asynclitism).
8. The station in the majority of cases is 0 to +1.
9. Molding and caput succedaneum may obscure the landmarks.

Orientation and Desired Application

1. The aim is for an ideal cephalic application (Figs 2, 7A, and 7B).
    a. The front of the forceps (the concave edges) is pointing toward the denominator (the occiput).
    b. The blades are over the parietal bones in an occipitomental application.
2. The pelvic application is not ideal.
    a. The diameter of the blades is in the anteroposterior diameter of the pelvis (instead of the transverse).
    b. The anterior blade (right) is between the pubis and the fetal head (instead of being next to the pelvic sidewall).
    c. The posterior blade (left) is between the sacrum and head.
    d. The concave edges of the blades point to the left side of the pelvis.
    e. The convex edges point to the right side.

Fig. 1. Left Occiput Transverse.

Fig. 2A. L. O. T. Orientation. Mid–Forceps, Simpson.

Fig. 2B. L. O. T. Orientation, Mid–forceps, Simpson.

Application of Forceps

1. We apply the anterior blade first, and for two reasons:
   a. Any difficulty in application will be with the anterior blade. Hence, there is no point in placing the posterior blade into the vagina until we are certain that the anterior one can be put in place correctly.
   b. The posterior blade occupies space, and, if put in first, it gets in the way and makes application of the anterior forceps more difficult.
2. The anterior blade (for LOT it is the right) is inserted into the vagina between the posterior parietal bone (left) and the sacrum (Fig. 3).
3. The next step is to make the forceps wander around the fetal head into position between the anterior parietal bone (right) and the pubis (Figs. 4 and 5). This is accomplished by manipulating the blade with the fingers in the vagina, and the handle with the other hand. There are two ways in which this maneuver can be accomplished:
   a. The blade can be moved over the baby's face. With the left hand in the vagina manipulating the blade and the right hand on the handle, the blade is moved over the baby's face into position between the anterior parietal bone and the pubis. The advantage of this method is that the smaller face offers less resistance than the bulky occiput and there is less danger of damaging the maternal tissues. The disadvantage is that should the head move with the forceps the occiput will be rotated posteriorly.
   b. The blade can be moved around the occiput. The right hand is placed in the vagina to manipulate the blade and the left hand is on the handle. The blade is moved gently around the occiput and into position between the anterior parietal bone and the pubis. The advantage of this method is that should the head turn with the forceps, the occiput is moved anteriorly, a desirable effect. The drawback is that the bulkiness and hardness of the occiput make less room for the blade, and there is greater danger of maternal lacerations than when the blade is wandered around the face.
4. The posterior blade (for LOT it is the left) is inserted into the vagina between the posterior parietal bone (left) and the sacrum (Fig. 6).

Fig. 3. L. O. T. Insertion of the anterior (right) blade between the posterior parietal bone and the sacrum.

Fig. 4. L. O. T. The blade is wandered anteriorly so that it lies between the face and the pelvic wall.

Fig. 5. L. O. T. The blade is wandered further until it lies between the anterior parietal bone and the pubis.

Fig. 6. L. O. T. The posterior (left blade) is inserted between the posterior parietal bone and the sacrum.

5. The forceps are locked, and the application is checked to be certain that a good biparietal application has been achieved (**Figs. 7A and 7B**).

Rotation and Extraction

1. With the handles making a wide arc the head is rotated 90 degrees to the anterior, LOT to LOA to OA (**Figs. 8 and 9**). Now the occiput is under the pubis, the face is next to the sacrum, and the sagittal suture is in the anteroposterior diameter of the pelvis. The ideal cephalic application has been maintained. The pelvic application is also good, since the diameter of the forceps is in the transverse diameter of the pelvis, the concave edges point to the pubis, the convex edges lie in the hollow of the sacrum, and the sides of the blades lie next to the side walls of the pelvis.
2. The head is extracted as an occipitoanterior. Traction is outward and posterior until the occiput comes under the pubis and the nape of the neck pivots in the subpubic angle. The direction is then changed to outward and anterior, so that by extension the forehead, face, and chin are born over the perineum.

Fig. 7A. L. O. T. The forceps are
locked in a cephalic application.

Fig. 7B. L. O. T. The forceps are
locked in a cephalic application.

Fig. 8. Anterior rotation: L. O. T.
to L. O. A. (45 degrees).

Fig. 9. Anterior rotation: L. O. A.
to O. A. (45 degrees). The head is
ready for extraction.

MANUAL ROTATION AND FORCEPS EXTRACTION: LOT

1. With the patient in the lithotomy position, the operator stands facing the perineum, and inserts the right hand into the vagina. The fetal head is grasped with the four fingers over the posterior parietal (left) bone and the thumb over the anterior parietal (right) bone (Fig. 10).
2. By pronating the arm, the operator turns the fetal head 90 degrees to the anterior, LOT to LOA to OA (Fig. 11).
3. Forceps are then applied in the OA position, and the head is extracted as an occiput anterior.
4. ROT is managed in the same way, except that the left hand is used, and the rotation is ROT to ROA to OA.

BIBLIOGRAPHY

Ahnquist, G. Delivery of the persistent transverse vertex utilising Barton forceps. West. J. Surg., 60:406, 1952.

Chalfant, G. O. Kjelland forceps in transverse arrest. Obstet. Gynec., 8:308, 1956.

Douglas, R. G., and Stromme, W. B. Operative Obstetrics, 2nd ed. New York, Appleton-Century-Crofts, 1960.

Wilson, J. R. Atlas of Obstetric Technic. St. Louis, C. V. Mosby Co., 1961.

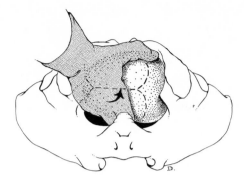

Fig. 10. L. O. T. Manual rotation. Grasping the head with the right hand.

Fig. 11. Manual rotation: L. O. T. to O. A. (90 degrees).

27 Arrested Posterior Positions of the Occiput

FORCEPS DELIVERY FACE TO PUBIS: OCCIPUT POSTERIOR

Occasionally the head seems to fit the pelvis better with the occiput posterior. This is so, for example, in some anthropoid pelves. When this is the case, and especially when the vertex is at or near the perineum, it is wiser to follow nature's lead and deliver the head face to pubis.

Orientation

Vaginal Examination (Fig. 1)

1. The presentation is cephalic.
2. The sagittal suture is in the anteroposterior diameter of the pelvis.
3. The posterior fontanelle and occiput are in the hollow of the sacrum.
4. The bregma and face are anterior, under the pubis.
5. The station is 0 to +3.

Orientation and Desired Application (Fig. 2A and 2B)

1. The cephalic application is not perfect but is satisfactory.
   a. The blades are over the parietal bones in an occipitomental application. The left blade is on the right parietal bone, and the right blade is on the left parietal bone.
   b. The front of the forceps (concave edges) point to the face. In an ideal cephalic application they point to the occiput.
   c. The convex edges point to the occiput. In the ideal application they point to the face.
2. The pelvic application is perfect.
   a. The diameter of the forceps is in the transverse diameter of the pelvis.
   b. The sides of the blades are next to the sidewalls of the pelvis, left blade near the left side, and right blade near the right side.
   c. The concave edges point to the pubis.
   d. The convex edges point to the sacrum.
   e. This may be low to mid forceps, depending on the exact station of the head.

Fig. 1. Occiput Posterior.

Fig. 2A. O. P. Orientation, Simpson forceps.

Fig. 2B. O. P. Orientation, Simpson forceps.

Application of the Forceps

1. The left blade is inserted gently into the vagina at about 5 o'clock.
2. It is then moved anteriorly so that it lies between the right parietal bone and the left side of the pelvis (Fig. 3).
3. The right blade is inserted (over the left) into the vagina at about 7 o'clock (Fig. 4).
4. It is then moved anteriorly so that it fits between the left parietal bone of the fetal head and the right side of the pelvis.
5. The forceps are locked, and vaginal examination is made to be certain that the application is correct and that there are no obstacles to extraction.
   The application is biparietal. The concave edges of the blades point to the pubis and the fetal face, while the convex edges point to the sacrum and the occiput (Figs. 5A and 5B).

O.P. APPLICATION OF FORCEPS

Fig. 3. O. P. Insertion of left blade between fetal head and left side of pelvis.

Fig. 4. O. P. Handle of left blade lowered and blade moved up over the right parietal bone. Insertion of the right blade between the fetal head and the right side of pelvis.

Fig. 5A. O. P. Forceps locked in biparietal application.

Fig. 5B. O. P. Forceps locked in biparietal application.

Extraction of the Head

1. Traction is made outward and posteriorly until the area between the bregma and the nasion lies under the pubic arch (Fig. 6).
2. Delivery is by one of two methods:
   a. The direction is changed to outward and anterior (Fig. 7), and as the handles of the forceps are raised, the occiput is born over the perineum by flexion. The forceps then slip off the head.
   b. The direction is then changed to outward and anterior until the occiput is on the perineum. The forceps are removed by raising first the right handle toward the left groin so that the blade slips around the head and out of the vagina. Then the left handle is raised toward the right groin so that the left blade slides out. By a modified Ritgen maneuver flexion is increased until the occiput has cleared the perineum completely.
3. The head then falls back in extension, and the nose, face, and chin are delivered under the pubis.
4. If the head cannot be delivered as a posterior presentation without the use of an excessive amount of force, this method of delivery should be abandoned and anterior rotation of the occiput carried out.
5. Since the diameter distending the perineum (biparietal of 9.5 cm) is larger than in anterior positions (bitemporal of 8.0 cm), lacerations are more extensive, and an adequate episiotomy should be made.

Fig. 6. O. P. Traction is made outward and posteriorly until the area between the bregma and nasion lies under the pubic arch.

Fig. 7. O. P. Traction is made outward and anteriorly to promote flexion.

FORCEPS ROTATION: ROP TO OP AND
EXTRACTION FACE TO PUBIS

Orientation

Vaginal Examination

1. The presentation is cephalic.
2. The sagittal suture is in the right oblique diameter of the pelvis.
3. The posterior fontanelle is in the right posterior quadrant of the pelvis (Fig. 8).
4. The bregma is in the left anterior quadrant.
5. The station is usually 0 to +2.

Orientation and Desired Application

1. The cephalic application is not perfect but is satisfactory (Fig. 9).
   a. The blades are over the parietal bones in an occipitomental application. The left blade is on the right parietal bone, and the right blade is on the left parietal bone.
   b. The front of the forceps (concave edges) point to the face. In an ideal cephalic application they point to the occiput.
   c. The convex edges point to the occiput. In the ideal application they point to the face.
2. The pelvic application is oblique.
   a. The diameter of the blades is in the left oblique diameter of the pelvis.
   b. The left blade is in the left posterior quadrant of the pelvis.
   c. The right blade is in the right anterior quadrant.
   d. The concave edges point anteriorly and to the left.
   e. The convex edges are posterior and to the right.

Fig. 8.   Right Occiput Posterior.

Fig. 9.   R. O. P.   Orientation.   Midforceps, Simpson.

Application of Forceps

1. The left blade is inserted gently into the vagina at about 5 o'clock, so that it lies between the right parietal bone and the left posterolateral wall of the pelvis (Fig. 10).
2. The right blade is inserted (over the left) into the vagina at about 7 o'clock (Fig. 11).
3. It is then moved anteriorly about 90 degrees around the fetal head so that it fits between the left parietal bone and the right anterolateral quadrant of the pelvis.
4. The forceps are now locked, and vaginal examination is performed to make sure that the application is correct. If it is not, the forceps are unlocked and the necessary   adjustments made (Fig. 12).

Rotation and Extraction*

1. The head is rotated 45 degrees from ROP to OP, so that the occiput is in the hollow of the sacrum and the face under the pubis (Fig. 13).
2. Traction is made outward and posteriorly until the area between the bregma and the nasion lies under the pubic arch.
3. The direction is then changed to outward and anterior, and as the handles of the forceps are raised, the occiput is born over the perineum by flexion. The forceps are then removed.

*The details of technic for extraction of the head are included in the previous section dealing with face to pubis delivery.

R.O.P.: FORCEPS ROTATION TO O.P.

Fig. 10. R. O. P. Insertion of the left blade between the fetal head and the left postero-lateral quadrant of the pelvis.

Fig. 11. R. O. P. Handle of the left blade is lowered. Insertion of the right blade between the fetal head and the right postero-lateral quadrant of the pelvis; followed by upward movement of the blade to the right antero-lateral quadrant of the pelvis.

Fig. 12. R. O. P. Locking of forceps in biparietal application.

Fig. 13. Posterior rotation R. O. P. to O. P. (45 degrees).

MANUAL ROTATION TO THE ANTERIOR

Orientation

Vaginal Examination

1. The presentation is cephalic.
2. The sagittal suture is in the right oblique diameter of the pelvis.
3. The posterior fontanelle is in the right posterior quadrant of the pelvis (Fig. 14).
4. The bregma is in the left anterior quadrant.
5. The station is usually 0 to +2.

Rotation is accomplished by one of two methods: 1, manual rotation of the head and shoulders: the Pomeroy maneuver; or 2, manual rotation of the head.

The Pomeroy Maneuver:
Manual Rotation of Head and Shoulders: ROP

1. The operator places his left hand into the posterior part of the vagina between the head and the sacrum and past the fetal head into the uterus, so that the finger tips grasp the anterior shoulder, and the head lies in the palm of the hand (Fig. 15).
2. By pressure upward on the anterior shoulder (as the hand is pronated), the body and head are turned anteriorly (Fig. 16).
3. The advantage of this maneuver is that since the body has been rotated, the head will not slip back to its original position. To insure against this happening the head may be overrotated, ROP to LOA.
4. The disadvantage is that the head must be dislodged to the point of disengagement to enable the hand to reach the shoulder. There is danger that the umbilical cord may prolapse or that the head may be extended and may not reengage properly.

Fig. 14. Right Occiput Posterior.

Fig. 15. R. O. P. Pomeroy maneuver: the fingers of the left hand are placed behind the anterior shoulder.

Fig. 16. Pomeroy maneuver: anterior rotation of the shoulders and head, R. O. P. to L. O. A.

ROP: Manual Rotation of the Occiput to the Anterior

1. After the patient is anesthetized the operator inserts the left hand in the vagina and grasps the fetal head, placing the thumb on the anterior parietal (left) bone, and the fingers on the posterior parietal (right) bone. The left hand is better for ROP and the right for LOP (Figs. 17 and 18).
2. First the head is flexed.
3. Then the head is rotated anteriorly to the occiput anterior position by pronating the hand in the vagina: ROP to ROT to ROA to OA (Figs. 19, 20, and 21).
4. At the same time the operator turns the body in the identical direction by applying pressure with his other hand on the shoulders or breech through the maternal abdomen.
5. This method is safe for the baby and for the mother. However, when the fit between baby and pelvis is snug, or when the head is impacted, it is difficult to obtain a good grasp of the head, and manual rotation may be impossible. Furthermore, the shoulders do not always rotate with the head, and sometimes when the head is released by the operator's hand it will return to the original posterior position. Despite these disadvantages manual rotation is so safe and so free from vaginal tears that it should be tried before resorting to more complicated methods.
6. Sometimes complete rotation to the OA position is not possible. In such cases forceps are applied to the head in the new position (ROT or ROA), rotation to OA is achieved with the forceps, and the head is extracted.

The Delivery

Once manual rotation of the head to the occipitoanterior has been accomplished two methods of delivery are available:

1. Originally the patient was permitted to awaken from the anesthetic and the onset of labor was awaited, the hope being that spontaneous delivery would take place.
2. Today we believe that, once the indications for interference are present, the baby should be born without delay. Hence, manual rotation is followed by extraction with forceps in the new position.

ROP MANUAL ROTATION TO OA

Fig. 17. R. O. P. Orientation. Manual rotation, left hand.

Fig. 18. R. O. P. Left hand grasping the head; thumb on the anterior parietal (left) bone, and fingers on the posterior parietal (right) bone.

Fig. 19. Manual rotation using left hand: R. O. P. to R. O. T. (45 degrees).

Fig. 20. Manual rotation using left hand: R. O. T. to R. O. A. (45 degrees).

Fig. 21. Manual rotation using left hand: R. O. A. to O. A. (45 degrees). Head ready for extraction.

DOUBLE APPLICATION OF FORCEPS: ROP
THE MODIFIED SCANZONI MANEUVER

A double application of forceps for the treatment of occipitoposterior positions was performed by William Smellie in the eighteenth century. In 1830 Scanzoni revived, improved, and popularized the maneuver which has since been associated with his name. Bill further modified the operation, and his technic is the one that we use today.

Orientation

Vaginal Examination

1. The presentation is cephalic.
2. The sagittal suture is in the right oblique diameter of the pelvis.
3. The posterior fontanelle is in the right posterior quadrant of the pelvis (Fig. 22).
4. The bregma is in the left anterior quadrant.
5. The station is usually 0 to +2.

Orientation and Desired Application (Fig. 23)

1. The cephalic application is not perfect but is satisfactory.
   a. The blades are over the parietal bones in an occipitomental application. The left blade is on the right parietal bone, and the right blade is on the left parietal bone.
   b. The front of the forceps (concave edges) point to the face. In an ideal cephalic application they point to the occiput.
   c. The convex edges point to the occiput. In the ideal application they point to the face.
2. The pelvic application is oblique.
   a. The diameter of the blades is in the left oblique diameter of the pelvis.
   b. The left blade is in the left posterior quadrant of the pelvis.
   c. The right blade is in the right anterior quadrant.
   d. The concave edges point anteriorly and to the left.
   e. The convex edges are posterior and to the right.

Fig. 22.   Right Occiput Posterior.

Fig. 23.   R. O. P.   Orientation.   Mid forceps, Simpson.

Application of Forceps

1. The left blade is inserted gently into the vagina at about 5 o'clock, so that it lies between the right parietal bone and the left posterolateral wall of the pelvis (Fig. 24).
2. The right blade is inserted into the vagina at about 7 o'clock (Fig. 25).
3. It is then moved anteriorly about 90 degrees around the fetal head so that it fits between the left parietal bone and the right anterolateral wall of the pelvis.
4. The forceps are now locked, and vaginal examination is performed to make sure that the application is correct. If it is not, the forceps are unlocked and the necessary adjustments made (Fig. 26).

Fig. 24. R. O. P. Insertion of the left blade between the fetal head and the left postero-lateral quadrant of the pelvis.

Fig. 25. R. O. P. Handle of the left blade is lowered. Insertion of the right blade between the fetal head and the right postero-lateral quadrant of the pelvis; followed by upward movement of the blade to the right antero-lateral quadrant of the pelvis.

Fig. 26. R. O. P. Locking of forceps in biparietal application.

Rotation: ROP to OA

1. After the forceps are locked, the handles are raised toward the opposite
groin, in ROP toward the left groin. This maneuver favors flexion of the
head (Fig. 27).

2. Without any traction the handles are carried around in a large circle so
that they point first to the left groin (ROP), next toward the left thigh (ROT),
then toward the left ischial tuberosity (ROA) (Fig. 29), and finally toward
the anus and floor (OA) (Fig. 30). With the wide sweep of the handles the
blades turn in a small arc and do not deviate from the same axis during the
process of rotation. The fetal head turns with the use of very little force
on the part of the operator.

3. The rotation is continued until the occiput lies under the symphysis pubis
and the sagittal suture is in the anteroposterior diameter of the pelvis. The
extent of the rotation is 135 degrees, and the sequence is ROP to ROT to
ROA to OA. The relationship of the forceps to the fetal head has not
changed, but now the concave edges of the blades are posterior and the convex edges are anterior. The forceps are upside down, and the pelvic curve
of the blades is the reverse of the curve of the maternal pelvis. This situation is not suitable for extraction of the head and adjustments are necessary.

Fig. 27. R. O. P. Head is flexed by raising the handles of the forceps.

Fig. 28. Anterior rotation by forceps: R. O. P. to R. O. T. (45 degrees).

Fig. 29. Anterior rotation by forceps: R. O. T. to R. O. A. (45 degrees).

Fig. 30. Anterior rotation by forceps: R. O. A. to O. A. (45 degrees).

Removal of Forceps

1. Removal of forceps
   a. Before removing the forceps a small amount of traction is made, not with the idea of delivering the head, but simply to fix it in its new position.
   b. The forceps are unlocked.
   c. The right forceps is removed first by depressing the handle further so that the blade slides around the head and out of the vagina (Fig. 31).
   d. Then the left forceps is removed in the same way (Fig. 32).
2. Vaginal examination in the new position: OA (Fig. 33)
   a. The sagittal suture is in the anteroposterior diameter of the pelvis.
   b. The occiput is under the pubis.
   c. The face is near the sacrum.

Fig. 31. Removal of right blade.

Fig. 32. Removal of left blade.

Fig. 33. New position: A. O.

Reapplication of Forceps

1. The left blade is inserted between the fetal head and the left posterolateral quadrant of the pelvis (Fig. 34).
2. The handle is lowered to the horizontal and the blade moved over the left parietal bone.
3. The right blade is inserted between the fetal head and the right posterolateral quadrant of the pelvis (Fig. 35).
4. The handle is lowered to the horizontal and the blade moved over the right parietal bone.
5. The forceps are locked in a biparietal cephalic and pelvic application (Fig. 36).
6. Then the head is extracted in the usual way.

Fig. 34. Reapplication of left blade between fetal head and left side of pelvis.

Fig. 35. Reapplication of right blade between fetal head and right side of pelvis.

Fig. 36. Locking of forceps in biparietal cephalic and pelvic application.

Alternate Method of Removing and Reapplying
the Forceps Using Two Sets

Occasionally the shoulders do not rotate with the head and there is a tendency for the head to turn back to the ROP position once the forceps are removed (Fig. 37).   This can be prevented by employing two sets of the forceps in the following way:

1. The right blade (upside down) is removed from the left side of the pelvis (Fig. 38).   An assistant holds the original left blade in place, and this prevents the head from turning back.
2. The left blade from the new set is then inserted right side up into the left side of the maternal pelvis, in the usual manner (Fig. 39).

Fig. 37. New position: O. A. Forceps upside down.

Fig. 38. Removal of the right Simpson forceps from left side of pelvis.

Fig. 39. Insertion of the left Tucker-McLane forceps between fetal head and left side of pelvis. The left Simpson is still in place.

3. The left upside down blade is then removed from the right side of the pelvis (Fig. 40). The head is prevented from turning back by the new left blade, which is held by an assistant.
4. The right blade of the new set is now inserted into the vagina (Fig. 41).
5. The forceps are now in a correct application, and are locked (Fig. 42).
6. Extraction is carried out in the usual way.

The risks of extensive vaginal lacerations, claimed by some authors to be inherent in the Scanzoni maneuver because of the long forceps rotation, have been exaggerated greatly. As long as the operation is performed gently and slowly a minimal amount of damage will occur. Many of the extensive vaginal tears, and vesical and rectal fistulae, occurred in cases of definite disproportion, where vaginal delivery should never have been carried out.

As the following translation of Scanzoni's article reveals, Scanzoni described the rotation of the head only as far as the ROT or ROA position.

The head stands with the forehead turned toward the front and left, so that the sagittal suture passes in the right oblique diameter; the left blade is applied in front of the left sacroiliac synchondrosis, the right behind the right obturator foramen: with this the transverse diameter of the forceps is placed in the left oblique diameter of the pelvis, their concave edges and tips are turned to the anterior circumference of the left lateral hemisphere of the pelvis, and so also with the forehead. An eighth of a circle is now described with the instrument, directed from left to right, whereby the right blade comes to rest under the symphysis, and the left in the hollow of the sacrum; and in this way, the head is rotated, the earlier standing forehead is moved to the middle of the left lateral wall of the pelvis, and the sagittal suture is placed parallel with the transverse diameter of the pelvis.

Now both blades of the forceps are removed, and again applied, so that the left blade comes to lie behind the left obturator foramen, the right in front of the right sacroiliac ligament, whereupon by the next rotation the occiput is brought completely under the pubic arch.

Fig. 40. Removal of the left Simpson forceps from the right side of the pelvis.

Fig. 41. Insertion of the right Tucker–McLane forceps between the fetal head and the right side of the pelvis.

Fig. 42. Locking of the Tucker–McLane forceps in biparietal cephalic and pelvic application.

THE MAUGHAN MANEUVER: ROP

1. The left forceps blade is placed upside down in the right posterolateral part of the vagina so that it lies over the occiput. The concave side of the blade points posteriorly and the convex side anteriorly (Fig. 43).
2. The blade is wandered anteriorly so that it sweeps by the occiput, catches the anterior fetal ear, and rotates the ear to a position directly behind the symphysis pubis. The sequence is ROP to ROT (45 degrees). The sagittal suture is now in the transverse diameter of the pelvis (Fig. 44).
3. The second blade is inserted between the fetal head and the sacrum so that it lies over the posterior ear (Fig. 45).
4. The forceps are then locked, each blade resting over an ear.
5. The head is rotated slowly 90 degrees so that the occiput is placed behind the symphysis. The sequence is ROT to ROA to OA.
6. The head is then extracted as an occipitoanterior.

This maneuver for rotation of the fetal head is primarily one of a single forceps blade application, applied upside down to the opposite side of the maternal pelvis (i.e., in right occipitoposterior, the left blade to the right side of the pelvis) in such fashion that, on anterior sliding movement, it sweeps over the occiput, and catching on the anterior fetal ear, rotates it to a position directly behind the symphysis pubis. The movement of this blade into place is, therefore, completely in the direction that rotation of the fetal head is intended, without upward displacement of the head.

Fig. 43. R. O. P. Left forceps blade inserted upside down over the occiput.

Fig. 44. Forceps blade moved anteriorly under the pubis; head rotates R. O. P. to R. O. T.

Fig. 45. Posterior blade inserted between parietal bone and sacrum. Forceps locked in biparietal cephalic application. Arrow shows direction of further rotation R. O. T. to O. A.

THE KEY IN LOCK MANEUVER OF DELEE

This is a multiple application method. The forceps are applied in the transverse diameter of the pelvis so that each blade lies next to the corresponding side of the maternal pelvis. Since the application to the fetal skull is often not ideal, this operation must be performed delicately, with the least possible compression being applied to the baby. The head is pushed up a short distance in the axis of the birth canal and rotated gently, so that the small fontanelle is brought anteriorly about 5 degrees. This is accomplished by sweeping the handles of the forceps through an arc of 10 degrees outside the pelvis. The head is then pulled down in the pelvis, a little less than it was pushed up, to fix it in its new position. The forceps are loosened and returned to the transverse diameter of the pelvis, but the head is maintained in its new position. The head is then pushed up and rotated another 5 degrees. These small rotations are continued until eventually the head is in the anterior position, and the front (concave side) of the forceps points properly to the symphysis pubis and also to the fetal occiput. The head is then extracted in the usual way.

BIBLIOGRAPHY

Bill, A. H. The treatment of the vertex occipito-posterior position. Amer. J. Obstet. Gynec., 22:615, 1931.

Danforth, W. C. The treatment of occipito posterior positions with especial reference to manual rotation. Amer. J. Obstet. Gynec., 23:360, 1932.

DeLee, J. B. The treatment of obstinate occipito-posterior positions. J. A. M. A., 75:145, 1920.

Douglas, R. G., and Stromme, W. B. Operative Obstetrics, 2nd ed. New York, Appleton-Century-Crofts, 1960.

King, E. L., Herring, J. S., Dyer, I., and King, J. A. The modification of the Scanzoni rotation in the management of persistent occipito posterior positions. Amer. J. Obstet. Gynec., 61:872, 1951.

Maughan, G. B. The safe and simple delivery of persistent posterior and transverse positions. Amer. J. Obstet. Gynec., 71:741, 1956.

Melhado, G. C. The occipito posterior position. Amer. J. Obstet. Gynec., 26:696, 1933.

Reddoch, J. W. The management of occipitoposterior positions with special reference to the Scanzoni maneuver. South. Med. J., 27:615, 1934.

Seides, S. A "two forceps maneuver" for persistent occipito-posterior position. Surg., Gynec. Obstet., 36:421, 1923.

28 Arrested Face Presentations

FORCEPS EXTRACTION: MENTUM ANTERIOR

Orientation

Vaginal Examination (Fig. 1)

1. The presentation is cephalic.
2. The long axis of the face is in the anteroposterior diameter of the pelvis.
3. The chin is under the pubic symphysis.
4. The forehead is toward the sacrum.

Orientation and Desired Application (Figs. 2 and 5)

1. The aim is for a biparietal cephalic application.
   a. The front of the forceps (concave edges) point toward the denominator (the chin).
   b. The blades are over the parietal bones in a mentooccipital (reverse occipitomental) application.
2. The pelvic application is correct.
   a. The diameter of the blades is in the transverse diameter of the pelvis.
   b. The sides of the blades are next to the corresponding sidewalls of the pelvis.
   c. The concave edges point to the pubis.
   d. The convex edges are in the hollow of the sacrum.

MENTUM ANTERIOR

Fig. 1. Face presentation: Mentum Anterior.

Fig. 2. M.A.: orientation. Kjelland forceps. (From Douglas and Stromme. Operative Obstetrics, Appleton-Century-Crofts, 1957.)

2. The pelvic application is correct.
   a. The diameter of the blades is in the transverse diameter of the pelvis.
   b. The sides of the blades are next to the corresponding sidewalls of the pelvis.
   c. The concave edges point to the pubis.
   d. The convex edges are in the hollow of the sacrum.

Application of Forceps

1. The left blade is inserted into the vagina at about 5 o'clock, and is moved around the face slightly until it lies between the right cheek and the left wall of the pelvis (Fig. 3).
2. The right blade is inserted into the vagina at about 7 o'clock, and is moved around the face until it lies between the left cheek and the right wall of the pelvis (Fig. 4).

Fig. 3. M.A.: insertion of left
blade to left side of pelvis. (From
Douglas and Stromme. Operative
Obstetrics, Appleton-Century-
Crofts, 1957.)

Fig. 4. M.A.: insertion of
right blade to right side of pelvis.
(From Douglas and Stromme. Operative Obstetrics, Appleton-Century-
Crofts, 1957.)

The forceps are locked, and vaginal examination is made to be sure that the application is correct and that no adjustment is necessary (Fig. 5).

Extraction of the Head

1. The handles of the forceps are depressed toward the floor to deflex the head completely.
2. Traction is made in an outward, horizontal, and slightly posterior direction until the chin appears under the symphysis pubis, and the submental region of the neck impinges in the subpubic angle (Fig. 6).
3. With further descent the face and forehead appear, and the direction of traction is changed to outward and anterior. This brings about both descent and flexion, and the vertex and occiput are born over the perineum (Fig. 7).
4. Since a large diameter is being born over the perineum, an episiotomy is advisable.

Fig. 5. M.A.: locking of forceps. Beginning traction in the axis of the birth canal. (From Douglas and Stromme. Operative Obstetrics, Appleton-Century-Crofts, 1957.)

Fig. 6. M.A.: horizontal traction. (From Douglas and Stromme. Operative Obstetrics, Appleton-Century-Crofts, 1957.)

Fig. 7. M.A.: delivery by flexion of the head. (From Douglas and Stromme. Operative Obstetrics, Appleton-Century-Crofts, 1957.)

FORCEPS ROTATION AND EXTRACTION: MENTUM POSTERIOR

Because the bulk of the head is in the anterior quadrant of the pelvis, the usual application is not practical, and the forceps are applied upside down. Because of their small pelvic curve the Kjelland forceps are valuable for this operation, but any instrument can be used.

Orientation

Vaginal Examination (Fig. 8)

1. The long axis of the face is in the anteroposterior diameter of the pelvis.
2. The chin is in the hollow of the sacrum.
3. The forehead is under the pubic symphysis.

Orientation and Desired Application (Figs. 9 and 12)

1. The cephalic application is biparietal.
   a. The front of the forceps (concave edges) points to the denominator (the chin).
   b. The blades are over the parietal bones.
2. The pelvic application is upside down.
   a. The diameter of the blades is in the transverse diameter of the pelvis.
   b. The sides of the blades are next to the opposite sidewalls of the pelvis: left blade next to the right wall, and right blade near the left wall.
   c. The concave edges point to the sacrum.
   d. The convex edges point to the pubis.

Fig. 8. Face presentation: Mentum Posterior.

Fig. 9. M. P.: orientation. Kjelland forceps upside down. (From Douglas and Stromme. Operative Obstetrics, Appleton–Century–Crofts, 1957.)

Application of the Forceps Upside Down

1. The right blade is inserted first. Its handle is grasped by the left hand and is held a little below the vagina and hear the mother's right thigh. The convex edge of the blade is anterior.
2. The right blade is inserted into the vagina between the left side of the face and the left wall of the vagina (Fig. 10).
3. The left blade is inserted next. Its handle is grasped by the right hand and is held a little below the vagina and near the mother's left thigh. The convex edge is anterior (upside down).
4. The left blade is introduced into the right side of the vagina, between the right side of the face and the right pelvic wall (Fig. 11).
5. The forceps are locked and vaginal examination is made to be sure that the application is correct (Fig. 12).

Fig. 10. M.P.: insertion of right blade, from below upward, to the left side of the pelvis. (From Douglas and Stromme. Operative Obstetrics, Appleton-Century-Crofts, 1957.)

Fig. 11. M.P.: insertion of left blade, from below upward, to the right side of the pelvis. (From Douglas and Stromme. Operative Obstetrics, Appleton-Century-Crofts, 1957.)

Fig. 12. M.P.: forceps locked, upside down. (From Douglas and Stromme. Operative Obstetrics, Appleton-Century-Crofts, 1957.)

Rotation to the Anterior: MP to MA

1. The face is then rotated 180 degrees with the forceps: MP to RMP to RMT to RMA to MA. The chin is now under the pubis and the forehead is in the hollow of the sacrum (Figs. 13 and 14).
2. The cephalic application has been maintained.
3. The pelvic application is now right side up, with the concave edges next to the pubis and the convex edges near the sacrum.

Extraction of the Head

1. Vaginal examination is made to check the application.
2. Traction is made in an outward and posterior direction until the chin appears under the symphysis and the submental region of the neck impinges in the subpubic angle.
3. With further descent the face and forehead appear, and the direction of traction is changed to outward and anterior. This brings about both descent and flexion, and the vertex and occiput are born over the perineum.
4. Because of the large diameter being delivered, an episiotomy is essential.

BIBLIOGRAPHY

Douglas, R. G., and Stromme, W. B. Operative Obstetrics, 2nd ed. New York, Appleton-Century-Crofts, 1960.

Fig. 13. Anterior rotation with forceps: M.P. to R.M.T. (From Douglas and Stromme. Operative Obstetrics, Appleton–Century–Crofts, 1957.)

Fig. 14. Anterior rotation with forceps: R.M.T. to M.A. (From Douglas and Stromme. Operative Obstetrics, Appleton–Century–Crofts, 1957.)

29 Breech: Delivery of the Aftercoming Head by Forceps

While any type of forceps can be used for this procedure, the Piper forceps, which was designed especially for this operation, is the best. The handles are depressed below the arch of the shanks, the pelvic curve is reduced, and the shanks are long and curved. These features make this instrument easier to apply to the aftercoming head.

Orientation

Vaginal Examination

1. The long axis of the head is in the anteroposterior diameter of the pelvis.
2. The occiput is anterior.
3. The face is posterior.

Orientation and Desired Application

1. The cephalic application is biparietal and mentooccipital, with the front of the forceps (concave edges) toward the occiput and the convex edges toward the face.
2. The pelvic application is good, with the diameter of the forceps in the transverse diameter of the pelvis, the concave edges pointing toward the pubis, and the convex edges toward the sacrum. The sides of the blades are next to the sidewalls of the pelvis (Fig. 4).

348

Fig. 1. Breech presentation: Piper forceps on the aftercoming head. Orientation. (From Douglas and Stromme. Operative Obstetrics, Appleton-Century-Crofts, 1957.)

Fig. 2. Insertion of the left blade. (From Douglas and Stromme. Operative Obstetrics, Appleton-Century-Crofts, 1957.)

Application of Forceps

1. An assistant lifts the baby's body slightly, but not too much or the structures in the neck will be damaged by excessive stretching. The lower and upper limbs and the umbilical cord are kept out of the way.
2. The handle of the left blade is grasped in the left hand.
3. The right hand is introduced between the head and the left posterolateral wall of the vagina.
4. The left blade is then inserted between the head and the fingers into a mentooccipital application.
5. The fingers are removed from the vagina, and the handle is steadied by an assistant.
6. The handle of the right blade is grasped with the right hand.
7. The left hand is introduced between the head and the right posterolateral wall of the vagina.
8. The right blade is introduced between the head and the fingers into a mentooccipital application.
9. The fingers are removed from the vagina.
10. The forceps are locked, and vaginal examination is made to be certain that the application is correct.

Extraction of the Head

1. Traction is outward and posterior until the nape of the neck is in the subpubic angle.
2. The direction is then changed to outward and anterior, and the face and forehead are born over the perineum in flexion.
3. An episiotomy should be used.

BIBLIOGRAPHY

Douglas, R. G., and Stromme, W. B. Operative Obstetrics, 2nd ed. New York, Appleton-Century-Crofts, 1960.

Fig. 3. Insertion of the right blade. (From Douglas and Stromme. Operative Obstetrics, Appleton-Century-Crofts, 1957.)

Fig. 4. Piper forceps locked in cephalic application. Beginning traction. (From Douglas and Stromme. Operative Obstetrics, Appleton-Century-Crofts, 1957.)

30   Version and Extraction

DEFINITIONS

Version is an operation by which the fetus is turned in utero for the purpose of changing the presentation.

Cephalic version: Results in a cephalic presentation

Podalic version: Results in a breech

External version: All the manipulations are done through the abdominal wall.

Internal version: The operation is performed by the hand or fingers inside the uterus. In most cases the intrauterine manipulations are furthered by the other hand acting through the abdominal wall.

Extraction is the operative and immediate forceful delivery of the child.

EXTERNAL VERSION

Indications

1. Cephalic
   a. To turn a breech to a cephalic presentation
   b. To change a transverse lie to a cephalic presentation
2. Podalic: To turn a transverse lie to a breech presentation. This is done only when cephalic version has failed.

Prerequisites

Certain conditions must be present before external version is attempted:

1. There must be a single pregnancy.
2. Accurate diagnosis of the fetal position is of prime importance.
3. Fetopelvic disproportion should be ruled out.
4. The presenting part must not be deeply engaged.
5. The fetus must be freely movable.
6. There must be intact membranes, with a good quantity of amniotic fluid.
7. Uterine relaxation is essential.
8. The maternal abdominal wall must be lax and thin enough to permit manipulations.
9. If possible the placenta should be located.

352

Contraindications

1. Deep engagement of the breech in the pelvis
2. Gross congenital abnormalities of the fetus
3. Intrauterine fetal death
4. Multiple pregnancy
5. Premature rupture of the membranes
6. Antepartum bleeding
7. Uterine scars, e.g., previous cesarean section
8. Cases in which vaginal delivery is not intended
9. Preeclampsia and hypertension

Dangers of External Version

1. There may be premature separation of the placenta from the uterine wall.
2. There is danger of injury to the umbilical cord and interference with the uteroplacental circulation.
3. The position achieved by the version may be worse than the original one. For example, little has been gained by changing a breech into a brow presentation.
4. Unexplained fetal death may follow version.
5. Induction of premature labor may take place.

Technic of External Version

Preparation

1. The patient lies on her back on a firm table with the abdomen uncovered. To help relax the abdominal wall muscles, a pillow is put under the head, and the hips and knees are flexed.
2. Placing the woman in slight Trendelenburg position (hips higher than the shoulders) for 15 or 20 minutes may help to dislodge the presenting part, and so make the version easier.
3. The bladder should be empty.
4. If the mother's abdomen or the operator's hands are moist, powder should be sprinkled on the abdomen.
5. The diagnosis must be precise. If there is any doubt x-ray should be used.

Anesthesia

There is considerable controversy about the use of an anesthetic agent in the performance of version. There is no doubt that it is easier to perform the operation when the patient is asleep and completely relaxed. On the other hand, it increases the danger of injury. When the patient is awake, her complaints of pain serve as an indication that the manipulations are too vigorous and that it is wise to be more gentle or to stop.

Procedure

1. The operator stands at the patient's side.
2. The fetal heart is checked frequently before, during, and after the procedure. If at any time there is irregularity, or a marked change in the rate, the operation is discontinued.
3. One hand is placed on the head and the other on the breech.
4. The presenting part is dislodged from the pelvis.
5. The head is moved toward the pelvis and the breech toward the fundus to achieve a transverse lie. This position is maintained while the fetal heart is auscultated.
6. If the fetal heart rate is slow or irregular, the baby is turned back to the original position.
7. If the heart is normal the version is continued until the head is over the pelvis and the breech is in the fundus.
8. If, at this point, the baby's heart is abnormal, the fetus must be returned to its primary position.
9. After the version is complete and the fetal heart is noted to be normal, the head should be pushed into the pelvis to try and prevent recurrence of the malpresentation. Unfortunately, and despite all efforts, this often happens.
10. Version must never be forced. If the procedure cannot be performed easily and gently, it should be abandoned or postponed.

Direction of Version

The fetus is turned in the direction which is easier, with either the occiput or the face leading the way. It is important that flexion of the head be maintained during the procedure. It is simpler to preserve flexion of the head by the backward somersault (occiput first), but there is more danger of the legs tangling with the umbilical cord. With the forward somersault (face first) there is less chance of the legs causing trouble, but it is more difficult to keep the head flexed.

Fig. 1. External version:
L. S. T. Dislodgement of breech.

Fig. 2. External version: forward somersault, L. S. T. to transverse lie.

Fig. 3. External version: forward somersault completed, transverse lie to R. O. T.

INTERNAL PODALIC VERSION

Internal version is always podalic. With a hand inside the uterus it is feasible to grasp the feet and turn the baby to a footling breech. When the feet have been brought through the introitus the version is complete.

Indications

1. When the situation of the mother or fetus is such that immediate rapid delivery is essential
2. Prolapse of the umbilical cord
3. In compound presentations where the arm is prolapsed below the head and cannot be pushed out of the way
4. Delivery of the second twin if it has not engaged within 30 minutes of the birth of the first
5. Transverse or oblique lie

Prerequisites

1. Accurate diagnosis of position of the child is essential.
2. The child must be alive. There is no point in submitting the mother to a dangerous procedure if the baby is dead.
3. The presenting part should not be deeply engaged.
4. The pelvis must be large enough to permit the passage of the fetal head, i. e., no disproportion.
5. The cervix must be open enough to admit the hand.
6. If extraction is to follow the version, the cervix must be dilated fully.
7. The uterus must not be in tetanus, nor be too tightly coapted around the child. The baby must be freely movable.
8. Membranes should be intact or recently ruptured. There must be sufficient amniotic fluid to permit the turning to be accomplished.

Contraindications

1. Contracted pelvis with fetopelvic disproportion. It is pointless to perform podalic version if there is not enough room for the head to come through.
2. An incompletely dilated or a rigid cervix
3. A spastic uterus, which will not relax even under anesthesia. A spastic uterus not only makes version difficult or impossible, but increases greatly the danger of uterine rupture.

4. Danger of uterine rupture. When the patient has been in labor for a long time, with the lower uterine segment thinned out and with a high retraction ring, any intrauterine manipulations carry a grave danger of uterine rupture.
5. Rupture of the membranes. Once the membranes have been ruptured for a long time (over one hour) and the amniotic fluid has drained away, version is difficult, and the attempt carries with it the risk of uterine rupture and fetal death.
6. Uterine scar from previous cesarean section or extensive myomectomy

Dangers of Internal Version

Maternal

1. Inherent dangers of deep anesthesia
2. Rupture of the uterus
3. Lacerations of the cervix
4. Abruptio placentae
5. Infection following the intrauterine manipulations

Fetal

1. Asphyxia from cord prolapse or compression
2. Anesthetic depression causes asphyxia
3. Asphyxia from placental separation
4. Intracranial damage and hemorrhage
5. General trauma from the difficult procedure

Technic of Internal Version

Preparation

1. The patient is placed in the lithotomy position with the buttocks a little past the end of the table.
2. The operator should wear long gloves extending well above the elbows. Rigid asepsis is observed.
3. The bladder is catheterized. The rectum should be empty.
4. An intravenous infusion with a large bore needle is set up.
5. Cross-matched blood should be available.

Anesthesia

The patient is anesthetized deeply.

Procedure

1. The introitus and vagina are lubricated with green soap or dettol.
2. One hand is placed on the uterine fundus to steady the uterus and the baby.
3. The other hand is placed through the cervix into the uterine cavity.
4. When the operator is ready for immediate action, the membranes are ruptured.
5. The fetal head is displaced upward out of the pelvis if the presentation is cephalic.
6. With the intrauterine hand both feet are grasped, if possible. If both feet are not attainable, then one foot is grasped. The operator must make sure that he has a foot and not a hand.
7. The feet are pulled slowly toward the pelvic inlet.
8. With the outer hand the head is pushed gently toward the fundus.
9. When possible the baby should be turned so that the back remains anterior and the head in flexion.
10. When the knees have reached the introitus, version is complete.
11. If there is no need for immediate delivery, the patient is permitted to recover from the anesthesia and to resume labor.

Fig. 4. Internal podalic version: vertex presentation. Grasping both feet.

Fig. 5. Internal podalic version: downward traction on feet. Upward pressure on head. Vertex presentation converted to footling breech.

EXTRACTION FOLLOWING VERSION

If there is an indication for immediate delivery, and this is so in most cases where internal version is performed, the baby is extracted as a footling breech. This procedure is described in Chapter 18.

CESAREAN SECTION OR VERSION AND EXTRACTION

In the days when cesarean section was fraught with great danger to the mother, version and extraction was employed frequently in the management of various obstetric difficulties. The improvement in surgical technics, the discovery of antibiotics, the advances in anesthesia, and the availability of blood for transfusion have decreased the fetal and maternal mortality and morbidity associated with abdominal delivery to a point where cesarean section is preferable by far to version and extraction. The use of the latter procedure is limited today to situations of an emergent nature, where immediate delivery of the baby is essential.

BIBLIOGRAPHY

Douglas, R. G., and Stromme, W. B. Operative Obstetrics, 2nd ed. New York, Appleton-Century-Crofts, 1965.

Erving, H. W. Internal podalic version and extraction. Amer. J. Obstet. Gynec., 57:333, 1949

_____ and Kenwick, A. N. An analysis of 1,146 cases of internal version and extraction. Amer. J. Obstet. Gynec., 67:315, 1954.

Friedlander, D. External cephalic version in the management of breech presentation. Amer. J. Obstet. Gynec., 95:906, 1966.

Thornhill, P. E. Changes in fetal polarity near term—spontaneous and external version. Amer. J. Obstet. Gynec., 93:306, 1965.

Trowbridge, E. W. The status of internal podalic version in obstetrics. Amer. J. Obstet. Gynec., 60:528, 1950.

31 Normal and Abnormal Uterine Action

DEFINITIONS

Contraction: Contraction is the shortening of a muscle in response to a stimulus, with return to its original length after the contraction has worn off.

Retraction: The muscle shortens in response to a stimulus, but does not return to its original length when the contraction has passed off. The muscle becomes fixed at a relatively shorter length, but the tension remains the same. In this way the slack is taken up and the walls of the uterus maintain contact with its contents.

Retraction is responsible for descent. Without this property the fetus would move down with the contraction, only to return to the original level once the contraction had ceased. With retraction, on the other hand, the fetus remains at a slightly lower level each time. During contraction it is as though three steps are taken forward and then three steps backward. With retraction three steps are taken forward, but only two steps are taken backward. In this way a little ground is gained each time. In the control of postpartum bleeding retraction is essential. Without it many patients might bleed to death.

Physiologic Retraction Ring: As labor and retraction proceed, the upper part of the uterus becomes progressively shorter and thicker, while the lower portion gets longer and thinner. The boundary between the two segments is the physiologic retraction ring.

Pathologic Retraction Ring: In cases of obstructed labor the physiologic ring becomes extreme, and is known as the pathologic retraction (Bandl's) ring.

Tonus: Tonus is the lowest intrauterine (intraamniotic) pressure between contractions. It is expressed in millimeters of mercury. The normal resting tension is 8 to 12 mm.

Intensity: Intensity or amplitude is the rise in intrauterine pressure brought about by each contraction. The normal is 30 to 50 mm of mercury.

Frequency: Caldeyro-Barcia has defined this as the number of contractions per 10 minutes. For the patient to be in good labor the frequency must be at least 2 per 10 minutes.

Uterine Activity: Uterine activity is described by Caldeyro-Barcia as the intensity multiplied by the frequency and is expressed in Montevideo units (millimeters of mercury per 10 minutes).

Polarity of the Uterus: When the upper segment contracts the lower segment relaxes. Actually the lower part does contract, but much less than the upper part. The effect is as though the lower portion did relax.

THE PAIN OF LABOR

Pain in labor is related to the contractions of the uterus. In normal labor the pain is intermittent. It starts as the uterus contracts, becomes more severe as the contraction reaches its peak, and, when the uterus relaxes, the pain disappears. The degree of pain varies in different patients, in the same patient in succeeding labors, and at different stages in the same labor. In some cases the contractions are painless.

Causes of Pain in Labor

1. Distension of the lower pole of the uterus
2. Stretching of the ligaments adjacent to the uterus
3. Pressure on or stretching of the nerve ganglia around the uterus
4. Contractions of the muscle while it is in a relatively ischemic state (similar to angina pectoris). This occurs especially when the uterine tonus is too high or when the contractions are too frequent and last too long. Adequate amounts of blood do not get to the muscles and they become anoxic.

Pain in the Lower Abdomen

Pain in the lower abdomen seems to be related to activity of the upper uterine segment, and is present during efficient labor.

Pain in the Back

Pain in the back is related to tension in the lower uterine segment and the cervix. In normal labor back pain is prominent only at the start of a contraction and in the early stages of cervical dilatation. When the cervix is abnormally resistant the backache is severe. Backache is prominent also in posterior positions. In general, the less the backache the more efficient the uterus.

Fig. 1. Normal and abnormal labor in the 1st stage. A. Average Multipara B. Average Primigravida C. Secondary arrest of dilatation D. Primary dysfunctional labor E. Prolonged latent phase.

Pain in the Incoordinate Uterus

1. An excessive amount of pain is felt in the back.
2. Because of persistent high tonus or spasm in some parts of the uterus the pain seems to be present even in the intervals between contractions.
3. The patient complains of pain before the uterus is felt to harden, and the pain persists even after the uterus relaxes and softens.

THE NORMAL UTERINE CONTRACTIONS

Caldeyro-Barcia has published a logical and understandable description of the normal uterine contraction wave.

Triple Descending Gradient (TDG) of Caldeyro-Barcia

Each contraction wave has three components:

1. The propagation of the wave is from above downward. It starts at the pacemaker and works its way to the lower part of the uterus.
2. The duration of the contraction diminishes progressively as the wave moves away from the pacemaker. During any contraction the upper portion of the uterus is in action for a longer period of time than the lower.
3. The intensity of the contraction diminishes from top to bottom of the uterus. The upper segment of the uterus contracts more strongly than the lower.

In order that normal labor may take place all parts of the triple descending gradient must perform properly. The activity of the upper part is greater than, and dominates, the lower part. All parts of the uterus contract, but the upper segment does so more strongly than the lower segment, and in turn the latter's contractions are stronger than those of the cervix. Were this not so there would be no progress. This is the modern interpretation of uterine polarity.

The normal contractions are regular and intermittent. There is contraction (systole) and relaxation (diastole). The most efficient uterus is one showing moderately low tonus and strong contractions.

Pacemakers

Normally there are two, one situated at each uterine end of the Fallopian tube. Since one pacemaker is responsible for the initiation of a contraction, their activities must be coordinated. In the abnormal uterus new pacemakers may spring up anywhere in the organ resulting in incoordinate uterine action.

Propagation

The wave begins at the pacemaker and proceeds downward to the rest of the uterus. A small wave goes up to the fundal portion of the uterus above the level of the pacemaker.

Coordination

Coordination is such that, while the wave begins earlier in some areas than in others, the contraction attains its maximum in the different parts of the uterus at the same time. The places where the contraction starts later achieve their acme more rapidly. Thus at the peak of the contraction, the entire uterus is acting as a unit. The relaxation, on the other hand, starts simultaneously in all parts of the uterus. For normal uterine action there must be good coordination between the two halves of the uterus as well as between the upper and lower segments.

Dilatation of the Cervix

Dilatation of the cervix is caused by two mechanisms:

1. The pressure on the cervix by the presenting part: When this part of the fetus is regular and well fitting, e.g., the flexed head, it favors effective uterine action and smooth cervical dilatation. The bag of waters does not play an important role in helping promote good contractions and rapid cervical opening.
2. The longitudinal traction on the cervix by the upper part of the uterus as it contracts and retracts: After each contraction
   a. The upper segment becomes shorter and thicker.
   b. The lower uterine segment becomes longer, thinner, and more distended.
   c. The cervix becomes more and more dilated.

Cervical dilatation is the result of a gradient of diminishing activity from the fundus through the lower uterine segment.

Round Ligament Contraction

These ligaments contain muscle, and they contract at the same time as the upper segment of the uterus. This anchors the uterus, prevents its ascending in the abdomen, and so helps force the presenting part down.

Uterine Contractions during Pregnancy

Some uterine activity goes on throughout pregnancy. During the first 30 weeks the frequency and strength of the contractions are low, less than 20 Montevideo units.

After 30 weeks, and especially after 35 weeks, the contractions become more frequent and may be noticed by the patient. Sometimes they are painful and are called false labor pains. Prelabor, as evidenced in the increasing activity of the uterus during the later weeks of pregnancy, is an integral part of the process of evacuation of the human uterus. The contractions of this period are associated with steadily increasing uterine activity, cervical ripening, and general readiness for true labor. Prelabor merges into clinically recognizable labor by such small degrees that the exact point at which so-called true labor begins is difficult to determine.

The onset of true labor occurs when the uterine activity reaches 80 to 120 Montevideo units.

CLASSIFICATION OF UTERINE ACTION

Clinical Conditions with Normal Contractile Waves

Normal Labor

The intensity or amplitude of the contractions varies from 30 to 50 mm of mercury, and the frequency is from 2 to 5 contractions per 10 minutes.

True Inertia

When the intensity of the contractions is less than 25 and the frequency is under 2 per 10 minutes, progress will be slow and labor prolonged. If the intensity is less than 15, labor will not begin, or if it has started, it will cease.

The uterine tonus is normal, the pattern of activity is coordinated, and the relaxation of the lower segment is adequate. The uterus, however, is inactive, and the expulsive efforts are weak, infrequent, or both. There is progress neither in descent of the presenting part nor in dilatation of the cervix. It is often difficult to be sure that the patient is in labor. Pain is mild or even absent entirely.

The force exerted on the fetus is small and no caput succedaneum is formed. No damage is done to either mother or child.

Precipitate Labor

Precipitate labor is one which lasts less than 3 hours. The amplitude of the contractions is over 50, and, hence, labor is rapid.

Conditions which predispose to, or contribute to the etiology of, precipitate labor include:

1. Multiparity
2. Large pelvis
3. Lax and unresistant soft tissues
4. Strong uterine contractions
5. Small baby in good position
6. Induction of labor by rupture of membranes and oxytocin infusion
7. Previous precipitate labor

The distinction must be made between precipitate labor and precipitate delivery. The latter, being sudden and unexpected, carries with it the dangers of an unattended birth.

While many authors have warned of the dangers of rapid labor, such as maternal lacerations, cerebral hemorrhage, brain damage in the fetus, and asphyxia from interference with the placental circulation, some recent studies have suggested that the risk to mother and child is not greater than in the average labor.

Cervical Dystocia

Cervical dystocia includes two main groups:

1. Primary
   a. Achalasia of the cervix: The failure or inability of the structurally normal cervix to relax and open
   b. Rigid cervix: An anatomic abnormality of the cervical tissue
   c. Conglutination of the external os: The sticking together of the lips of the cervix
2. Secondary
   a. Post delivery
   b. Postoperative scarring
   c. Cancer

If the condition is not treated the cervix may rupture or annular detachment may take place. The constant and prolonged pressure on the cervix leads to anoxia and devitalization of the tissue, which eventually separates and comes away as a ring. Usually there is thrombosis in the vessels at the site of separation, so bleeding is rarely a problem.

In some cases the cervix becomes well effaced and the external os very thin, but dilatation does not take place. In this situation incision of the rim of cervix is followed by easy delivery.

Obstructed Labor

Etiologic factors range from fetopelvic disproportion through malpresentations to neoplasms blocking the birth canal.

As labor proceeds and the uterus tries to overcome the obstruction, the contractions become more frequent and stronger, and the tonus rises. There is progressive retraction of the upper segment with stretching and thinning of the lower part of the uterus. The physiologic retraction ring becomes the pathologic (Bandl's) ring. The round ligaments are tense and may be palpable through the abdomen. The pain is severe and felt in the abdomen.

If the obstruction is not relieved and the contractions go on, rupture of the lower segment is the final outcome. In some cases the myometrium becomes exhausted and inertia sets in before rupture occurs.

While the uterus itself does not impede the descent and birth of the baby, the strong, frequent contractions and high tonus may cut off the placental circulation, and kill the baby.

Rapid Overdistension of the Uterus

Acute polyhydramnios is an example. The rapidly accumulating amniotic fluid leads to a rise in tonus and a fall in the intensity of the contractions.

Slow Distension of the Uterus

Slow distension of the uterus is seen in multiple pregnancy or in chronic polyhydramnios. The increase in the intrauterine volume is slow and gradual, and so there is time for compensatory hypertrophy and hyperplasia of the uterine muscles. For this reason the tonus and intensity of the contractions are normal.

Contractile Waves with Inverted Gradient

Caldeyro-Barcia described the normal contraction wave as having three properties:

1. The propagation of the wave is from above downward.
2. The duration of the contraction diminishes progressively as the wave moves away from the pacemaker.
3. The intensity of the contraction decreases from the top of the uterus to the lower part.

One of the varieties of inefficient uterine action takes place when the gradients of the normal contraction are inverted. The inversion may be total or partial.

1. Total: All three gradients are affected. The uterine contractions are completely ineffective. There is no progress—neither dilatation of the cervix nor descent of the fetus.
2. Partial: One or two of the gradients are involved. Some cervical dilatation may take place, but it is very slow.

Inversion of the Gradient of Propagation

The contraction begins in the lower segment and moves upward. Normally it goes the other way.

Inversion of the Gradient of Duration

The contraction lasts longer in the lower than in the upper segment. This is the opposite of the normal wave.

Inversion of the Gradient of Intensity

The lower segment contractions are stronger than the upper. This is the hypertonic lower segment of Jeffcoate. Normally the opposite is true.

When these conditions are present the polarity of the uterus is reversed. The contractions are of no value in furthering progress. They produce no effacement or dilatation of the cervix. They are the type of contraction seen often in false and prelabor.

Clinically, as compared with true inertia, these patients do have pain, and it may be severe. Backache is often the main complaint. Typically, the fetus remains high, and the cervix stays thick, uneffaced, and poorly applied to the presenting part.

Incoordination of the Uterus: Localized Contraction Waves

Asymmetrical Uterine Action

The pacemakers do not work in rhythm, and each half of the uterus acts independently. Small contractions alternate with large ones. The minor contractions are entirely ineffective. The major ones do bring about some cervical dilatation, but much less effectively than normal waves. Progress is painfully slow.

Uterine Fibrillation: the Colicky Uterus

In this condition new pacemakers appear all over the uterus. The myometrium contracts spasmodically, frequently, irregularly, and purposelessly. The tonus is elevated slightly but the action is not effectively expulsive. The fetus is not pushed down, and the cervix does not dilate well.

Pain is present all the time—before, during, and after contractions. The pain is out of proportion to the intensity of the contractions.

Constriction Ring

A constriction ring is a localized phenomenon. A ring of myometrium goes into tetanic contraction. The most common site is 7 to 8 cm above the external os of the cervix. A constriction ring can develop rapidly. Causes include:

1. Intrauterine manipulations
2. Failed forceps
3. The use of oxytocin when the uterus is hypertonic
4. Spontaneous constriction ring which usually occurs in a colicky uterus

The constriction ring grips the fetus tightly and prevents its descent. It is the cause of the obstruction. In the pathologic contraction ring of Bandl, on the other hand, the obstruction to the passage of the fetus comes first and it is the cause of the ring.

The area of spasm is thick, but the lower segment is neither stretched nor thinned out. Constriction rings never lead to uterine rupture. The patient experiences severe pain, and the tenderness of the uterus makes her resist palpation of the abdomen.

While deep surgical anesthesia is needed to relax the major rings, lesser degrees of anesthesia, sedation, or adrenalin chloride may be effective in the milder forms.

Diagnosis is made by abdominal, vaginal, and intrauterine examinations:

1. The ring may be felt on abdominal examination.
2. There is no change in the station of the presenting part during a contraction.
3. The fetal head is loose in the pelvic cavity both during and between uterine contractions.
4. The portion of the uterus between the external os and the ring is lax during the contraction.
5. The cervix is floppy and is not well applied to the presenting part.
6. Because of the laxity of the cervix a hand can be passed into the uterine cavity and the ring palpated.
7. By placing a finger between the cervix and the head, the impact on the finger during a strong contraction will be found to be quite weak.

DIFFERENTIAL DIAGNOSIS

Constriction Ring	Pathologic Retraction Ring
A localized ring of spastic myometrium	Formed by excessive retraction of upper segment
May occur in any part of the uterus	Always at junction of upper and lower segments
The muscle at the ring is thicker than above or below it	Myometrium is much thicker above than below the ring
Uterus below the ring is neither thin nor distended	Wall below is thin and overdistended
Uterus never ruptures	If uncorrected, uterus may rupture
Uterus above ring is relaxed and not tender	Uterus above ring is hard
Round ligaments are not tense	Round ligaments are tense and stand out
May occur in any stage of labor	Usually occurs late in the second stage
The position of the ring does not change	The ring gradually rises in the abdomen
Presenting part is not driven down	Presenting part is jammed in the pelvis
Fetus may be wholly or mainly above the ring	Part of the child must be below the ring
Patient's general condition is good	Patient's general condition is poor
Uterine action is inefficient	Uterine action is efficient or overefficient
Abnormal polarity	Normal polarity
It results in obstructed labor	It is caused by an obstruction

Spasm of the Internal or External Os of the Cervix

The cervix does not relax and does not dilate. The contractions of the cervix are stronger than those of the lower uterine segment, and no progress is made.

Abnormal Uterine Action in the Third Stage of Labor

The separation and expulsion of the placenta and the control of hemorrhage are dependent on normal uterine action. Abnormal uterine contractility can lead to the following complications:

1. Uterine inertia may cause delayed separation of the placenta and postpartum hemorrhage.
2. The colicky uterus interferes with normal separation.
3. A constriction ring prevents normal expulsion.
4. Cervical spasm may trap the placenta in the uterus.
4. Incoordinate uterine action may lead to inversion of the uterus.

INCOORDINATE UTERINE ACTION

Etiology of Incoordinate Uterine Action

The great majority of cases occurs in primigravidas, and the uterus is, with rare exception, more efficient in subsequent labors.

The quoted incidence varies from 1 to 7 percent, but it is doubtful that the real syndrome occurs in more than 2 percent of labors.

Mild disproportion and malpresentations predispose to abnormal uterine action.

Age and Parity

This is mainly a condition of primigravidas. About 95 percent of severe cases occur in first labors, and the uterus is almost always more efficient in the next pregnancy. The incidence in elderly primigravidas is only a little higher than in young women.

Constitutional Factors

Especially prone to have incoordinate uterine action is the thickset, obese, masculine, relatively infertile woman. There appears to be a familial tendency. It is not associated with general debility or malnutrition.

Nervous and Emotional Conditions

We do not know how nervous and emotional problems act in causing or aggravating incoordination of the uterus in labor. It has been claimed that fear increases the tension of the lower uterine segment. However there are placid women who have difficult labors, and highly emotional ones who have easy deliveries. Most grave disorders of the central nervous system do not affect labor adversely.

Errors of the Uterus

While some workers believe that overdistension, fibroids, and scars of the uterus predispose to poor uterine contractions, others deny it.   Certainly the uterus which is congenitally abnormal, incompletely fused, or bicornuate does not behave well in labor.

Rupture of the Membranes

Rupture of the membranes under proper conditions stimulates the uterus to better contractions, and speeds up progress.   However rupture of the bag of waters when the cervix is unripe, that is, uneffaced, hard, thick, and closed, does lead to a prolonged and inefficient type of labor.

Mechanical Errors in the Relation of Fetus to Birth Canal

A close and even application of the presenting part to the cervix and lower uterine segment in the first stage of labor and to the vagina and perineum in the second stage results in good reflex stimulation of the myometrium.   Anything which prevents this good relationship causes the reflex to fail, and poor contractions may be the result.

The relationship of posterior positions, extended attitudes, and transverse arrest to faulty uterine action is well known.   The malposition precedes the uterine disturbance, and if it can be corrected, good contractions often return.

Late engagement and incomplete formation of the lower uterine segment may be an early sign of an incoordinate uterus.   Mild degrees of cephalopelvic disproportion predispose to incoordinate uterine action.

Irritation of Uterus

Improper stimulation of the uterus by drugs or intrauterine manipulations may bring about incoordination.

The Clinical Picture of Incoordinate Uterine Action

Labor

The clinical picture is of prolonged labor in the absence of fetopelvic disproportion.   There is hypertonus, increased tension, and spasm in some areas of the uterine muscle which persist even between the contractions.   The resting intrauterine pressure is increased.   The contractions may be frequent and are usually irregular in strength and periodicity.   Despite uterine contractions which are often strong and always painful, progress is slow or absent.   The cervix dilates slowly, and the presenting part advances little or not at all.   This condition occurs in all degrees, from the mildest to the most severe.

Labor may be normal at first or it may be incoordinate from the beginning. Premature rupture of the membranes while the cervix is closed and uneffaced is seen frequently. The patient complains bitterly of pain, and when examination shows no progress, the assumption is made that she is making more fuss than the condition warrants. The experienced obstetrician will recognize the condition and will order sedation. After a rest the contractions may resume in a normal pattern, or they may still be incoordinate. As time passes the colicky nature of the pain increases. The patient holds her hands over the sensitive uterus to protect it. Eventually more sedation is needed.

Labor is long, especially the first stage, because with incoordinate uterine action the cervix fails to dilate normally. After a long period: 1, the cervix may dilate fully, and the baby may be born spontaneously or by forceps; 2, some method of promoting cervical dilatation may have to be used before the baby can be extracted; or 3, vaginal delivery may be abandoned and cesearean section performed.

It is characteristic of this condition that the patient complains of the pain before the uterus is felt to harden, and the pain persists after the uterus softens. Sometimes there is continual pain, especially severe in the back. The patient realizes that she is not making progress, and her anxiety and loss of morale aggravate the situation. Eventually she becomes exhausted, dehydrated, and the pulse and temperature rise.

The cervix may be thick or thin, it may be applied tightly to the presenting part or hang loosely in the vagina. It dilates very slowly and may never reach full dilatation. In most cases dilatation stops at 6 to 7 cm. Sometimes a thick edematous anterior lip is caught between the pubis and the fetal head.

The patient often experiences the acute desire to bear down before the cervix is fully dilated. The attendant must stop the patient from doing this, for it exhausts her without furthering progress. There is a tendency to retention of urine. Vomiting is common and adds to the dehydration.

Diagnosis

Diagnosis is based on the following:

1. The patient's subjective impression of the strength and duration of the pains
2. The physician's objective impression of the duration of the contractions, and his partly objective opinion of their strength
3. Observation of the effectiveness of the contractions in promoting progress, especially cervical dilatation

Dangers to the Mother

1. Exhaustion
2. Hemorrhage and shock
3. Infection
4. Lacerations of the vagina during difficult deliveries
5. Annular detachment or lacerations of the cervix

After 24 hours the dangers to the mother and fetus rise sharply. Many women suffer so much that they refuse to have more children. Maternal mortality is under 1 percent.

Dangers to the Fetus

1. Asphyxia from prolonged labor and from interference with uteroplacental circulation during long, hard uterine contractions
2. Injury during traumatic delivery
3. Pulmonary complications from aspiration of infected amniotic fluid

The fetal mortality is under 15 percent. The prognosis used to be bad, especially because of traumatic forceps deliveries performed often before the cervix was fully dilated and with the head not engaged. The improvement in the results are due to:

1. Earlier diagnosis of ineffective uterine action
2. More timely forceps extractions
3. Increased use of cesarean section
4. Better anesthesia
5. Antibiotics and blood transfusions

False Labor

False labor is attended by irregular contractions. There is no progress, no dilatation of the cervix, and no descent of the presenting part. No damage is done to the fetus. The contractions may be painful and prevent the patient from resting. Sometimes they do have an effect in effacing the cervix, and are called prelabor contractions. Treatment is by sedation and rest.

Secondary Uterine Inertia

Secondary uterine inertia is a condition of myometrial and general fatigue. It is often associated with prolonged obstructed labor. The contractions become feeble, infrequent, irregular, and may stop altogether. Progress ceases. Treatment is by hydration and rest.

Management of Incoordinate Uterine Action

Investigation and Diagnosis

1. The patient is observed as to her general condition, the amount of pain, and the degree of progress.
2. The uterus is palpated to try to determine the type and severity of the contractions.
3. Vaginal examination shows the position, the station, the size of the caput, the condition of the cervix, the presence of a constriction ring, and any disproportion.
4. In cases of doubt, x-rays are taken to rule out fetopelvic disproportion or abnormal position.

5. Questions to be answered include:
   a. Is there disproportion?
   b. Is the fetus placed badly?
   c. Is the woman in true labor?
   d. Is the uterus hypertonic or hypotonic?
   e. Is the uterine action incoordinate?
   f. Is the basic problem at the cervix?

Prevention

1. Fear is counteracted by good prenatal care.
2. Analgesia is used when necessary to prevent loss of control.
3. Heavy sedation is prescribed for false labor, so that the patient will not be exhausted when she goes into true labor.

General Measures

1. The morale of the patient should be maintained.
2. Intravenous infusions are given for hydration. Glucose in water provides nourishment and prevents acidosis.
3. The bladder and bowel should be emptied when necessary.
4. Antibacterial measures are used when indicated.

Sedation and Analgesia

While an excessive amount of sedation can inhibit uterine contractions, properly used it will not interfere with true labor. The patient needs sedation to relieve her anxiety and analgesia to make the pain less severe. Often sedation and rest will change poor labor into a better variety.

Stimulation of the Uterus

The uterus should be stimulated only in hypotonic conditions. If the uterus is hypertonic, stimulation will make the situation worse. Methods include:

1. Keeping the patient walking around to maintain the presenting part against the cervix
2. Enemas
3. Oxytocin, given best as a dilute intravenous infusion
4. Artificial rupture of the membranes

Operative Measures

1. When the head is low and the cervix is thin, the cervix may be dilated manually or an anterior rim pushed over the fetal head.
2. Dührssen's incisions of the cervix at 2, 6, and 10 o'clock can be performed when the head is presenting and the cervix is effaced, thin, and at least half dilated.

3. Forceps rotation and extraction can be performed when the cervix is fully dilated. The operation should not be delayed until the mother and fetus are in poor condition.
4. Cesarean section is used more often today. It is safer for mother and child than a traumatic vaginal delivery.

Constriction Ring

1. Relaxing drugs and deep anesthesia can be tried. If these succeed in releasing the constriction, the fetus is extracted with forceps.
2. Cesarean section is probably the method of choice.

Bandl's Pathologic Retraction Ring

Since the basic problem here is cephalopelvic disproportion, cesarean section is the proper therapy. If the baby is dead craniotomy may be considered.

Cervical Dystocia

1. Manual dilatation
2. Incision of the cervix
3. Cesarean section

BIBLIOGRAPHY

Caldeyro-Barcia, R., Alvarez, H., and Reynolds, S. M. R. A better understanding of uterine contractility through simultaneous recording with an internal and a seven channel external method. Surg. Gynec. Obstet., 91:641, 1950.

———— Alvarez, H., and Poseiro, J. J. Normal and abnormal uterine contractility in labour. Triangle, 2:41, 1955.

Conger, G. T., and Randall, J. R. Precipitate labor. Amer. J. Obstet. Gynec., 73:1321, 1957.

Jeffcoate, T. N. A., Baker, K., and Martin, R. H. Inefficient uterine action. Surg., Gynec. Obstet., 95:257, 1952.

Johnson, J. W. The clinical diagnosis of varying degrees of uterine contraction rings. Amer. J. Obstet. Gynec., 52:74, 1946.

Kaern, T. Anomalies of uterine action and their treatment. Acta obstet. gynec. scandinav., 37:26, 1958.

Kennedy, C. Uterine inertia. Brit. Med. J., 1:1522, 1955.

32   Prolonged Labor

Definition: Labor which lasts longer than 24 hours is classified as prolonged. However, when adequate progress is not being made, the situation must be assessed immediately. Problems should be recognized and treated before the 24-hour limit has been reached.

Most prolonged labors represent extensions of the first stage. Whatever the reason, the cervix fails to become fully dilated within a reasonable length of time.

The Onset of Labor: Because it is difficult, in many cases, to be certain as to exactly when labor began, there is no unanimously accepted definition of the onset of labor.

The definition based on the frequency, regularity, and duration of uterine contractions ignores the fact that patients with dysfunctional labor do have painful, though irregular, contractions.

The definition which insists on progressive effacement and dilatation of the cervix as an essential feature of real labor fails to recognize the important latent phase or preliminary stage of labor. During this period, despite regular uterine contractions, little recognizable change may take place in the cervix.

Perhaps, therefore, the imprecise definition of the onset of labor as being when the patient experiences uterine contractions which lead toward the birth of a baby, may be the best one available.

Incidence: This varies from 1 to 7 percent. Modern methods of diagnosis and treatment have reduced the frequency of this complication.

Etiology: The principal causes of prolonged labor are:

1. Fetopelvic disproportion
2. Malpresentations and malpositions
3. Inefficient uterine action, including the rigid cervix

Accessory factors are:

1. Primigravidity
2. Premature rupture of the membranes when the cervix is uneffaced, closed, and hard
3. Excessive analgesia or anesthesia in the latent phase
4. The dependent, anxious, frightened girl whose parents accompany her to hospital is a candidate for prolonged labor. Another type is the masculine masochistic woman who seems almost to be enjoying her pain.

377

These agents may act alone or in concert. A marked abnormality of one, or a minor deviation in several, can prevent successful termination of the labor. Whereas normal delivery is impossible in the presence of absolute cephalopelvic disproportion, a mild disparity between the size of the pelvis and that of the fetus can be overcome by strong and effective uterine contractions. The pelvis may be sufficiently large to accommodate an occipitoanterior presentation, but may be too small for an occipitoposterior one. It is a matter of balance.

Rupture of the membranes in the presence of a ripe cervix and strong contractions will never prolong labor. If, however, the bag of waters breaks when the cervix is long, hard, and closed, there is often a long latent period before progressive labor sets in.

Inefficient uterine action includes the inability of the cervix to dilate smoothly and rapidly, as well as ineffective uterine contractions.

GRAPHIC ANALYSIS OF LABOR

By correlating the duration of labor with the rate of cervical dilatation, Friedman has described a graphic analysis of labor. On graph paper the cervical dilatation in centimeters is placed on the ordinate, and hours of time on the abscissa. Joining the points of contact makes a sigmoid curve. The rate of cervical dilatation, as shown by the slope of the curve, is described in centimeters per hour.

The first stage of labor (from the onset of labor to full dilatation of the cervix) is divided into two periods, the latent phase and the active phase.

By studying a large series Friedman obtained figures for the lengths of the various phases. The upper normal limits represent the longest time that labor went on and still terminated normally. However, in slowly or nonprogressing cases (as shown by a low rate of cervical dilatation) investigation must be instituted long before the maximum time limit has been reached.

Latent Period

This phase begins with the onset of labor and lasts until the beginning of the active phase of cervical dilatation as shown by the upswing of the curve. The uterine contractions become orientated and the cervix softened and effaced. The slope of the cervix is nearly flat, the cervical dilatation averaging only 0.35 cm per hour. At the end of the latent phase the cervix is 2 to 2.5 cm in diameter.

In primigravidas the average length of the latent phase is 8.6 hours, with the upper limit of normal at 20 hours. For multiparas the figures are 5.3 and 14 hours. Wide variations occur, and a prolonged latent period does not mean that the active phase will be abnormal.

Active Period

The active period lasts from the end of the latent phase to full dilatation of the cervix. The curve changes from the almost horizontal slope of the latent phase to a nearly vertical incline. As the second stage is being reached the curve flattens again. Effective labor begins with the active phase, the period of steady and rapid cervical dilatation.

The vertical linearity of the curve makes possible the early recognition of deviations from the average. Premature flattening of the curve (indicating a reduction in the rate of cervical dilatation) calls for immediate investigation of the cause.

In the primigravidas of Friedman's series the average length of the active phase was 5.8 hours, and the upper limit of normal was 12 hours. The rate of cervical dilatation ranged from 1.2 to 6.8 cm per hour. A rate under 1.2 cm per hour is below normal and suggests dysfunctional labor.

In multiparas the average length of the active phase was 2.5 hours with the upper normal limit at 6 hours. A rate of cervical dilatation less than 1.5 cm per hour is abnormal.

In the primigravidas the maximum duration of the normal first stage of labor (latent and active phases combined) was 28.5 hours (average 13.3), with the second stage maximum at 2.5 hours (average 57 minutes). In multiparas the figures were 20 hours (average 7.5) for the first stage, and 50 minutes (average 18 minutes) for the second stage.

LENGTHS OF THE PHASES OF LABOR

	PRIMIGRAVIDA		MULTIPARA	
	Average	Upper Normal	Average	Upper Normal
Latent Phase	8.6 hr	20 hr	5.3 hr	14 hr
Active Phase	5.8 hr	12 hr	2.5 hr	6 hr
First Stage of Labor	13.3 hr	28.5 hr	7.5 hr	20 hr
Second Stage of Labor	57 min	2.5 hr	18 min	50 min
Rate of Cervical Dilatation During Active Phase	Under 1.2 cm/hr is abnormal		Under 1.5 cm/hr is abnormal	

CLASSIFICATION OF PROLONGED LABOR

Prolonged Latent Phase

A latent phase which exceeds 20 hours in the primigravida or 14 hours in the multipara is abnormal.

Causes of a prolonged latent phase include: 1, an unripe cervix at the onset of labor; 2, abnormal position of the fetus; 3, fetopelvic disproportion; 4, dysfunctional labor; and 5, the administration of excessive sedation.

The unripe cervix prolongs only the latent phase, and most cervices will open normally once effacement is achieved. Even when the latent phase lasts over 20 hours, many patients will advance to normal cervical dilatation when the active phase begins. While a long latent phase is worrisome, it does not endanger the mother or the child.

Prolonged Active Phase in the Primigravida

In the primigravida an active phase longer than 12 hours is abnormal. More important than the length of this phase is the speed of cervical dilatation. A rate less than 1.2 cm per hour is evidence of some abnormality, and should alert the attendant.

Prolongation of the active phase is associated with 1, malpositions of the fetus; 2, fetopelvic disproportion; 3, injudicious use of sedation and analgesia; and 4, rupture of membranes before the onset of labor. It is followed by an increase in mid forceps, cesarean section, and fetal damage or death.

The prolonged active period can be divided into two main clinical groups: 1, where there is a progressing, albeit slow, dilatation of the cervix; and 2, where there is actual arrest of dilatation.

Primary Dysfunctional Labor: The rate of cervical dilatation is less than 1.2 cm per hour. Spontaneous increase in the rate of dilatation occurs rarely, and little can be done to speed up progress.

In the absence of other complications the risk to the mother and child is small. Hence, as long as progress is being made and there is no fetal distress, the phenomenon of slow cervical dilatation must be accepted.

Two thirds of these patients deliver normally, 20 percent require mid forceps, and 10 percent come to cesarean section. A few women will go into secondary arrest of dilatation, where the prognosis is more serious.

Secondary Arrest of Dilatation: During the active phase, previously advancing dilatation of the cervix stops. On the graph a flattening of the curve is noted. Two hours of arrest is diagnostic.

There are two subgroups: 1, the uterine contractions become insufficient to maintain progressive dilatation of the cervix; and 2, cervical dilatation ceases in spite of strong and efficient uterine contractions.

While this is a different entity from the primary protracted active phase, both can occur in the same patient and the etiology may be related. Thus, either a slowly dilating cervix or one that had been opening normally may stop advancing.

Accurate assessment of the situation and diagnosis of etiology is vital. Keeping in mind that inefficient uterine action is often associated with disproportion and abnormal position of the fetus, one must not blame the lack of progress on poor contractions until mechanical factors have been ruled out.

When ineffective labor (often myometrial fatigue) is the sole cause, half the patients will resume progress after no more treatment than rest and an infusion of glucose in water. In this group amniotomy and oxytocin stimulation works well.

When there are complications such as disproportion or abnormal position, the treatment must be directed in their direction.

Prolonged Active Phase in the Multipara

An active phase in the multipara lasting over 6 hours (average 2.5 hours), and a rate of cervical dilatation of less than 1.5 cm per hour is abnormal.

The prolonged active phase is a disorder primarily of primigravidas and occurs rarely in the multipara. The etiology is similar to that in the primigravida. Disproportion, when it occurs, is often caused by a large baby or a malposition.

INVESTIGATION OF PROLONGED LABOR

Graphic Analysis of Labor

By charting the progress of labor on a graph, we can ascertain whether cervical dilatation is occurring at a normal rate or too slowly, or has ceased altogether. The type of abnormality can be diagnosed, and the point at which detailed investigation should be carried out is indicated.

Fetal Condition

The condition of the baby is evaluated by listening to the fetal heart to observe rate and rhythm and by seeing if meconium is being passed or whether agonal movements are being made.

Maternal Status

The patient's general physical and mental condition is assessed with respect to fatigue, morale, hydration, and nourishment.

Vaginal Examination

Vaginal examination is performed under sterile conditions, with the patient in the lithotomy position and the bladder and rectum empty. Sometimes an anesthetic is necessary to ensure adequate assessment. Rectal examinations have no place in problem cases when a decision must be made as to definite treatment. Errors are made too often as to the condition and dilatation of the cervix, a large caput is mistaken for the skull, and the position and station are diagnosed inaccurately. During the vaginal examination the following points are noted.

The State of the Cervix

Is it open or closed, soft or hard, effaced or long, dilatable or resistant? Has any progress been made since the last examination? Is an anterior lip caught between the head and the symphysis? In the majority of cases the cervix ceased dilating when it was one half to three quarters open. In many of these instances it had been considered erroneously to be fully dilated on rectal examination.

The Station of the Presenting Part

The station of the bony presenting part is determined. Is it at, above, or below the spines? Has engagement taken place? Is there a caput?

Position

The position must be diagnosed accurately. In all cases of prolonged labor malpositions, such as brow presentation and occiput posterior, should be kept in mind.

Failure of Descent

What seems to be holding up the presenting part? Can it be pushed down?
Is the cause of arrest in the bony pelvis or is it the cervix? Is the head too big
for the pelvis? Or, does one get the impression that the problem is not the pelvis or the cervix but that a few hours of really good labor will achieve progress
to successful delivery?

The Uterine Contractions

The uterine contractions are assessed. Is the basic problem in the type of
labor, or is the main problem elsewhere and the poor uterine action a secondary
complication? If the contractions are judged to be efficient, then the reason for
the failure of progress must be in another field. Since inefficient uterine action
is almost entirely a disorder of primigravidas, multiparas with prolonged labors must be investigated for other factors carefully before a diagnosis of poor
labor is made. A woman who has delivered a 7 pound baby with no trouble may
not be able to do the same with a 9 pound baby.

X-ray Examination

X-ray examination is performed to:

1. Estimate the size and type of the pelvis
2. Determine the size of the baby with respect to the capacity of the pelvis
3. Determine the station of the presenting part
4. Discover fetal abnormalities which may affect the management of the case

MANAGEMENT OF PROLONGED LABOR

Prevention of Prolonged Labor

1. Good prenatal care and preparation for childbirth will reduce the incidence
   of prolonged labor.
2. Labor should not be induced or forced when the cervix is not ripe. A ripe
   cervix is less than half an inch in length, effaced, patulous to admit at
   least a finger, and soft and dilatable.
3. False labor is treated by rest and sedation.

Supportive Measures

1. During labor the patient's morale should be bolstered. Encouragement is
   offered, and remarks that may worry the patient are avoided.
2. A fluid intake of at least 2,500 ml daily is essential. In all prolonged labors this is maintained by intravenous infusions of glucose in water. Dehydration, of which acetone in the urine is a sign, must be prevented.
3. Food taken during labor is not digested well. It remains in the stomach
   with danger of vomiting and aspiration. Hence, in long labors nourishment
   is given by intravenous feeding.

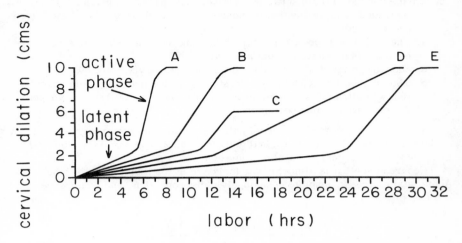

Fig. 1. Normal and abnormal labor in the 1st stage. A. Average Multipara   B. Average Primigravida   C. Secondary arrest of dilatation   D. Primary dysfunctional labor   E. Prolonged latent phase.

4. Elimination of bladder and bowel must be adequate. A full bladder and rectum not only cause discomfort and impede progress but are more liable to injury than empty ones.
5. While women in labor must be rested with sedation and relieved of pain by analgesia, this must be administered judiciously. An excessive amount of narcosis may interfere with contractions and can harm the baby.
6. When the membranes have been ruptured for over 12 hours antibiotics are given to reduce the danger of infection in mother and child.
7. The number of rectal or vaginal examinations should be kept to a minimum. It hurts the patient and it increases the risk of infection. Each examination must be done for a definite purpose.
8. Should the findings at examination suggest that progress is being made, that delivery may be expected within a reasonable time, and if there is no fetal or maternal distress, supportive therapy is given and labor is allowed to go on.

<u>Prolonged Latent Phase</u>

First the mechanical factors must be ruled out. Further treatment depends on the condition of the cervix.

1. Ripe cervix: Effaced, soft, and 2.5 to 3.0 cm dilated.
   a. Amniotomy
   b. Oxytocin

2. Unripe cervix: Treatment is supportive. The patient is given nourishment, reassurance, and medication to induce sleep. Following this, one of three courses will follow:
   a. The patient will be out of labor (indicating that she had been in false labor) and is discharged from hospital.
   b. She will go into efficient labor and dilate the cervix.
   c. The original type of labor will resume. In this event oxytocin stimulation will often push the patient into good labor. Once the cervix ripens the membranes may be ruptured.

The prognosis is good. 1, most patients proceed into the progressive labor of the active phase leading to vaginal delivery; and 2, some will develop dysfunctional labor or secondary arrest of dilatation.

Cesarean section is almost never indicated in the latent stage of labor. Acute fetal distress, absolute cephalopelvic disproportion, and transverse lie are exceptions.

Primary Dysfunctional Labor

1. Mechanical factors must be ruled out.
2. In some cases there is fetopelvic disproportion, and cesarean section is indicated.
3. For the rest, medical management is carried out as long as the fetus and mother are in good condition. Nothing is done which will complicate the situation further. Premature and traumatic vaginal operations are contra-indicated. Slow progress is accepted.
4. Support, reassurance, rest, fluids, and electrolytes are provided.
5. Amniotomy. The results are not predictable, nor is there agreement as to whether it is a wise procedure in this situation.
   a. In some cases the progress of labor is improved.
   b. In others the arrest of labor seems to begin following artificial rupture of the membranes.
   c. In many, amniotomy has no effect on the course of labor.
   d. In prolonged labor the incidence of ascending infection is increased once the membranes are ruptured, and this danger must be kept in mind when amniotomy is being considered.
6. Oxytocin. Reports concerning the value of an oxytocin infusion vary. Many workers feel it is ineffective in improving the progress of labor. However we have had good results in some cases and feel it should be given a trial in managing this problem.
7. Results of medical treatment:
   a. Two thirds of the patients will dilate the cervix slowly and proceed to vaginal delivery spontaneously or with the help of low forceps.
   b. About 20 percent require mid forceps.
   c. Some 10 percent come to cesarean section because of arrest of progress or fetal distress.

Secondary Arrest of Dilatation

1. It is vital that mechanical factors are ruled out carefully. This includes malpositions and malpresentations as well as disproportion.
2. In a large group there is disproportion and cesarean section must be performed.
3. A few women are exhausted and are given support, rest, fluids, and electrolytes.
4. The majority of patients in whom there is no disproportion and no fetal distress are given an oxytocin infusion and the membranes are ruptured artificially. One of four courses will follow:
   a. Rapid progress to full dilatation and vaginal delivery.
   b. Slow progress to full dilatation and vaginal delivery.
   c. Too slow progress so that after 4 to 6 hours cesarean section is done.
   d. No progress at all. At the end of 2 hours cesarean section is carried out.

Fetal And/Or Maternal Distress

1. Fetal or maternal distress calls for early intervention.
2. If the prerequisites are present and there is no disproportion, the baby should be delivered by forceps, if a cephalic presentation, and by extraction or cesarean section if a breech.
3. Preparations should be at hand for the treatment of postpartum hemorrhage and fetal distress.

Cervical Dystocia

The cervix may be holding up progress:

1. A thick anterior lip may be caught between the head and the symphysis pubis. This can be pushed over the head during a contraction.
2. There may be a thin, soft rim of cervix. This can also be pushed gently over the head.
3. If the cervix is 6 to 7 cm dilated and well effaced, Dührssen's incisions may be considered.
4. If the cervix is less than half open, vaginal delivery is impossible at that time. If immediately delivery is indicated, cesarean section may be necessary.

DANGER OF PROLONGED LABOR

Maternal Dangers

Prolonged labor exerts a deleterious effect on both the mother and child. The severity of the damage increases progressively with the duration of the labor, the risk rising sharply after 24 hours. There is a rise in the incidence of uterine atony, lacerations, hemorrhage, infections, maternal exhaustion, and shock. The high rate of operative deliveries aggravates the maternal dangers.

Fetal Dangers

The longer the labor, the higher the fetal mortality and morbidity, and the more frequently do the following conditions occur:

1. Asphyxia from the long labor itself
2. Cerebral damage caused by pressure against the fetal head
3. Injury as a result of difficult forceps rotations and extractions
4. Rupture of the bag of waters long before delivery: This may result in the amniotic fluid's becoming infected, and, in turn, may lead to pulmonary and general infection in the fetus.

Even when there is no obvious damage these babies require special care. While any type of prolonged labor is bad for the child, the danger is greater once there has been cessation of progress. This is especially true when the head has been arrested on the perineal floor for a long time, with continual pounding of the skull against the mother's pelvis.

Some workers feel that while prolonged labor increases the risk to the child during labor and in the neonatal period, it has little effect on the infant's subsequent development. Others claim to have found that children born after extended labor were deficient intellectually as contrasted with babies born after normal delivery.

PROLONGED LABOR IN THE SECOND STAGE

Once the cervix has reached full dilatation, a limit until birth of 2 hours in a primigravida and 1 hour in a multipara has been set. Experience has shown that after this period fetal and maternal morbidity rises. Should fetal or maternal distress occur, immediate treatment is indicated.

Etiology

1. Fetopelvic disproportion
   a. Small pelvis
   b. Large child
2. Malpresentation and malposition
3. Ineffective labor
   a. Primary inefficient uterine contractions
   b. Myometrial fatigue: secondary inertia
   c. Constriction ring
   d. Inability or refusal of the patient to bear down
   e. Excessive anesthesia
4. Soft tissue dystocia
   a. Narrow vaginal canal
   b. Rigid perineum

Management

1. When there is disproportion or an irreversible constriction ring, cesarean section should be performed.
2. When there is no disproportion
   a. An oxytocin drip will improve the uterine contractions.
   b. Artificial rupture of the membranes is indicated if the bag of waters is intact.
   c. The patient should be placed on the delivery table and urged to bear down with each contraction.
   d. Forceps are used to further descent and rotation of the head.
   e. An episiotomy will overcome the unyielding perineum.
3. When these methods of treatment fail or when operative vaginal delivery is considered to be too traumatic for safe delivery, cesarean section is indicated.

The detailed descriptions of these procedures are found in the chapters concerned with each problem.

BIBLIOGRAPHY

Davis, M. E. Prolonged labor. Post grad. Med., 18:264, 1955.

Evans, T. N. Prolonged labor. Obstet. Gynec., 6:522, 1955.

Friedman, E. A. The graphic analysis of labor. Amer. J. Obstet. Gynec., 68:1568, 1954.

_____ and Sachtleben, M. R. Dysfunctional labor. A comprehensive program for diagnosis, evaluation, and management. Obstet. Gynec., 25:844, 1965.

Jeffcoate, T. N. A. Causes of prolonged labour. Lancet, 2:61, 1961.

Keettel, W. C., and Pettis, G. S. Prolonged labor. Obstet. Gynec., 7:15, 1956.

Schulman, H. Prolonged and abnormal labor. Amer. J. Obstet. Gynec., 95:732, 1966.

Thompson, E. W. L. Prolonged labour: Its management and prognosis. Irish J. Med. Sc., July, 1963, p. 327.

33 Premature Labor

Because of the unreliability of the menstrual history, prematurity is defined by infant weight rather than by gestational age. A premature infant is one weighing less than 2,500 g (5 pounds, 8 ounces). The average gestation for a baby whose birthweight is 2,500 g is 34 weeks.

Included in the premature group are small infants whose weight corresponds to the duration of the pregnancy, and children born near term whose intrauterine growth has been retarded. Whether birthweight or gestational age is the more important consideration is not clear. While a larger baby does have a better chance of survival, a higher birthweight does not abolish entirely the risks of being born before term. Newborns of the same weight may have varying degrees of maturity, and require different handling.

The incidence of prematurity in the United States is between 7 and 8 percent. The rates of prematurity tend to be higher when calculated on the basis of gestational age rather than of weight.

ETIOLOGY OF PREMATURE LABOR

1. Idiopathic. In almost half the cases of premature labor no cause is found.
2. Medical complications such as toxemia, diabetes, anemia, and chronic kidney disease. In some cases the prematurity is caused directly by the illness. In others the treatment of the disease necessitates the early termination of the pregnancy.
3. Acute febrile illnesses, such as influenza, pneumonia, and pyelitis, may bring on premature labor.
4. Abnormalities of the pelvic organs include uterine fibromyomata, congenital malformations of the uterus, and incompetent, or amputated cervix.
5. Among obstetric conditions are placenta previa, abruptio placentae, and previous cesarean section.
6. Trauma such as falls, blows on the abdomen, and surgical operations
7. Fetal factors include multiple pregnancy, congenital anomalies, polyhydramnios, and rising anti-Rh titer.
8. Premature rupture of the membranes is the first episode in 20 percent of cases.
9. Repeat cesarean section performed too early
10. Factors which seem to be associated with prematurity include:
    a. Lower socioeconomic status

b. Certain ethnic groups
c. Small women
d. Smoking during pregnancy, according to some investigators
e. Bacteruria
f. Poor prenatal care

PREMATURE RUPTURE OF THE MEMBRANES

Definition: The spontaneous rupture of the membranes one hour or more before the onset of labor

Incidence: This is between 10 and 12 percent. In about 20 percent the infant is premature.

Etiology: In most cases the reason is not known. In 20 percent rupture of the membranes is the first sign of impending onset of labor.

Diagnosis

Diagnosis may be difficult. Methods include: 1. History as to the time of rupture, and the color, odor, and volume of the fluid 2. Seeing the fluid escaping from the vagina, or from the cervix on speculum examination 3. The passage of meconium 4. Grasping fetal hair with forceps 5. The Nitrazine test for alkalinity of the normally acid vaginal fluid 6. Quinaldine blue stain of vaginal fluid—vaginal cells stain darkly, fetal cells lightly 7. Arborization test of vaginal fluid. (See Ch. 11 for details of the diagnosis of ruptured membranes.)

Onset of Labor

Between 50 and 70 percent of patients will go into labor spontaneously within 48 hours. This depends on the following:

1. Length of time the membranes are ruptured
2. Gestational age. If the pregnancy is beyond 36 weeks most will go into labor.
3. The earlier the pregnancy the longer will be the latent period (time between the rupture of the membranes and the start of contractions).
4. Fetal weight
5. Intrauterine infection tends to start labor sooner.
6. Presentation
7. Gravidity. Primigravidas are slower to go into labor after premature rupture of the membranes than multiparas.

Maternal Danger

The risk to the mother is small compared to that to the infant. The morbidity is low if the latent period is less than 48 hours. After this interval the incidence of infection rises. Maternal morbidity is between 11 and 12 percent.

Fetal Danger

Prolapse of the Umbilical Cord: This depends on the presentation and station at the time the membranes rupture.

Infection: The leading cause of fetal death is infection. The longer the latent period, the longer the first stage of labor, the greater the incidence of infection. The incidence rises significantly after a latent period of over 48 hours. The fetus can be infected even when there are no signs of sepsis in the mother. The commonest site is the respiratory tract. Most pneumonias in the first 2 weeks of life have an intrauterine origin.

Fetal Prognosis: This depends on:

1. Fetal maturity. Babies weighing under 2,500 g do less well than larger ones.
2. Presentation. Breeches have a worse prognosis, especially, when premature.
3. Intrauterine infection increases fetal mortality.
4. The longer the pregnancy is carried with ruptured membranes, the higher the incidence of infection.

Management of Premature Rupture of Membranes

The problem of prematurity must be weighed against the danger of the long latent period and potential infection. In marked prematurity the gestational age transcends other considerations, and maintaining the pregnancy may give the infant a better chance.

Hospitalization: All patients should be in hospital for a few days at least. Occasionally, if the head is well engaged and the cervix thick and closed, the patient may go home on restricted activity.

Antibiotics: Many doctors feel that, as prophylaxis, a wide spectrum antibiotic should be given to the mother. However, most recent reports suggest that antibiotics given to the mother during the latent period are of no value in protecting the child.

Active Labor: No special treatment is needed unless the baby is premature.

Induction of Labor: This should be carried out in the following situations:

1. In the presence of intrauterine sepsis, regardless of the period of gestation
2. When the pregnancy is 37 weeks or more, the baby is judged to be a good size, and the latent period has reached 48 hours

Inactive Treatment: Labor should not be induced:

1. When the pregnancy is less than 36 weeks
2. When the fetus is so small that it could not survive outside the uterus
3. In the presence of a hard, thick, closed cervix

INCOMPETENT INTERNAL OS OF THE CERVIX

Some women with a history of repeated midtrimester abortions have an incompetent cervix. The internal os undergoes painless dilatation and is unable to maintain the pregnancy.

Etiology: The exact etiology is not known. The condition may be congenital, but most women have a history of previous pregnancy, dilatation of the cervix beyond the ability of the internal os to remain intact, or cervical amputation.

Diagnosis: The condition is suspected when there have been abortions in second trimester for which no other cause can be found. During pregnancy, premature shortening, effacement, and dilatation of the cervix point to the diagnosis.

Clinical Picture: The first sign is usually spontaneous rupture of the membranes. The cervix shortens and dilates, and a part of the membranes bulges through and eventually ruptures. Rapid labor often follows.

Treatment: A suture is placed around the cervix near the internal os to narrow the canal thereby preventing the descent and rupture of the bag of waters. The suture is placed at the junction of the smooth mucosa of the portio and the rugose mucosa of the vagina. Many technics have been described. Some operations are done before and some during pregnancy. Afterward the patient may be ambulatory and active.

Time of Suture: We prefer suturing the cervix between the fourteenth and sixteenth weeks of pregnancy for these reasons:

1. The first trimester has passed, the pregnancy is established, and the danger of abortion because of a defective ovum is small.
2. The operation is easier to perform during pregnancy.
3. At this stage the cervix is not yet so effaced or dilated that it interferes with the technic.
4. If one waits until the membranes begin to protrude through the cervix, the chance of success is small and the danger of infection great.

Delivery: Two or three weeks before term the suture is removed and the onset of labor awaited. Vaginal delivery is permitted unless there is some other indication for cesarean section.

Contraindications: Included are: 1, infection; 2, ruptured membranes; 3, labor; 4, bleeding per vaginam.

Complications: 1, infection; 2, hemorrhage; 3, accidental rupture of membranes; 4, stimulation of labor. These are rare.

PREVENTION OF PREMATURE LABOR

Most attempts at prevention of premature labor are futile. There are, however, several general and a few specific measures which can be taken.

General Measures

1. Prenatal care, diet, vitamins, and hygiene
2. Restriction of activity (work, travel, coitus) for patients with a history of premature labor
3. Acute febrile illnesses must be treated promptly and actively.
4. Medical conditions such as toxemia and diabetes need careful control.
5. Elective abdominal surgery and extensive dental work are postponed.

Specific Measures

1. Patients with multiple pregnancy should be at bed rest from the twenty-eighth to the thirty-sixth or thirty-eighth week.
2. Uterine fibromyomata, when symptomatic, are managed by bed rest and analgesia. Surgery is avoided as long as possible.
3. Placenta previa is treated by confinement to bed and blood transfusion to delay the birth of the baby until it has reached a viable size. Profuse hemorrhage, of course, calls for immediate surgery.
4. The incompetent cervix should be sutured in the early part of the second trimester, as long as all precepts have been fulfilled.
5. Elective and repeat cesarean section is done only when one is certain that the child is of good size. The danger of too early operation is the delivery of a small baby which does not survive.
6. Isoxsuprine has the property of reducing uterine activity. It is sometimes effective in stopping contractions in the prelabor phase or in the early part of the first stage of labor. However, once active labor is established, the cervix is effaced and dilating, or the membranes have ruptured, this drug has little or no value. Administration is by intravenous drip until the contractions have ceased, and then the patient is maintained on intramuscular and oral medication. An occasional complication is hypotension.
7. Some success has been achieved in reducing premature labor by the treatment of bacteruria, even when asymptomatic, with appropriate antibiotics.

MANAGEMENT OF PREMATURE LABOR AND DELIVERY

Labor

Gentleness is of paramount importance. The premature baby, with its soft skull and low resistance, stands trauma poorly. When possible, excessively strong contractions and precipitate labor should be avoided. Unfortunately neither the baby nor the uterus is prepared for normal labor. Often an unripe cervix adds to the difficulties.

Analgesia and Anesthesia

The premature baby is hypersensitive to drugs given to the mother for relief of pain. Even a small dose may so depress the vital centers that the onset of respiration is delayed and asphyxia results. During labor it is wisest to

avoid narcotics of any kind. Delivery is safest under local infiltration or pudendal block. If more anesthesia is necessary a conduction technic, such as
epidural block, is used.

The Delivery

1. Birth should be gentle and slow to avoid rapid compression and decompression of the head.
2. Oxygen is given to the mother by mask during the delivery.
3. The membranes should not be ruptured artificially. The bag of waters acts
   as a cushion for the soft premature skull with its widely separated sutures.
4. An episiotomy reduces pressure on the baby's cranium.
5. Low forceps may help in dilating the maternal soft parts, and in guiding the
   head over the perineum. We prefer spontaneous delivery when possible.
6. Breech extraction should not be performed. An added danger in premature
   births is that the buttocks may not dilate the birth canal enough to make
   room for the relatively large head.
7. Precipitous and unattended births are dangerous for the premature baby.
8. Vaginal delivery gives better results than cesarean section for premature
   infants.

Care of the Premature Infant

1. The head-down position (at an angle of about 30 degrees) is maintained to
   promote drainage of the respiratory tract. If there is suspicion of intracranial hemorrhage the baby should lie in the horizontal plane.
2. The secretions are aspirated from the throat and nose by gentle suction.
3. An incubator is useful so that the temperature, humidity, and oxygen can
   be controlled. A warm atmosphere is best. To prevent retrolental fibro-
   plasia the oxygen concentration should be below 40 percent.
4. The apneic infant must be oxygenated within 1 to 2 minutes of birth. Adequate ventilation is essential. We have found the bag and mask technic to
   be efficient and safe.
5. Resuscitation measures must be gentle. Slapping and rubbing are to be
   discouraged. The least amount of handling is best.
6. Occasionally laryngoscopy is necessary to remove debris from the respiratory tract and intubation to get oxygen in.
7. Persistent labored respiration may indicate a pneumothorax or a diaphrag-
   matic hernia.
8. When the baby has been narcotized by drugs administered to the mother,
   Nalline is given to the infant to counteract the effects of the depressing
   drugs. The dose is 0.2 mg into the umbilical vein. If the baby weighs less
   than 1,000 g the dose is 0.1 mg. Stimulatory drugs are not used.
9. While there is disagreement as to whether umbilical cord should be clamped
   early, or whether the baby should be held below the level of the placenta until the cord pulsations cease, there is agreement that the cord should not be
   milked toward the infant, as the sudden extra blood infused into the circulation may overload it and put a strain on the heart.

10. Because of the association of prematurity with congenital malformation, the baby should be examined thoroughly.
11. When possible a pediatrician should attend the birth.
12. A separate premature nursery with a specially trained staff is invaluable.

PROGNOSIS OF PREMATURITY

1. Prematurity is today the most frequently recurring factor involved in infant death and morbidity. Most babies who die within the first 28 days of life weighed less than 2,500 g at birth.
2. Anoxia is 12 times more common in premature infants.
3. Respiratory distress causes 44 percent of deaths under one month. If the fetus weighs under 1,000 g this figure rises to 74 percent.
4. Because of the softness of the skull bones and the immaturity of the brain tissue, the premature infant is more vulnerable to compression of the head.
5. Intracranial hemorrhage is 5 times more frequent in the premature than in the full term infant. Much of this results from anoxia.
6. Cerebral palsy is more common in premature infants.
7. The prognosis in low birthweight infants for physical and intellectual health is not clear despite numerous investigations. There seems to be a higher incidence of organic brain damage in premature babies. Yet many men of genius were born before term.

BIBLIOGRAPHY

Abramowicz, M., and Kass, E. H. Pathogenesis and prognosis of prematurity. New Eng. J. Med., 275:878, 938, 1001, 1053, 1966.

Cosgrove, R. A. Premature labor. J. Louisiana State Med. Soc., 116:283, 1964.

Ekvall, L. D., Wixted, W. G., and Dyer, I. Spontaneous premature rupture of the fetal membranes. Amer. J. Obstet. Gynec., 81:848, 1961.

Raphael, S. I. Incompetent internal os of the cervix. Obstet. Gynec., 28:438, 1966.

Speert, H. Premature labor. Bull. Sloane Hosp. Women, 10:7, 1964.

Stander, R. W. Phenethanolamines and inhibition of human myometrium. Amer. J. Obstet. Gynec., 94:749, 1966.

34 Prolonged Pregnancy

In calculating the expected date of confinement Naegele's rule is that term is reached 40 weeks after the first day of the last normal menstrual period. This is based on the belief that conception takes place on about the fourteenth day of the cycle. In most instances the exact date of conception is not known.

Postterm pregnancy has been described as one having reached 42 weeks. Because this would include 12 percent of all pregnancies, a more acceptable definition is 43 weeks. Here the incidence is 4 percent.

Reasons for errors associated with Naegele's rule include: 1, the menstrual history is unreliable. Many women do not remember when the last menstruation began; 2, women whose cycle is longer than 28 days, or whose ovulation is late, may deliver after the expected date; 3, even under normal conditions the length of pregnancy varies; 4, women have been known to falsify the menstrual history for social reasons.

Assuming that the expected date of confinement is known accurately, the following questions need to be answered:

1. Does postterm pregnancy add any risk to mother and child?
2. At what stage do these dangers play a part?
3. How do they compare with the problems of artificial termination of the pregnancy?

There are two opposite views as to the implications of postterm pregnancy:

1. This is a physiological variation. In itself it poses no danger to the fetus. Hence, no routine interference is indicated.
2. Prolongation of gestation carries with it an increased fetal mortality, and termination of the pregnancy should be considered in all cases.

FETAL SIZE AND CONDITION

There are variations in the size of infants born after the expected date of confinement.

1. Most babies are within normal limits.
2. The number of children weighing over 4,000 g is increased in prolonged pregnancy. The disproportion and dystocia caused by the oversized fetus can lead to fetal damage or death. Some obstetricians advise induction of labor to obviate this problem.

3. Fetal dysmaturity. Some postterm babies are small and undernourished.
Presumably because of placental insufficiency, either the infant's stage of
development does not correspond to the period of gestation, or he shows
the regressive changes and signs of intrauterine hypoxia. This syndrome
is seen as often before term as after it. The problem is thus placental
malfunction, and not postmaturity. It may be that placental efficiency decreases after term, and when the placenta is not functioning well to start
with, prolongation of the pregnancy may result in the fetal dysmaturity syndrome. The need is for accurate methods of determining placental function.
The appearance of the child is characteristic
a. The weight is reduced in relation to length.
b. The limbs are long and lean.
c. The baby looks undernourished and has only a small amount of subcutaneous fat.
d. The vernix is absent or scanty and when present is yellow or green.
e. The hair is abundant.
f. The nails are long.
g. The skin hangs in folds. There is a tendency to desquamation, especially on the palms and soles. The skin dries after birth and becomes
parchment like.
h. There is meconium staining of the skin, nails, umbilical cord, and amniotic fluid.
i. In advanced cases the amniotic fluid becomes scanty and thick with
meconium. There is a tendency to aspiration of this fluid with subsequent pulmonary complications.

FETAL MORTALITY

Most obstetricians and pediatricians agree that perinatal fetal mortality is
increased in prolonged pregnancy. The exact reason for this has not been established. Browne found that, as compared with term births, the perinatal
mortality doubles at 43 weeks, trebles at 44 weeks, and quintuples at 45 weeks.
Evans and others noted that most babies that died after postterm pregnancy suf-
fered from specific conditions which could not have been avoided by earlier delivery.

The increased fetal mortality is seen in all groups—before the onset of labor, during labor and delivery, and in the neonatal period. However, antepartum and intrapartum deaths are more frequent than those of the newborn.
There is a higher incidence in primigravidas and in older women.

There is disagreement as to the etiology of fetal death in association with
prolonged pregnancy:

1. One group believes that anoxia resulting from placental insufficiency is the
main cause.
2. The other group feels that while anoxia is probably the chief factor, it is
the result of the prolonged labor and difficult delivery so often seen in postterm pregnancy.

Walker's studies of cord blood suggested that the supply of oxygen to the fetus decreases slowly in term and rapidly thereafter. He postulated that the well-oxygenated baby can withstand the trauma of labor, but the fetus who is deficient in oxygen is likely to experience distress during labor and to manifest this by passing meconium in utero. Other findings are that the permeability of the placenta increases up to 36 weeks and then decreases steadily. The oxygen consumption of the placenta is reduced as term is approached. It has been suggested that the uterine circulation becomes less efficient at term, and that neither the placenta nor the fetus can compensate for this.

Other investigators have been unable to substantiate these findings. They noted no decrease in oxygen saturation of fetal blood in prolonged pregnancy, no increase in fetal hemoglobin, and no reduction in uterine blood flow. They feel that hypoxia alone does not explain the increased perinatal mortality.

MANAGEMENT

There are two schools of thought. One believes that every pregnancy that passes term should be terminated; the time of interference varies with the individual case. The other group feels that the spontaneous onset of labor should be awaited in most cases.

Termination of Pregnancy

In the belief that prolonged pregnancy is detrimental to the fetus, Browne and others suggest the following plan:

1. At every antepartum visit the accuracy of the expected date of confinement is checked.
2. At 42 weeks the membranes are ruptured artificially, regardless of the condition of the cervix. The amniotic fluid is examined for volume, appearance, and consistency.
3. If the fluis is abundant and clear, the onset of labor is awaited. Oxytocin is not used because the strong contractions which it could produce might kill a baby who is already hypoxic.
4. Should the amniotic fluid be scanty, stained with meconium, and thick, cesarean section is performed either immediately or at the first sign of change in the fetal heart.
5. When induction fails, cesarean section is done after 48 hours.
6. Fetal distress at any time during labor demands immediate cesarean section.
7. In older women, and in those with hypertension or preeclampsia, induction is started at 40 to 41 weeks.

Noninterference

Opposed to the interventionists are those who feel that routine induction of labor is not indicated for every postterm pregnancy, and they point out the following:

1. One must be certain that the risks of treatment are not greater than those of postmaturity.
2. It is probable that the hazards of prolonged pregnancy are less than those of induction in the presence of an unripe cervix.
3. Prolonged labor is especially harmful to the fetus in postterm pregnancy, and induction when conditions are not perfect often leads to a long inertic type of labor.
4. In the presence of placental insufficiency induction may hasten the death of the fetus.
5. The original ideas of Walker that hypoxia is the main factor have not been substantiated by other investigators.

There seems to be fetal danger in postterm pregnancy if labor is prolonged or complicated, if delivery is difficult, and if an elderly primigravida is still pregnant at 42 or 43 weeks. One answer to the problem lies in the realization that it exists, that postmaturity causes trouble mainly during labor, and that the careful management of labor and delivery is more important than routine induction at a given date.

The following is a suggested plan of management:

1. If the cervix is ripe and the fetus is engaged and in good position, labor should be induced at 42 or 43 weeks.
2. In elderly primigravidas cesarean section is considered at 41 weeks and is performed no later than 42 weeks.
3. In other cases the spontaneous onset of labor is awaited.
4. Because of the increased fetal mortality of the postterm baby, labor must be supervised especially carefully, keeping in mind these features.
    a. Prolonged labor is more hazardous for the postterm baby, and if good progress is not being made, cesarean section is done sooner than under normal conditions.
    b. Some of these babies are large, and disproportion, difficult delivery, and shoulder dystocia must be anticipated.
    c. Signs of fetal distress are more ominous in prolonged pregnancy.
    d. The postterm baby is hypersensitive to excessive sedation, narcosis, and anesthesia. Conduction technics are probably safest.
    e. Older women and those with hypertension or preeclampsia warrant special care.
    f. Prompt and expert neonatal care should be available.

Perhaps the final answer lies in the discovery of accurate methods of diagnosing placenta insufficiency and fetal distress, enabling us to select those fetuses for whom further intrauterine existence is dangerous.

BIBLIOGRAPHY

Browne, J. C. M. Postmaturity. Amer. J. Obstet. Gynec., 85:574, 1963.

Cushner, I. M. Postmaturity. Sinai Hosp. J., 12:39, 1964.

Evans, T. N., Koeff, S. T., and Morley, G. W. Fetal effects of prolonged
   pregnancy. Amer. J. Obstet. Gynec., 85:701, 1963.

Lucas, W. E., Anctil, A. O., and Callagan, D. W. The problem of post term
   pregnancy. Amer. J. Obstet. Gynec., 91:241, 1965.

Nesbitt, R. E. L. Prolongation of pregnancy. Obstet. Gynec. Survey, 10:311,
   1955.

35   Induction of Labor

<u>Definition</u>: Induced labor is labor started by artificial methods.

INDICATIONS FOR THE INDUCTION OF LABOR

Maternal Indications

1. Toxemia of pregnancy: When medical therapy is unable to control toxemia, the pregnancy must be terminated.
2. Polyhydramnios: Polyhydramnios is the accumulation of an excessive amount of amniotic fluid. Pressure symptoms and dyspnea may be so severe that the patient is unable to carry on.
3. Intrauterine fetal death: In selected cases labor is induced to relieve the mother of the strain of carrying a dead child and to prevent the development of afibrinogenemia.
4. Antepartum bleeding: Included here are cases of low-lying placenta and mild placental separation, where the bleeding is not controllable by bed rest, or when the baby is dead.
5. Cancer: The termination of the pregnancy is for the purpose of permitting surgical, radiation, or chemical treatment of the lesion, or simply to remove a drain on the patient's resources and powers of resistance.
6. Spontaneous rupture of membranes: If the pregnancy is within 2 weeks of term and labor does not begin after 24 hours, induction with oxytocin should be considered.
7. History of rapid labors: The aim is to avoid birth of the baby at home or en route to hospital.
8. Patients living far from hospital
9. Elective: Here the procedure is being carried out for the convenience of the patient, the doctor, or both. Because there is no pressing medical reason for the induction, great care must be taken in selecting the patient, and no risks should be taken. The labor must be supervised constantly. If there is the least doubt about the procedure it should not be instituted. It is almost never warranted in primigravidas.

Advantages of elective induction include:

a. The patient is admitted to hospital the previous night and a hypnotic is prescribed to assure her of sleep.
b. No food is given by mouth, the stomach is empty, and this decreases the anesthetic risk.
c. The rush to hospital is avoided.
d. It is a daytime procedure when full staff is available.
e. The doctor chooses a day when he has no other duties and can remain in hospital with the patient.
f. The length of labor is shortened.

Fetal Indications

1. Maternal diabetes: The babies tend to be large and often die in utero in the latter weeks of pregnancy. Hence, the pregnancy should be terminated at around the thirty-seventh week.
2. Rhesus incompatibility: When the fetus is being sensitized or when there has been fetal death in utero in previous pregnancies, premature induction of labor is sometimes indicated.
3. Recurrent intrauterine death: Intrauterine death near term in past pregnancies is a rational reason for premature induction of labor.
4. Excessive size of the fetus
5. Postterm pregnancy: There is some evidence that there is a progressive decrease in placental function and in the oxygen content of fetal blood as pregnancy proceeds past term. Occasionally there is fetal death in utero, or often the baby is born with poor nutrition and has difficulty in the postnatal period.

PREREQUISITES AND CONDITIONS

1. The presentation: The presentation should be vertex. Labor is never induced in the presence of attitudes of extension, transverse lies, or compound presentations, and almost never when the breech presents.
2. Stage of the pregnancy: The closer to term the easier will be the induction.
3. Station: The head must be engaged. The lower the head the easier and safer the procedure.
4. Cervical ripeness: The cervix must be effaced, less than half an inch in length, soft, dilatable, and open to admit at least one finger and preferably two. The firm ring of the internal os should not be present. It is advantageous for the cervix to be in the center of the birth canal or anterior. When the cervix is posterior conditions for induction are less favorable.
5. Parity: It is much easier and safer to induce a multipara than a primipara, and the success rate increases with parity.
6. Fetal maturity: In theory the fetus becomes viable at the end of the twenty-eighth week. However, the chances of survival before 32 weeks are reduced, and if possible, labor should not be induced before then. In general the nearer the pregnancy is to term the better the fetal results.

DANGERS

1. Prolapse of the umbilical cord: This may occur if artificial rupture of the membranes is performed when the presenting part is not well engaged.
2. Fetal death, unexplained
3. Prolonged labor
4. Prematurity as a result of miscalculation of the expected date of confinement
5. Genital and fetal infection following a long period of ruptured membranes
6. Failure of induction, which sometimes necessitates cesarean section: As long as the prerequisites are observed scrupulously the rate of success with induction of labor is over 95 percent. Unfortunately there is a tendency on the part of even the experienced obstetrician to stretch the indications and conditions, and this may lead to trouble.

Should anything go wrong, even if it has nothing to do with the induction, the doctor will be blamed for interfering.

METHODS OF INDUCING LABOR

Medical

1. Castor oil, two ounces, followed by soap suds enema
2. Quinine: We no longer employ quinine. It has not proved to be effective, it may have toxic effects, and better methods are available.

Hormonal

Oxytocin is used to achieve two purposes:

1. To induce labor when conditions are correct
2. To ripen the cervix: When induction is necessary but the cervix is not ripe, intravenous oxytocin is given for several hours daily until the cervix is ripe, when induction can be carried out. (For details of technic see Ch. 36.)

Artificial Rupture of the Membranes

1. The fetal heart is checked carefully.
2. Sterile vaginal examination is made to determine that the necessary conditions and prerequisites are present.
3. With a finger placed between the cervix and the bag of waters, the cervix is rimmed, stripping the membranes away from the lower uterine segment.
4. Pressure is maintained on the uterine fundus through the abdomen to keep the head well down.
5. Using a uterine dressing forceps, an Allis forceps, a Kelly clamp, or a membrane hook, the bag of waters is torn or punctured.
6. A gush of fluid from the vagina or the grasping of fetal hear in the clamp is proof of success.
7. The fetal heart is checked carefully.
8. While the head may be pushed upward slightly to allow the escape of the amniotic fluid, this must be done with caution, for there is danger of prolapse of the umbilical cord.

In most cases labor will follow within 24 hours. If it does not, other procedures must be instituted.

Contraindications to artificial rupture of the membranes include:

1. High presenting part
2. Presentation other than vertex
3. Unripe cervix
4. Irregular or slow fetal heart

Mechanical Technics

The use of bougies, inflatable bags, and packing of the lower uterine segment were once popular methods for the induction of labor. Because these technics were attended by a high rate of infection and because better procedures are available today, mechanical methods for the induction of labor are used rarely.

Intraamniotic Injection of Hypertonic Solutions

The intraamniotic installation of a hypertonic solution will result in the onset of labor within 24 hours. In most cases the entire products of conception are delivered within 30 hours. The solutions in current use are 20 percent saline and 50 percent glucose.

There are four hypotheses as to the mechanism of action:

1. Normally progesterone blocks the onset of labor. The hypertonic solution disrupts the placenta and releases the local progesterone block, and labor follows.
2. Uterine volume is an important factor in controlling the onset of labor. The body attempts to equilibrate the hypertonic solution, the volume of intraamniotic fluid is increased, and uterine contractions begin.
3. The hypertonic solution has a direct effect on the myometrium and fetal membranes.
4. This theory postulates an action of the saline on the hypothalamus and pituitary glands, releasing oxytocin.

Technic: The technic of intraamniotic injection is as follows:

1. Premedication consists of a barbiturate and, if necessary, Demerol is administered.
2. The patient is placed on an operating table in moderate Trendelenburg position.
3. An intravenous infusion is instituted.
4. Transabdominal amniotomy is performed, using a 4 inch spinal needle with stylet. The needle is inserted (under local anesthesia) half way between the symphysis pubis and the umbilicus, 1 inch from the midline, toward the side of the small parts of the fetus.
5. Amniotic fluid (100 to 300 ml) is removed and replaced with an equal amount of the hypertonic solution.
6. The patient is then placed in bed and the onset of labor awaited.

Indications: The above method is used for the induction of labor when the fetus is dead or when the termination of pregnancy is so essential in the interests of the mother that the fetus is being disregarded. This technic is useful in missed abortions. It works even when the cervix is unripe. This procedure is not employed to induce labor in a normal pregnancy or when the fetus is viable.

Advantages: Advantages of this method include: 1, it is an effective way of emptying the uterus and 2, it obviates the need for hysterotomy after the twelfth week when the pregnancy must be terminated.

Dangers: Dangers of this procedure include:

1. Maternal death
2. Infection may be introduced by the procedure.
3. Damage to placental vessels during amniotomy may allow fetal erythrocytes to enter the maternal circulation.
4. Injury to bladder or bowel.

In Japan there have been numerous maternal deaths following this procedure, and the technic is no longer in widespread use. Recent similar reports from other countries are such that the original enthusiastic opinions as to the safety of saline or glucose induced abortions are being questioned seriously.

Deaths: Deaths are of several types:

1. Infection, more common with glucose
2. Direct injection into the blood stream
3. Aggravation of such conditions as toxemia, chronic nephritis, and hypertension
4. Postpartum hemorrhage, cervical laceration, and uterine rupture
5. Death following shock-like symptoms or vascular collapse. In a few cases of this type autopsy revealed brain damage with widespread infarction, caused probably by cerebral dehydration. It is thought that the saline enters the maternal circulation by way of the intervillous space or a vein.

Since this procedure is not the inocuous procedure it was once thought to be, its use must be restricted.

Preferred Method of Induction

We favor the following routine:

1. The patient is admitted to hospital the night before.
2. Secobarbital, 100 or 200 mg, is given at bedtime.
3. The patient is advised to inform the nurse should labor begin.
4. Vulvar preparation is carried out on admission.
5. Breakfast is withheld.
6. Next morning a soap suds enema is given.
7. An intravenous drip using 5 units of oxytocin in 500 or 1,000 ml of 5 percent glucose in water is set up in the labor room (see Ch. 36).

8. At the proper time the membranes may be ruptured artificially. Generally this speeds the progress of labor. However, a long delay between the breaking of the bag of waters and the onset of progressing labor promotes infection in mother and child. Once the membranes are ruptured there is no turning back. Therefore, during an oxytocin induction, the membranes should be ruptured artificially when regular contractions have started, the cervix has begun to dilate, and the presenting part is through the inlet.
9. The fetal heart is checked carefully before and after the start of the oxytocin infusion and the rupture of the membranes.

BIBLIOGRAPHY

D'Esopo, D. A., Moore, D. B., and Lenzi, E. Elective induction of labor. Amer. J. Obstet. Gynec., 89:561, 1964.

Gochberg, S. H., and Reid, D. E. Intra-amniotic injection of hypertonic saline for termination of pregnancy. Obstet. Gynec., 27:648, 1966.

Johnson, J. W. C., Cushner, I. M., and Stephens, N. L. Hazards of using hypertonic saline for therapeutic abortion. Amer. J. Obstet. Gynec., 94:225, 1966.

Niswander, K. R., and Patterson, R. J. Hazards of elective induction of labor. Obstet. Gynec., 22:228, 1963.

Wagatsuma, T. Intra-amniotic injection of saline for therapeutic abortion. Amer. J. Obstet. Gynec., 93:743, 1965.

Weingold, A. B., Seigal, S., and Stone, M. L. Intra-amniotic hypertonic solutions for induction of labor. Obstet. Gynec., 26:622, 1965.

36 The Use of Oxytocin in Obstetrics

To fill the need for an agent to stimulate uterine contractions in selected obstetric situations, posterior pituitary extract has been available for over 50 years. The history of the use of this powerful drug may be divided into three phases.

The first phase, one of complete acceptance, began in 1909 when Blair Bell used posterior pituitary extract in the treatment of postpartum hemorrhage caused by uterine atony. Dale had shown that pituitrin has an oxytocic effect on uterine muscle. Others took up the use of this hormone in all stages of labor. Imprudent use, excessive dosage, and improper clinical indications led to frequent and tragic accidents, including fetal and maternal death. The second phase, after 1920, was characterized by condemnation and abandonment.

The need for a reliable oxytocic agent continued, and in 1946 the reevaluation of pituitrin was undertaken. Rare accidents were reported in some series, and none in others. The present phase is characterized by widespread use and favorable reports, as long as proper indications are adhered to strictly, minute amounts of the hormones are used, and the patient is observed carefully and continuously. In institutions where posterior pituitary extract was used correctly the incidence of mid forceps and prolonged labor was reduced. Indiscriminate use of this drug is to be condemned. It is not a panacea for all obstetric problems.

PITUITRIN, PITOCIN, AND PITRESSIN

At first, whole posterior pituitary extract (pituitrin) was used. It contains mainly an oxytocic agent and an antidiuretic hypertensive factor. The extract has been divided into its two main components: an almost pure oxytocic (pitocin) and its hypertensive counterpart (pitressin).

In the early 1950's DuVigneaud and his colleagues succeeded in the purification, chemical identification, and synthesis of oxytocin and vasopressin. In their action on the myometrium the efficiency of the natural and synthetic products is the same. Synthetic oxytocin is a chemically pure substance and is free from the danger of reaction to the animal protein.

At the present time all commercial preparations of oxytocin used in the United States and Canada are synthetic. These include Syntocinon (Sandoz), Pitocin (Parke-Davis), and Uteracon (Lloyd).

In response to certain stimuli, oxytocin (an octopeptide) is released from the hypothalamic nuclei. It travels via the hypothalamohypophyseal tract to arrive in the posterior lobe of the pituitary gland where it is stored.

In causing the uterus to contract oxytocin is believed to act on the myometrial cell membrane. It increases the normal excitability of the muscle but adds no new properties to the muscle cell.

ADMINISTRATION

Routes of administration in common use today are:

1. Intramuscular injection of large or small, single or repeated doses
2. The placing in the nostril of a cotton pledget soaked in 5 or 10 units of oxytocin. From here the drug is absorbed in varying concentrations and speeds.
3. The intravenous infusion by Murphy drip (or ideally by a pump) of a dilute solution of oxytocin in 5 percent glucose in water. The popular dilutions are 5 or 10 units of oxytocin in 1 liter of glucose in water. Recently a mixture of 2 units per liter has been used successfully. The more dilute the solution the safer it is. It is sufficiently effective, and, in addition, it is much easier to regulate the speed of a drip at 40 drops per minute than at 10, and yet the same amount of the drug is administered. Most patients in labor need the extra fluid.
4. However, because of the antidiuretic effect of intravenous oxytocin, it is imperative (when large doses are used, or when the infusion is to run for a long period of time) that a high concentration is employed, so that the intake of fluid is limited to 2,500 cc per day. This precaution is necessary to avoid water intoxication.

Advantages of the Intravenous Drip Method

1. The amount of oxytocin entering the blood stream can be regulated. With other technics the amount given to the patient is known, but there is no control over the rate of absorption. It can be fast or slow, regular or intermittent, and it may accumulate in the tissues, to be released later in a large amount and high concentration.
2. Minute amounts are effective.
3. The blood level and the activity of oxytocin are constant as long as the rate of the drip is maintained. It can be speeded up or slowed down with instant changes in effect.
4. The plasma of pregnant women near term contains an enzyme, pitocinase, in such high concentration that half of an intravenously given dosage of pitocin is destroyed in about 90 seconds. Thus, within 2 or 3 minutes of the shutting off an intravenous infusion, the oxytocic activity has ceased.
5. The contractions brought on by this technic seem to be mainly of the normal triple descending gradient type.

Technic of Intravenous Drip Administration

The two bottle method is preferable. One bottle contains a liter of 5 percent glucose in water. The other contains a liter of 5 percent glucose in water to which the oxytocin has been added; this labeled clearly. The two tubes leading from the bottles are connected by a "Y" adapter which connects to the needle in the vein. The "Y" adapter should be as close to the needle as possible, so that change from one solution to the other will have an immediate effect.

The drip is started with the pure glucose solution, and when it is running at 10 to 15 drops a minute, the switch is made to the oxytocin solution. Careful observation is made as to the type, strength, and duration of the contractions and to their effect on the fetal heart. If no untoward reactions are noted, the drip is continued. If excessive uterine contractions occur, or if there is fetal bradycardia (under 100), tachycardia (over 160), or irregularity of the heart, the oxytocin is stopped, and plain glucose is infused. Oxytocin is one of the most potent drugs known. It may vary a hundredfold in its actions on different people. The dosage is regulated by the effect on the individual who is receiving it. The speed of the drip is determined by, and correlated to, the frequency, intensity, and duration of the resulting contractions, rather than by any arbitrary number of drops per minute. The aim is to bring about strong uterine contractions lasting 40 to 50 seconds, and recurring every 2 to 3 minutes. Care must be exercised to avoid tumultuous contractions so frequent and prolonged that there is no interval between them. This carries the danger of uterine rupture, placental separation, and fetal asphyxia.

It is advisable to keep the drip running through the delivery and for at least 1 hour post partum to reduce the danger of postpartum hemorrhage from uterine atony.

INDICATIONS FOR THE USE OF OXYTOCIN

Management of Abortions

1. To stimulate the uterus to pass retained tissue
2. To control bleeding

Inevitable Abortion

The symptoms are bleeding and cramps. The cervix is partly open, but the products of conception have not been passed. Oxytocin will stimulate the uterus to contract and expel its contents after the cervix has been opened widely. Curettage is easier through an open cervix. The oxytocin will keep the uterus firm, will make it easier to avoid perforation of the uterine fundus, and will help control hemorrhage.

Incomplete Abortion

The fetus has been passed, but part or all of the placenta is in situ. Oxytocin helps expel what is left, makes curettage easier, and controls hemorrhage.

Complete Abortion

Oxytocin is used to reduce postabortal bleeding.

Missed Abortion

While most missed abortions will terminate spontaneously, in some instances (e.g., danger of hypo- or afibrinogenemia) one can wait only so long, and then steps must be taken to empty the uterus. Oxytocin is valuable to soften the cervix, to open it sufficiently so that dilatation and curettage can be performed safely, and to keep the uterine tone high so that bleeding is controlled.

Induction of Labor

Elective Induction of Labor

Elective induction of labor is performed for a variety of reasons including the following:

1. Convenience to the mother and doctor
2. Patients with a history of precipitate labors
3. Patients who live a long distance from the hospital

As long as the cervix is ripe (soft, less than 1/2 inch long, effaced, open to admit at least one finger, and easily dilatable) and the head is well in the pelvis induction of labor is feasible. Artificial rupture of the membranes increases the efficiency of inducing labor with oxytocin.

Spontaneous Rupture of the Membranes

If the membranes rupture prematurely, much before term, an attempt is made to prolong the pregnancy to a point where the baby is big enough to survive. On the other hand, most patients who rupture the membranes near or at term will go into spontaneous labor. If this does not take place within 24 hours induction of labor is indicated.

Fetal Salvage

In certain instances where the pregnancy has gone past the date of expected confinement by two or more weeks, induction is indicated. Rupture of the membranes and an oxytocin drip are the methods of choice, providing the cervix is ripe and the head engaged. In diabetic mothers and in those who are sensitized to the Rhesus factor, induction of labor before term may be necessary. If conditions are right this can be done with oxytocin and rupture of the membranes. If the cervix is not ripe and the presenting part is high, cesarean section may be safer.

Maternal Indications

In conditions such as preeclampsia, premature separation of the placenta, and fetal death in utero, the time comes when medical management or watchful expectancy is no longer indicated, and the pregnancy must be terminated artificially in the interests of the mother.   This is especially true if her condition is deteriorating.   Often simple rupture of the membranes will start labor.   If it does not, oxytocin will do so in most cases.

Ripening of the Cervix

As a general rule, induction of labor by artificial rupture of the bag of waters is not attempted unless the cervix is ripe and the head is in the pelvis. Should induction be essential in the presence of an unripe cervix, an attempt is made to ripen it.   The patient is given an oxytocin drip for several hours daily for a few days.   This will, in most instances, not institute true labor, but the oxytocin induced contractions will often bring the head down into the pelvis and ripen the cervix so that the membranes can be ruptured and good labor instituted.

Improved Efficiency of Uterine Contractions

Prolonged Labor due to Hypotonic Uterine Inertia

In prolonged labor due to hypotonic uterine inertia oxytocin is most valuable.   The effect is to increase the type of contraction already present.   In true hypotonic inertia the pattern is normal, but the contractions of the upper segment are weak and progress is not made.   Before using oxytocin in these conditions one must be sure that there is no disproportion or malpresentation, since these abnormalities and poor uterine action go together.

In hypotonic uterine action an oxytocin drip may result in an immediate improvement of the labor, with steady progress to successful delivery of the child. The proper use of pitocin in these cases has resulted in:

1.   Successful termination of the labor
2.   Reduction in the incidence of mid forceps, cervical lacerations, cesarean section, Dührssen's incisions, and traumatic deliveries
3.   Shortening of prolonged labor

Treatment of Postpartum Hemorrhage

In postpartum hemorrhage caused by uterine atony an oxytocin drip is a good method of treatment.   Other causes of the bleeding must, of course, be ruled out.   The drip is effective in improving the tone of the uterus, and it can be kept running as long as necessary.

Prevention of Postpartum Hemorrhage

Such conditions as uterine inertia, twin pregnancy, polyhydramnios, difficult delivery, and excessive anesthesia predispose to uterine atony and postpartum hemorrhage.   The complication should be anticipated and guarded against by starting an oxytocin drip before the hemorrhage takes place.

Normal Management of the Third Stage

To hasten delivery of the placenta and to reduce the bleeding of the placental stage, oxytocin may be given before or after the delivery of the placenta.

PREREQUISITES FOR THE USE OF OXYTOCIN

1. In all cases consultation is sought.
2. The presenting part should be well engaged.
3. The cervix must be ripe, effaced, soft, and partially dilated.
4. There must be a normal obstetric history and the absence of an abnormal one.
5. There must be no fetopelvic disproportion.
6. The fetus should be in normal position.
7. The fetus should be in good condition with normal fetal heart.
8. Adequate personnel must be available to watch the patient.
9. The patient must be examined carefully before the oxytocin is started.
10. The doctor in charge of the case should:
    a. Examine the patient himself before the drip is set up
    b. Be present when the infusion is started
    c. Observe the patient and the fetal heart for the first few contractions. He should then regulate the speed.
    d. Not order the drip by telephone
    e. Be in hospital and available while the drip is running
11. The response of the human uterus to intravenous oxytocin increases with the length of pregnancy, reaching a peak in the thirty-sixth week. After this the reactiveness changes little. Induction is as successful in the thirty-sixth to thirty-ninth weeks as later. However in the earlier period the induction takes longer, and more oxytocin is needed.

CONTRAINDICATIONS TO THE USE OF OXYTOCIN

1. Absence of proper indication
2. Absence of the prerequisites
3. Disproportion, generally contracted pelvis, and obstruction by tumors
4. Grand multiparity: There is too great a chance of uterine rupture.
5. Previous cesarean section
6. Hypertonic or incoordinate uterus: The hypertonic or incoordinate uterus will be made worse by oxytocin and may lead to a constriction ring.
7. Maternal exhaustion: This condition should be treated by rest and fluids, not by oxytocin stimulation.
8. Fetal distress: Not only should oxytocin not be given, but the appearance of an irregular or slow heart while the drip is running demands that it be stopped.
9. Abnormal presentation and position of all types
10. Unengaged head
11. Congenital anomalies of the uterus

DANGERS OF OXYTOCIN

Maternal

1. Uterine rupture
2. Cervical and vaginal lacerations
3. Hemorrhage from lacerations

4. Hemorrhage from uterine atony post partum
5. Death

The danger lies in the fact that if the patient is sensitive to the drug, she may get hard and even tetanic contractions which will be enough to rupture the uterus, where ordinary contractions would do no harm. So, too, the excessively rapid passage of the baby through the pelvis may cause extensive lacerations.

Fetal

1. Anoxia caused by contractions that are too hard, too frequent, and last too long: The uterus never relaxes enough to maintain adequate circulation. In some cases separation of the placenta has taken place.
2. Damage to the baby from too rapid propulsion through the pelvis
3. Forcing the fetus through a pelvis which is too small for it
4. In a large series it was shown that the signs of fetal distress are more common in patients receiving an oxytocin drip than in those without stimulation of labor. In almost all instances slowing or stopping the oxytocin infusion resulted in the rapid return to normal of the fetal heart. The incidence of emergency obstetric intervention was no higher, and the final fetal results were comparable.

SPARTEINE SULFATE

Sparteine sulfate is an alkaloid derived from the plant Cytisus scoparius (Scotch broom). It has the property of increasing the intensity, frequency, and duration of uterine contractions.

For induction of labor the dosage is 150 mg given intramuscularly every hour to a maximum of three doses or 450 mg. Once labor has started, no more is given. Because some patients react strongly to the drug, it has been suggested that the first dose be only 75 mg.

The original claims that the drug has no side effects, that the margin of safety is wide, that it poses no danger to mother and child, and that constant supervision is not required during its administration, have not been borne out by further experience. Sparteine sulfate is not a safe oxytocic. The same care must be exercised as with any other oxytocic drug.

Advantages of sparteine sulfate include:

1. Administration to the patient is easy.
2. Induction is successful in many cases.
3. Labor is shortened.
4. It is a simple way of getting labor into the active phase.

Disadvantages and dangers include:
1. Uterine hypertonus and tetanic contractions
2. Tumultuous labor and delivery
3. Rupture of uterus and lacerations of the cervix
4. Separation of the placenta from the uterus
5. Fetal distress
6. The intramuscular injection is unpredictable and potentially dangerous.

7. There is great variability in the effect of sparteine, not only in different patients, but in the same patient from one injection to the next.

Sparteine sulfate may be used under these conditions:

1. It is an efficient oxytocic drug.
2. Its use requires the same constant and careful supervision as any other oxytonic drug.
3. The prerequisites and contraindications to its administration are the same as those given for oxytocin.
4. The safest time for its use is during the latent phase when the cervix is effaced and dilated to 3 cm. By giving one injection of 150 mg the labor can be lifted into the active phase in many cases.
5. Sparteine should never be given when the patient is in active labor. Sudden tumultuous contractions may ensue.
6. Sparteine sulfate must not be given concomitantly with oxytocin. At least 2 hours must elapse before a change is made from one agent to the other.
7. There is no advantage in using sparteine rather than oxytocin. On the contrary we have found oxytocin to be more efficient, more reliable, and more predictable.

BIBLIOGRAPHY

Cromer, D. W., Reeves, B. D., and Danforth, D. N. Sparteine sulfate in the conduct of labor. Amer. J. Gynec., 89:268, 1964.

Donnelly, J. F. The proper use of posterior pituitary extract in pregnancy. North Carolina Med. J., 18:191, 1957.

Engström, L. Induction of labour around full term especially by means of synthetic oxytocin in intravenous drip. Acta Obstet Gynec. Scandinav., 38:suppl. 3, 1959.

Munsick, R. A. The pharmacology and clinical application of various oxytocic drugs. Amer. J. Obstet. Gynec., 93:442, 1965.

Newton, B. W., Benson, R. C., and McCorriston, C. C. Sparteine sulfate: A potent, capricious oxytocic. Amer. J. Obstet. Gynec., 94:234, 1966.

Page, E. W. The usefulness of intravenous pitocin infusions in obstetrics. West. J. Obstet. Gynec., 62:125, 1954.

Schulman, H., and Ledger, W. Sparteine sulfate: A clinical study of 711 patients. Obstet. Gynec., 25:542, 1965.

Silva, P., and Allan, M. S. Water intoxication due to high doses of synthetic oxytocin. Obstet. Gynec., 27:517, 1966.

Sogolow, S. R. An historical review of the use of oxytocin prior to delivery. Obstet. Gynec. Survey, 21:155, 1966.

Stewart, R. H., and Slezak, R. M. Synthetic and natural oxytocins. Obstet. Gynec., 11:295, 1958.

Stone, M. L., and Tanz, A. Intravenous administration of posterior pituitary extract before and during labor. Obstet. Gynec., 1:346, 1953.

37 Fetopelvic Disproportion

Definition: This term refers to the inability of the fetus to pass through the pelvis. Disproportion may be absolute or relative. It is absolute when under no circumstances can the baby pass safely through the birth canal. Relative disproportion is present when other factors contribute to the problem. Minor degrees of pelvic contraction can be overcome by efficient uterine contractions; dilatability of the soft tissues; favorable attitude, presentation, and position of the fetus; and moldability of the fetal head. On the other hand, poor contractions, rigid soft parts, abnormal position, and inability of the head to mold properly can make vaginal delivery impossible.

THE PASSAGE

Pelvic Size

While the important question is the relationship between a given pelvis and a particular fetus, in some cases the contraction of the pelvis is such that no normal fetus can pass through. The reduced size may be at any level: the inlet, midpelvis, or outlet. Sometimes the pelvis may be small in all planes—the generally contracted pelvis.

Inlet Contraction

Inlet contraction is present when the anteroposterior diameter (obstetric conjugate) is less than 10.0 cm, or the transverse diameter is less than 12.0 cm. Inlet contraction may result from rickets or from generally poor development.

Effect on the fetus:

1. Failure of engagement
2. Increase in malpositions
3. Deflexion attitudes
4. Exaggerated asynclitism
5. Extreme molding
6. Formation of a large caput succedaneum
7. Prolapse of the umbilical cord: This becomes a complication since the presenting part does not fit the inlet well.

Effect on labor:

1. Dilatation of the cervix is slow and often incomplete.
2. Premature rupture of the membranes is common.
3. Inefficient uterine action is a frequent accompaniment.

Midpelvic Contraction

Midpelvic contraction is basically a reduction in the plane of least dimensions, the one that passes from the apex of the pubic arch, through the ischial spines, to meet the sacrum usually at the junction of the fourth and fifth segments.

When the distance between the ischial spines is less than 9.0 cm, or when the sum of the interspinous (normal is 10.5 cm) and the posterior sagittal (normal is 4.5 to 5.0 cm) distances is less than 13.5 cm (normal is 15.0 to 15.5 cm), contraction of the midpelvis is probably present. To obtain accurate measurement of these diameters x-ray pelvimetry is essential. Clinical suspicion of a small midpelvis is aroused by the finding on manual examination of a small pelvis, the palpation of large spines which jut into the cavity, and the observation that the distance between the ischial tuberosities is less than 8.5 cm.

Midpelvic contraction is a common cause of dystocia and operative delivery. It is more difficult to manage than inlet contraction. For, if the fetal head cannot even enter the inlet there is no doubt that abdominal delivery is necessary. But once the head has descended into the pelvis one is loathe to perform cesarean section, and hope that the head will come down to a point where it can be extracted with forceps. A danger here is that with molding and caput formation one may believe that the head is lower than it actually is. Instead of the projected midforceps delivery one is engaged in a high forceps operation, often with disastrous results for both patients.

Midpelvic contractions may prevent anterior rotation of the occiput and may direct it into the hollow of the sacrum. Failure of rotation and deflexion attitudes are associated frequently with a small pelvic cavity.

Outlet Contraction

Outlet contraction is present when the distance between the ischial tuberosities is less than 8.0 cm. Dystocia may be expected when the sum of the intertuberous diameter and the posterior sagittal diameter is much less than 15.0 cm. Diminution of the intertuberous diameter and the subpubic angle will force the head backward, and so the prognosis depends on the capacity of the posterior segment, the mobility at the sacrococcygeal joint, and the ability of the soft tissues to accommodate the passenger. The sides of the posterior triangle are not bony.

While outlet contraction causes an increase in perineal lacerations and a greater need for forceps deliveries, only in the rare instance of the absence of inlet or midpelvic dystocia is it an indication for cesarean section. Because, however, the bituberous diameter can be measured manually and since it may warn us that there is contraction higher in the pelvis, it should always be assessed as part of the routine examination.

Delay at the outlet may be caused by a rigid perineum. The tissues do not stretch well, and when they tear, a large uncontrolled laceration results. Treatment is by mediolateral episiotomy as soon as the problem is recognized.

The Influence of Pelvic Shape

The obstetric capacity of the female pelvis is governed by: 1, the size and 2, the shape or configuration. By radiologic technics accurate classification by shape is more reliable than precise measurement of diameters. Hence, with the exception of cases of extreme contraction, we feel that in attempting prognosis, the type of pelvis is more important than the size. These factors complement each other. A poor class of pelvis may be compensated for by being large. Or, a relatively small pelvis may function well because of a favorable shape.

The Gynecoid Pelvis

The gynecoid or normal female pelvis offers the best diameters in all three planes for the uncomplicated passage of the fetus.

The Android Pelvis

The android or male pelvis has a bad obstetric reputation. With reduced posterior segments in all pelvic planes, the occiput has a tendency to enter the inlet posteriorly, is impeded in rotation in the midpelvis, and is forced posteriorly at the outlet. The results are arrest of descent, failure of rotation, and lacerations of the perineum and the rectum.

The Anthropoid Pelvis

In the anthropoid pelvis the reduced transverse measurements in the various planes are only relative and are compensated for by large anteroposterior diameters. The head descends often in the occipitoposterior position with surprising ease and is born frequently face to pubis. In general the prognosis is better than that of the android or platypelloid types.

The Platypelloid Pelvis

In the platypelloid pelvis there is interference with entry of the presenting part into the inlet, and there may be difficulty at the lower levels as well. In this group is found the highest incidence of cesarean section.

Mixed Types

A gynecoid or anthropoid pelvis may have an android-like narrowing at the midpelvis or the outlet. Thus the head will enter the pelvis but will become arrested lower down. Minor forms of funnelling are common and are frequent causes of forceps extractions. In these situations the size of the fetal head, the degree of flexion, and the capacity for molding are critical factors. Even a slight variation in the presenting dimensions will make a great difference in the ease or difficulty of the delivery.

Abnormal Pelves

There are numerous varieties of grossly abnormal pelves which are associated with deformity and contraction. Fortunately these are not common and
do not play a prominent part in the problem of fetopelvic disproportion.

Kyphosis

With rare exception women with kyphosis of the spine have poor pelves,
and need delivery by cesarean section. Every pregnant kyphotic should be examined by x-ray pelvimetry. Many of these women have associated heart disease and require careful management.

Scoliosis

With scoliosis of the lower part of the spine the sacrum is affected, and
asymmetry of the pelvis results.

Bony Disease of the Femurs and Acetabula

Bony disease of the femurs and acetabula, by causing abnormal pressures
on the pelvis during development, may result in asymmetry and reduction of
pelvic capacity.

Extremely Rare Abnormalities

Naegele pelvis: There is absence or imperfect development of one wing of
the sacrum. The pelvis is contracted obliquely.

Robert pelvis: Both wings of the sacrum fail to develop, so the transverse
diameter is contracted markedly.

Split pelvis: There is failure of union between the pubic bones. This is often associated with nonunion of the walls of the bladder and the anterior abdomen.

Assimilation pelvis: This is an elongated pelvis in which the last lumbar
or first coccygeal vertebra resembles a sacral vertebra, and seems to be part
of the sacrum rather than the lumbar spine or the coccyx.

Osteomalacic pelvis: There is softening of the bones which bend into the
cavity of the pelvis. This reduces all the diameters greatly.

Spondylolisthetic pelvis: The last lumbar vertebra is displaced forward and
downward over the sacral promontory. Pregnancy may aggravate the condition
to the extent that symptoms appear for the first time. Prolonged labor and operative delivery are common.

The Soft Tissues

While poor dilatability of the muscles and fascia of the pelvis rarely causes
severe disproportion in itself, in cases of borderline bony disproportion or poor
uterine action it may make the difference between vaginal delivery or cesarean
section. The rare case has been reported of a septum in the vagina causing
obstruction. It must be excised before the baby can be born.

Neoplasms

Uterine fibromyomata or ovarian cysts may block the birth canal and prevent the passage of the fetus through the pelvis. A large fibromyoma of the vagina can block the passage of the child. It should be removed before or during the pregnancy. If this is not feasible, cesarean section is necessary.

THE PASSENGER

Fetal Size

Fetal size is important. Rarely a baby is too large for any pelvis. The essential problem is the relationship of the child to the pelvis. The question which must be answered is: Can this baby pass through this pelvis?

Oversized Fetus

Definition: The excessively large fetus is defined as one weighing either 4,500 g (9 pounds, 15 ounces) or 10 pounds (4,545 g).

Incidence

The incidence varies between 0.5 to 1.8 percent.

Etiology

The following factors are associated with the oversized fetus:

1. It is more common in white women.
2. There is a familial tendency.
3. In 80 percent the patient is multiparous.
4. There is a slightly higher incidence in older women.
5. Maternal weight gain is often excessive.
6. The incidence of overt or subclinical diabetic mothers is high.
7. Toxemia of pregnancy is a little more common.
8. Often the pregnancy is longer than 40 weeks.
9. Two thirds of the babies are male.

Diagnosis

There is no accurate way of determining fetal size in utero. Estimation of fetal size by abdominal palpation is inexact. In most cases the diagnosis is made at delivery and the problem arises as an emergency.

Labor

1. In over 90 percent the presentation is cephalic.
2. The length of labor is not prolonged.
3. There is usually no trouble delivering the head.
4. Shoulder dystocia occurs frequently.

Delivery

1. Many babies are born spontaneously or by low forceps.
2. There is an increased incidence of mid forceps, cesarean section, and operations to relieve shoulder dystocia.
3. Destructive operations (craniotomy and cleidotomy) were used many years ago, but with modern diagnosis and x-ray pelvimetry, cesarean section has obviated the need for these procedures.
4. To improve maternal and fetal results cesarean section may be performed more often.

Maternal Complications

1. Lacerations of the genital tract
2. Postpartum hemorrhage from uterine atony and lacerations
3. Separation of the pubic symphysis

Fetal Complications

1. Infant mortality is increased.
2. There is a higher incidence of serious injury.
3. Among central nervous system complications are fractured skull, intracranial hemorrhage, and brain damage by compression.
4. Peripheral neurologic damage includes Erb's and brachial palsy, as well as nonspecific paralyses.
5. Fractures of the humerus, femur, and clavicle are seen.

Attitude and Position

In borderline pelves a well-flexed head in a good occipitoanterior position may deliver normally, while face presentation or an occipitoposterior will become arrested.

Moldability

Moldability of the fetal head may be critical. The ability of the head to change its shape to fit the pelvis may enable it to negotiate safely the birth canal. Excessive molding can damage the brain, and this must be considered in deciding whether vaginal delivery is to be awaited. A reduction of more than 0.5 cm in the biparietal diameter is considered dangerous.

Fetal Abdominal Enlargement

This rare condition may cause dystocia. The diagnosis is made after the head is born, and the trunk cannot be delivered. The fetal mortality is high because: 1, intrauterine death may take place; 2, the causal condition is incompatible with extrauterine life; and 3, the trauma of a difficult birth may be lethal. There are several varieties:

1. Generalized edema of all organs and cavities. This is associated with diabetic mothers, erythroblastosis, and toxemia of pregnancy.
2. Ascites (3 to 4 liters) is often associated with abnormalities of the urinary tract and is more common in males. Perforation of the abdomen or thorax is usually necessary before birth can be effected.

3. Distention of the urinary tract caused by vesical neck obstruction
4. Polycystic kidneys may cause dystocia.
5. Fluid collection in and distention of the female genital tract as a result of vaginal atresia
6. Cystic or tumerous liver

UTERINE CONTRACTIONS

Strong uterine contractions should not be allowed or relied upon to push a baby through a pelvis where there is absolute disproportion. In borderline cases, however, where there are minor degrees of disproportion, uterine efficiency may be the essential difference between success and failure.

INVESTIGATION OF DISPROPORTION

In attempting to determine whether a given baby can be born per vaginam without serious injury to itself or to the mother, the following investigative procedures are carried out: 1, history; 2, abdominal palpation; 3, vaginal examination; 4, radiologic studies; and 5, trial labor.

History

To an extent the information which is sought varies with the parity of the patient. If there have been previous pregnancies and labors the details of these are of great help in determining the prognosis. In patients who are pregnant for the first time other information is elicited to aid in making the decisions.

Multipara

1. The number of children and the number of pregnancies
2. The size of the babies at birth, especially the largest. Many women tend to have progressively larger babies, and the knowledge that a 6 pound child was delivered with no difficulty does not guarantee the same success with an 8 pound baby.
3. The condition of the children at birth, including any damaged children or intrapartum deaths
4. The length of labor
5. The method of delivery
6. Maternal lacerations

Most labors and deliveries subsequent to the first are easier. The pelvic joints and soft tissues, once stretched, offer less resistance.

Primigravida

1. The age of the patient: For the purpose of childbearing a woman is said to be as old as her cervix. While some clinics consider that a woman is not an elderly primigravida until she reaches 40, in many institutions 35 years of age is taken as the dividing line. Many elderly primigravidas will ripen the cervix well, will push the presenting part into the pelvis even before labor has started, and will have an easy, spontaneous delivery. An equal number, however, will have difficulties. Hence, all older women who are pregnant for the first time merit careful investigation.

2. The type of menstrual cycle: The type of menstrual cycle is important. Women whose menses were late in starting, were irregular, and were attended with severe dysmenorrhea, have a tendency toward difficult labor.
3. Sterility: Women with a history of involuntary sterility for seven or eight years often have worrisome labors with uterine dysfunction, soft tissue dystocia, and operative deliveries.
4. Familial history: Information about the patient's mother and sisters is important. A history of dystocia with injured or dead babies calls for an especially careful investigation.

Failure of Engagement

While any doubt as to the pelvic adequacy must be resolved by thorough examination, one of the most common problems is the unengaged head in the primigravida near term. In the majority of primigravidas with normal pelves the head engages about three weeks before term. Breeches, on the other hand, often do not engage until good labor has set in.

In about 5 percent of primigravidas the head will be unengaged at term. Since most of these will deliver per vaginam there is no need to panic, but the persistence of nonengagement is an indication for complete study to determine the cause for the failure of descent.

Abdominal Palpation

The patient lies on her back on the examining table in as relaxed a condition as possible. First the position is ascertained. Then with one hand the examiner presses the head gently but firmly into the pelvic brim. The fingers of the other hand are applied to the area of the abdomen above the pubic symphysis. As pressure is being applied the examiner determines whether the head will enter the inlet of the pelvis, or whether it overrides the pubis and fails to enter the superior strait. If the head can be pushed into the pelvis it suggests that there is no disproportion at the inlet. If it does not go in, further investigation must be carried out.

Causes of failure to descend or overriding include:

1. Disproportion
2. Malpresentation or malposition
3. Underdeveloped lower uterine segment
4. Polyhydramnios
5. Placenta previa
6. Soft tissue tumor blocking the pelvis
7. Full bladder or rectum
8. Patient not close enough to term, a situation often associated with an underdeveloped lower segment

Vaginal and Combined Abdominopelvic Examination

This is the most important procedure in the assessment of fetopelvic disproportion. The patient should be positioned on a table in the lithotomy position to ensure adequate examination. Sometimes the discomfort is such that a short anesthetic is necessary. (See Ch. 9 for details of procedure.)

The inner walls of the inlet, cavity, and outlet of the pelvis are palpated to estimate their capacities and to search for abnormalities. The length, dilatation, and consistency of the cervix are determined. The elasticity of the soft tissues (muscles, fascia, and ligaments) are checked to see whether they are likely to stretch or prevent the head from descending.

The position of the presenting part is noted, as well as its ability to flex. Extreme asynclitism is a bad sign. Pressure is applied to the presenting part over the pubis and to the fundus of the uterus to see whether it can be forced down to the level of the ischial spines, or further. If this can be accomplished by manual pressure, then one can assume that strong uterine contractions will have no difficulty in doing the same.

These examinations should allow the patient to be placed into one of three categories:

1. No disproportion is present. This infant should go through this pelvis.
2. Absolute fetopelvic disproportion
3. The fetopelvic relationship is borderline. X-ray pelvimetry and a trial of labor are indicated.

Radiographic Examination

In all doubtful cases x-ray pelvimetry is performed to obtain additional valuable information (see Ch. 42).

Trial Labor

This is a clinical attempt to evaluate the extent of cephalopelvic disproportion. The patient is allowed to labor under close supervision to see if the natural forces of labor can overcome real or suspected disproportion. It is also an excellent measure of the labor mechanism, which will often determine the success or failure of the trial.

First a careful study is made of the pelvic adequacy in the light of the size and presentation of the baby. If gross disproportion is encountered cesarean section should be elected.

The patient is allowed to go into labor spontaneously. Trial labor is never induced either by artificial rupture of the membranes or by oxytocin infusion. Once the cervix is half dilated the membranes may be ruptured to see if progress can be improved.

During the labor the following factors are evaluated:

1. The mental and physical condition of the mother
2. The fetal heart rate as well as other signs of fetal distress, such as the passage of meconium
3. The force and coordination of the uterine contractions
4. The dilatation of the cervix
5. The descent of the presenting part
6. The degree of molding and the formation and size of the caput succedaneum

There are no satisfactory arbitrary time limits for trial labor. It may last from 6 to 18 hours, rarely to 24 hours. This is sufficient time to decide the degree of disproportion and, what is equally important, to demonstrate the effectiveness of the uterine mechanism. Good labor will often overcome small degrees of disproportion. The exact length of a trial labor for a specific case is a matter of judgment, and can be determined only by the attending obstetrician and his consultant.

Needless rectal or vaginal examinations should be avoided. They are painful and predispose to infection. At the end of a reasonable period of labor a careful vaginal examination is made under aseptic conditions to evaluate the state of the cervix, the fetal position and presentation, and the station of the presenting part. On the basis of these findings the decision is made as to the success or failure of the trial.

Favorable progress of cervical effacement and dilatation, descent of the head into the pelvis, and the demonstration that the lower part of the pelvis is adequate, are the criteria for continuing the trial.

A poor labor mechanism with irregular, desultory, and ineffective contractions, the lack of effacement and progressive dilatation of the cervix, and the failure of the head to enter the inlet and descend to the ischial spines are evidences that the trial of labor has failed and that other means of delivery are to be sought.

The old time test of labor, which is no longer used, lasted long enough for the cervix to become fully dilated, followed by a sufficiently long second stage with the membranes ruptured to demonstrate beyond a doubt that the head would not progress down the pelvic canal. Common complications were infection of the amniotic cavity, formation of a pathologic contraction ring, and uterine rupture. The fetal loss was 25 percent. Fetal and maternal damage could never be evaluated accurately. Thus while a patient should be given the opportunity to achieve a safe vaginal delivery, the trial of labor must not be carried to a dangerous extreme.

TREATMENT OF FETOPELVIC DISPROPORTION

Cesarean Section

Cesarean section is the method of choice where a marked degree of disproportion is present. The low transverse incision in the uterus is preferred by most.

Forceps

When the disproportion is minor, when the arrest is caused by failure of flexion or rotation, and when the obstetrician has experience, low or mid forceps may be used to effect delivery. If, however, extraction by forceps would entail a difficult and traumatic procedure, it is wiser to turn to cesarean section.

Other Procedures

Rarely used procedures:

1. Induction of premature labor, to try to deliver the baby while it is smaller, was once a popular procedure to overcome disproportion. The drawbacks are:

    a. Prematurity with its attendant complications

    b. A poorly formed lower uterine segment with its resistant tissues

    c. The unripe cervix

    d. Inefficient function of the uterus which is stimulated into labor before its polarity and coordinate action have been established

    e. Prolonged labor

    For these reasons we feel that it is preferable to allow the patient to have a trial of labor at term and to perform cesarean section, if necessary, rather than induce labor prematurely.

2. Symphysiotomy or pubiotomy has been used, especially in cases of severe outlet contraction, to make the pelvic diameters larger and so to enable the vaginal delivery of a head which is impacted low in the pelvis. Because of injury to the bladder, disruption of the urethra, urinary fistulas, local sepsis, and permanent weakening of the pelvic girdle, this procedure is almost never used today in western countries. In places where cesarean section is not available because of local conditions, surgical separation of the pubic symphysis is employed with good results.

3. Craniotomy has no place in the planned treatment of disproportion. It is permissible only for dead babies in situations where the fetus is not deliverable intact, and its aim is to spare the mother an operative abdominal delivery.

BIBLIOGRAPHY

Collin, H. A., Ellis, A. H., and Evans, E. F. The problem of the oversized fetus. Amer. J. Obstet. Gynec., 75:742, 1958.

Greig, D. S. Symphysiotomy. J. Obstet. Gynaec. Brit. Emp., 61:192, 1954.

Nathanson, J. N. The excessively large fetus as an obstetric problem. Amer. J. Obstet. Gynec., 60:54, 1950.

Radman, H. M. Dystocia due to fetal abdominal enlargement. Obstet. Gynec., 19:481, 1962.

Seedat, E. K., and Crichton, D. Symphysiotomy: Technique, indications and limitations. Lancet, March: 554, 1962.

Trelford, J. D. Spondylolisthesis and pregnancy. Amer. J. Obstet. Gynec., 91:320, 1965.

38 Obstetric Trauma, Accidents, Operations

EPISIOTOMY

Definition: An episiotomy (perineotomy) is an incision into the perineum to enlarge the space at the outlet, thereby facilitating the birth of the child.

Advantages to the Mother: Advantages of this procedure are:

1. A straight incision is simpler to repair and heals better than a jagged, uncontrolled laceration.
2. By making the episiotomy before the muscles and fascia are stretched excessively, the strength of the pelvic floor can be preserved and the incidence of uterine prolapse, cystocele, and rectocele reduced.
3. The structures in front are protected as well as those in the rear. By increasing the room available posteriorly, there is less stretching of and less damage to the anterior vaginal wall, the bladder, the urethra, and the periclitoral tissues.
4. Tears into the rectum can be avoided.

Advantages to the Child: A well-timed episiotomy not only makes the birth easier but lessens the pounding of the head on the perineum and so helps avert brain damage. This is true for any baby, but is especially important for those who have a low resistance to trauma, such as premature infants, babies born to diabetic mothers, and those with erythroblastosis.

Indications for Episiotomy: Indications are:

1. Prophylactic: To preserve the integrity of the pelvic floor
2. Arrest of progress by a resistant perineum
   a. Thick and heavily muscled tissue
   b. Operative scars
   c. Previous well-repaired episiotomy
3. To obviate uncontrolled tears, including extension into the rectum
   a. When the perineum is short, there being little room between the back of the vagina and the front of the rectum
   b. Where large lacerations seem inevitable
4. Fetal reasons
   a. Premature and infirm babies
   b. Large infants
   c. Abnormal positions such as occipitoposteriors, face presentations, and breeches
   d. Fetal distress, where there is need for rapid delivery of the baby and dilatation of the perineum cannot be awaited

The Proper Time to Make the Episiotomy: Made too late, the procedure fails to prevent lacerations and to protect the pelvic floor. Made too soon, the incision leads to needless loss of blood.

The episiotomy is made when the perineum is bulging, when a 3 to 4 cm diameter of fetal scalp is visible during a contraction, and when the presenting part will be delivered with the next 3 or 4 contractions. In this way lacerations are avoided, overstretching of the pelvic floor is prevented, and excessive bleeding is obviated.

Types of Episiotomy: Classification is made into:

1. Midline
2. Mediolateral, left or right
3. Lateral episiotomy, which is no longer used

Midline Episiotomy

Technic of the Midline Episiotomy

In making the incision two fingers are placed in the vagina between the fetal head and the perineum. Outward pressure is made on the perineum, away from the fetus, to avoid injury to the baby. The scissors* are placed so that one blade lies against the vaginal mucosa and the other on the skin. The incision is made in the midline from the fourchette almost to, but not through, the external fibers of the anal sphincter. The cut is in the central tendinous portion of the perineal body to which are attached the bulbocavernosus muscle in front, the superficial transverse perineal and part of the levator ani muscles at the sides, and the anal sphincter behind. This is an excellent anatomic incision.

Advantages of the Midline Episiotomy

1. The muscle belly is not cut.
2. It is easy to make and easy to repair.
3. The structural results are excellent.
4. Bleeding is less than with other incisions.
5. Postoperative pain is minimal.
6. Healing is superior and dehiscence is rare.

Disadvantages of the Midline Episiotomy

The one drawback is that should there be extension of the incision as the head is being born, the anal sphincter will be torn and the rectum entered. Although most bowel injuries heal well if repaired properly, this accident should be avoided. Median episiotomies are not ideal in the following situations:

1. Short perineum
2. Large baby
3. Abnormal positions and presentations
4. Difficult operative deliveries

*Some operators prefer using the scalpel.

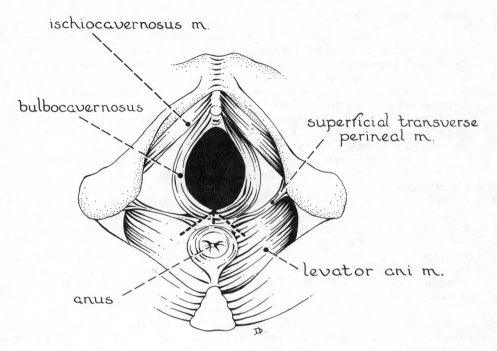

Fig. 1. The muscles of the pelvic floor and perineum. The sites of median and mediolateral episiotomy are shown.

Fig. 2. The incision of the midline episiotomy.

Repair of Midline Episiotomy

Since in most cases the third stage is completed soon after the birth of the child, the repair of the episiotomy is performed after the placenta is delivered, the uterus contracted, and the cervix and vagina found to be uninjured. Not only are intrauterine procedures, such as manual removal of the placenta, and intravaginal procedures more difficult to perform after the episiotomy has been closed, but the repair may be broken down.

Except for the subcuticular layer a medium round Ferguson needle is employed. In the deep tissues a cutting edge needle may lacerate a blood vessel and cause a hematoma. Our preference is for 000 chromic catgut.

First the vaginal mucosa is sewn together. The procedure is begun at the top of the incision, the first bite being taken a little above the apex to include any retracted blood vessel. The suture is tied leaving one end long. The edges of the wound are then approximated, but not strangulated, using a simple continuous or a lock stitch to assure hemostasis. Each bite includes the mucous membrane of the vagina and the tissue between the vagina and rectum. This reduces bleeding, eliminates dead space, and makes for better healing. The repair is carried past the hymenal ring to the skin edges. The last two bites include the subcutaneous tissue at the base of the episiotomy, but do not come through the skin. This end of the continuous suture may be tied, or it may be left untied and held with a hemostat.

The second stitch near the base of the wound is the crown suture. The needle passes under the skin deeply enough to catch and bring together the separated and retracted ends of the bulbocavernosus muscle and fascia. The crown suture is important. For, if these tissues are approximated too tightly coitus will be painful. If the repair is too loose, the introitus will gape.

Next the transverse perineal and levator ani muscles and fascia are approximated in the midline anterior to the rectum with three or four interrupted sutures. One layer is enough in most cases.

Finally the incision is closed by one of several methods:

1. The skin edges are united by interrupted, or mattress, sutures which pass through the skin and subcutaneous tissue. These are tied loosely to prevent strangulation as postpartum swelling takes place (Fig. 3D).
2. The skin edges are approximated using a continuous subcuticular stitch on a small cutting needle, starting at the lower end of the incision. The first bite is taken in the subcuticular tissue, just under, but not through, the skin, going from side to side until the base (upper end) of the wound is reached. Here it is tied separately, or if the suture used to repair the vaginal mucosa has been left untied, this suture and the subcuticular one are tied together. This completes the repair (Fig. 4D).

A.

A. Closure of the vaginal mucosa by a continuous suture.

B.

B. The crown suture, reuniting the divided bulbocavernous muscle.

C.

D.

C. Drawing together the perineal muscles and fascia with interrupted sutures.

D. Approximation of the skin edges with interrupted sutures.

Fig. 3. Repair of the midline episiotomy.

Aftercare of the Episiotomy

Aftercare of the episiotomy is essentially a matter of cleanliness. The perineum is cleaned with a mildly antiseptic solution after each urination and bowel evacuation. Heat, as from an electric bulb, may be used to dry the area and to reduce the swelling. Daily showers and washing with mild soap and water are excellent ways of keeping the perineum clean and free from irritating discharges. Several investigators have used oral proteolytic enzymes with success in reducing pain and edema.

Mediolateral Episiotomy

When a large episiotomy is needed, or when there is danger of rectal involvement, the mediolateral variety is advised. Included here are patients with short perineum, contracted outlets, large babies, face to pubis deliveries, attitudes of extension, breech births, and midforceps operations.

Technic

The incision is made from the midline of the posterior fourchette toward the ischial tuberosity, far enough laterally to avoid the anal sphincter. The average episiotomy is about 4 cm long and may reach the fatty tissues of the ischiorectal fossa. Whether it is placed on the left or right side is unimportant.
The following structures are cut:
1. Skin and subcutaneous tissue
2. Bulbocavernosus muscle and fascia
3. Transverse perineal muscle
4. Levator ani muscle and fascia. The extent to which this structure is involved is determined by the length and depth of the incision.

Repair of the Mediolateral Episiotomy

The technic is essentially the same as for the median perineotomy. The vaginal mucosa is repaired starting at the apex, and bringing together the mucous membrane and the underlying supporting tissue. The crown suture is placed carefully.
The muscles and fascia which were cut are approximated with interrupted sutures. The tissues on the medial side tend to retract, and care must be taken not to enter the rectum. Some operators prefer to place these sutures, leaving them untied, before the vaginal mucosa is repaired. In many patients a single layer of four or five stitches is sufficient. When the wound is deep or when there is much bleeding two layers may be necessary, one in the muscles, and one to bring together the overlying fascia. The skin edges are joined by a subcuticular stitch, beginning at the apex, or by interrupted sutures through skin and subcutaneous tissue.

A.

B.

B. The crown suture.

A. Closure of the vaginal mucosa by a continuous suture.

C.

D.

C. Drawing together the perineal muscles and fascia with interrupted sutures.

D. Approximation of the skin edges with a continuous subcuticular suture.

Fig. 4. Repair of left mediolateral episiotomy.

Disruption of the Episiotomy

Etiology

Like incisions in other parts of the body, an episiotomy may dehisce. Predisposing factors include:

1. Poor healing powers
   a. Nutritional deficiencies
   b. Anemia
   c. Exhaustion after a long and difficult labor
   d. Avascular scarred tissue
2. Failure of technic
   a. Careless approximation of the wound
   b. Incomplete hemostasis leading to hematoma formation
   c. Failure to obliterate dead space
3. Devitalization of tissue
   a. The use of crushing instruments
   b. Strangulation of tissue by tying sutures too tightly
   c. The employment of too heavy catgut
4. Infection
   a. Infected lochia in puerperal sepsis
   b. Poor technic and neglect of aseptic standards
   c. Proximity of the rectum
   d. Extension of the incision into, or passage of the needle through, the bowel
   e. Sepsis in a hematoma
   f. Improper postpartum cleanliness

Clinical Course

The episiotomy becomes extremely painful, tender, swollen, red, and indurated. The patient may or may not have fever. Sometimes there is a discharge from the incision. By the fourth or fifth day the edges of the wound separate.

Management of Disruption

Management of disruption is either supportive or operative.

Supportive: The area is kept clean and free from irritating discharge and debris by warm sitz baths twice daily for 20 minutes. If this procedure is not feasible warm compresses of saline or magnesium sulphate are used. Following this the perineum is lamped for 30 minutes. The wound granulates in and heals from the deep layers up. The patient may go home at the usual time and continue the treatment there. Unless there has been damage to the rectum this management has always been successful in our experience. The wound heals well, no aftereffects are noted, and prolonged hospitalization is avoided.

Secondary Repair: Supportive treatment is carried on until the area is clean. This takes five or six days. Then the patient is anesthetized, the devitalized tissue is debrided, and the episiotomy is repaired.

In our experience supportive therapy alone has given the best results and is the simplest to carry out.

A late complication of an infected episiotomy is a rectovaginal fistula. This results from an unrecognized tear of the rectum or from a suture being passed through the rectal wall and left there.

LACERATIONS OF THE PERINEUM

Many women suffer tears of the perineum at the birth of the first child. In about half the cases these tears are extensive. Lacerations must be repaired carefully.

Maternal Causes

1. Precipitate, uncontrolled, or unattended delivery. This is the most frequent cause.
2. The patient's inability to stop bearing down
3. Hastening the delivery by excessive fundal pressure
4. Edema and friability of the perineum
5. Vulvar varicosities weakening the tissue
6. Narrow pubic arch with outlet contraction, forcing the head posteriorly
7. Extension of midline episiotomy

Fetal Factors

1. Large baby
2. Abnormal positions of the head, e.g., occipitoposterior and face presentations
3. Breech deliveries
4. Difficult forceps extractions
5. Shoulder dystocia
6. Congenital anomalies, such as hydrocephaly

Classification of Perineal Lacerations

First Degree Tear

First degree tear involves the vaginal mucosa, the fourchette, and the skin of the perineum just below it.

Repair of First Degree Lacerations: These tears are small and are repaired as simply as possible. The aim is the reapproximation of the divided tissue and hemostasis. In the average case a few interrupted sutures through the vaginal mucosa, the fourchette, and the skin of the perineum are enough. If bleeding is profuse, figure of 8 stitches may be used. Interrupted sutures, loosely tied, are best for the skin because they cause less tension and less discomfort to the patient.

Second Degree Tears

Second degree lacerations are deeper. They are mainly in the midline and extend through the perineal body. Often the transverse perineal muscle is torn and the rent may go down to, but not through, the rectal sphincter. Usually the tear extends upward along the vaginal mucosa and the submucosal tissue. This gives the laceration a doubly triangular appearance with the base at the four-chette, one apex in the vagina, and the other near the rectum.

Repair of Second Degree Lacerations: Repair of second degree lacerations is in layers:

1. Interrupted, continuous, or lock stitches are used to approximate the edges of the vaginal mucosa and submucosa.
2. The deep muscles of the perineal body are sewn together with interrupted sutures.
3. A running subcuticular suture or interrupted sutures, loosely tied, bring together the skin edges.

A.

A. Closure of the rent in the vaginal mucosa with a continuous suture.

B.

B. Drawing together the perineal muscles and fascia with interrupted sutures.

C.

C. Closure of the skin edges with interrupted sutures tied loosely.

Fig. 5. Repair of a second degree laceration.

Third Degree Tears

Third degree tears extend through the perineal body, the transverse perineal muscle, and the rectal sphincter. In partial third degree tears only the
rectal sphincter is torn; in complete tears the rectal sphincter is severed, and
the laceration extends up the anterior rectal wall for a variable distance. Some
authors refer to this as a fourth degree tear.

Repair of Complete Third Degree Tear: Complete third degree tear is repaired in layers:

1. The anterior wall of the rectum is repaired with fine 000 or 0000 chromic
   catgut on a fused needle. Starting at the apex, interrupted sutures are
   placed submucosally so that the serosa, muscularis, and submucosa of the
   rectum are apposed. Some authors advise that the knot be tied in the lumen
   of the bowel. Others approximate the edges of the rectum with a continuous suture going through all layers. This part of the repair must be performed meticulously.
2. The line of repair is oversewn by bringing together the perirectal fascia
   and the fascia of the rectovaginal septum. Interrupted or continuous sutures are used.
3. The torn ends of the rectal sphincter (which have retracted) are identified,
   grasped with Allis forceps, and approximated with interrupted sutures or
   two figures of 8 sutures.
4. The vaginal mucosa is then repaired as in a midline episiotomy, with continuous or interrupted sutures.
5. The perineal muscles are sewn together with interrupted stitches.
6. The skin edges are sewn together with a continuous subcuticular suture or
   loosely tied interrupted sutures.

Repair of Partial Third Degree Tear: Repair of partial third degree tear
is similar to that of the complete variety, except that the rectal wall is intact,
and the repair starts with the reapproximation of the torn ends of the rectal
sphincter.

Aftercare of Third Degree Tears: Aftercare of third degree tears includes:

1. General perineal asepsis
2. Low residue diet
3. Encouragement of soft bowel movements with mild laxatives
4. Suppository or carefully given enema on the fifth or sixth day

A. Third degree laceration showing the torn and retracted ends of the rectal sphincter, the laceration of the anterior wall of the rectum, and the torn vagina and perineum.

B. Closing the tear in the anterior wall of the rectum with interrupted sutures tied in the lumen.

C. The retracted ends of the rectal sphincter are grasped with Allis forceps, and the first figure of 8 suture is being placed.

D. Reunion of torn rectal sphincter completed with two figure of 8 sutures.

Fig. 6. Repair of a third degree laceration.

LACERATIONS OF THE ANTERIOR PART OF THE VULVA
AND THE LOWER ANTERIOR VAGINAL WALL

Various areas may be involved. Superficial tears are not serious, but when deep the bleeding may be profuse.

Locations of the Lacerations

1. The tissue on either side of the urethra
2. The labia minora
3. The lateral walls of the vagina
4. The area of the clitoris: With deep tears the corpora cavernosa may be torn. Because of the general vascularity of this structure, as well as the presence of the deep and dorsal blood vessels of the clitoris, these lacerations are accompanied by severe bleeding.
5. The urethra, under the pubic arch
6. The bladder: The bladder is close to the anterior vaginal wall and may be damaged. Vesicovaginal fistula can occur. The main causes of fistula are:
   a. Prolonged labor with pressure necrosis of the wall of the bladder
   b. Instrumental damage in difficult deliveries

Repair of Lacerations

Superficial Lacerations: Superficial small lacerations do not need repair in many cases. When the legs are brought together the torn edges are approximated and will heal spontaneously. Larger tears should have the edges brought together with interrupted sutures to promote healing.

Deep Lacerations: Deep lacerations must be repaired. Profuse bleeding is controlled best by figure of 8 sutures, placed to include and shut off the torn and bleeding vessels. Unfortunately in many cases the lacerated area is the site of varicosities, and the passage of the needle through the tissue provokes fresh bleeding. If the sutures do not stop the bleeding, a firm pack should be applied against the bleeding site, and the hemorrhage controlled by tamponade.

Often the area of bleeding is near the urethra, and when the priclitoral region is involved, the hemorrhage can be excessive. Repair is difficult because of the proximity of the urethra. To prevent damaging the urethra a catheter should be inserted to guide the needle away from it.

Tears of the Urethra and Bladder: Tears of the urethra and bladder are repaired in three layers to approximate the bladder mucosa, bladder wall, and anterior wall of the vagina. An indwelling catheter should be inserted into the bladder for drainage.

Fig. 7. Anterior paraurethral laceration: placing of fine interrupted sutures. A catheter is in the urethra.

LACERATIONS OF THE UPPER VAGINA

These lacerations may take place during spontaneous delivery, but are more common with operative deliveries, and are associated with a variety of conditions.

Predisposing factors include congenital anomalies of the vagina, a small or infantile vagina, loss of tissue elasticity in elderly primigravidas, scar tissue following the use of caustic substances in attempting to induce abortions, and unhealthy tissues which tear like wet blotting paper.

Forceps rotations and extractions following deep transverse arrest, persistent occipitoposteriors, or face presentations often cause vaginal tears. The fact that these malpositions are frequently associated with small or male type pelves aggravates the situation and increases the incidence and extent of the lacerations. During the rotation the edge of the blades may shear off the vaginal mucosa. Improper traction tends to overstretch the tissues and may result in a large tear. A large infant increases the danger of extensive lacerations.

The majority of vaginal tears are longitudinal and extend in the sulci along the columns of the vagina. In many cases the lacerations are bilateral.

Technic of Repair

Lacerations of the upper vagina bleed profusely; the bleeding must be controlled as soon as possible. As the tear is often high and out of sight, good exposure, good light, and good assistance are essential. Bleeding from the uterus may obscure the field. The placenta should be removed and oxytocics given before the repair is begun. The operator must be certain that the apex of the tear is included in the suture, or hemorrhage may take place from a vessel which has retracted. If the apex cannot be reached several sutures are placed below it, and traction on these will then expose the apex of the laceration. Figure of 8 sutures are preferable if bleeding is profuse, or a continuous lock stitch may be employed.

In some instances the sutures do not control the bleeding adequately. The vagina should be packed tightly with a 5 yard gauze. This will reduce the oozing and help prevent the formation of hematomas. The pack is removed in 24 hours.

Fig. 8. Right mediolateral episiotomy with high left vaginal sulcus tear. A, introduction of first suture at highest point visible. B, traction on first suture exposes the apex of the laceration and enables top suture to be placed. The remainder of the vaginal laceration is closed with continuous or interrupted sutures.

HEMATOMAS OF VULVA AND VAGINA

Puerperal hematoma

1. Vulvar.   The bleeding is limited to the vulvar tissue and is readily apparent.
2. Vulvovaginal.   The hematoma involves the paravaginal tissue and the vulva, perineum, or ischiorectal fossa.   The extent of the bleeding is only partially revealed on inspection of the vulva.
3. Vaginal or concealed.   The hematoma is confined to the paravaginal tissue and is not visible externally.
4. Supravaginal or subperitoneal.   The bleeding occurs above the pelvic fascia and is retroperitoneal or intraligamentous.

These result from the rupture of the blood vessels, especially veins, under the skin of the external genitals and beneath the vaginal mucosa.   The causal trauma occurs during delivery or repair.   In rare cases the accident takes place during pregnancy or in very early labor, in which case a large hematoma can obstruct progress.   Damage to a blood vessel may lead to its necrosis, and the hematoma may not become manifest for several days.

Most hematomas are small and are located just beneath the skin of the perineum.   While they cause pain and discoloration of the skin, they are not important.   Since the blood is absorbed spontaneously no treatment is required beyond ordinary perineal care.

Rupture of the vessels under the vaginal mucosa is serious, since large amounts of blood can collect in the loose submucosal tissues.   Many vaginal hematomas contain over half a liter of blood by the time the diagnosis is made.   The mass may be so large that it occludes the lumen of the vagina, and pressure on the rectum is intense.   When the bleeding occurs at the base of the ligament the blood may extend in the retroperitoneal space even as far as the kidneys.

Many hematomas occur after easy spontaneous deliveries as well as in association with traumatic deliveries.   The hematoma often is located on the side opposite the episiotomy.   Stretching of the deep tissues can result in the rupture of a deep vessel without any visible external bleeding.   Varicosities play a predisposing role.

Diagnosis

The diagnosis is made within 12 hours of delivery.   Classically, the patient's complaints of pain are dismissed as being part of the usual postpartum perineal discomfort.   After a time it is realized that the pain is out of proportion to that associated with the ordinary trauma of delivery.   Sedatives and analgesics do not alleviate the pain.   Careful examination of the vulva and vagina reveals the swelling, discoloration, extreme tenderness, rectal pressure, and the large fluctuant mass palpable per rectum or vaginam.   Where large amounts of blood have been lost from the general circulation there is pallor, tachycardia, hypotension, and even shock.   If the hematoma is high and ruptures into the peritoneal cavity, sudden extreme shock may occur and the patient may die.

Treatment

Active treatment is not needed for small hematomas and those which are not getting larger. The area should be kept clean, and since tissue necrosis may be followed by infection, antimicrobial agents are prescribed.

Big hematomas and those which are enlarging require surgical therapy. The wound is opened, the blood clots are evacuated, and if bleeding points can be found, these are ligated. The area is packed with sterile gauze and a counter pack is placed in the vagina. This is left in situ for 24 to 48 hours. Antibiotics are given, blood transfusion is used as needed, and the patient is observed carefully for fresh bleeding. An indwelling catheter should be placed.

Most cases do well, but several weeks pass before the wound heals and the perineum looks normal.

HEMATOMAS OF THE BROAD LIGAMENT

The danger of broad ligament hematomas is that they can rupture into the general peritoneal cavity and cause sudden and extreme shock.

Diagnosis

Diagnosis is made by vaginal examination. Rupture of the lower uterine segment must be ruled out. If the hematoma is large the uterus will be pushed to the opposite side.

Treatment

Treatment depends on the degree of bleeding. Conservative therapy consists of bedrest, antibiotics, blood transfusion, and observation. Serial blood counts are done.

In the event of continued bleeding or progressive anemia, surgical intervention is carried out. The abdomen is opened, and the blood clots are evacuated. Where possible the bleeding points are tied off, care being taken to avoid the ureter. An extraperitoneal drain may be inserted. In older women hysterectomy is considered, and this operation may be necessary in young women to control the situation.

LACERATIONS OF THE CERVIX

As a result of its dilatation, superficial lacerations of the cervix occur in almost every confinement. They are partly responsible for the bloody show. These small tears heal spontaneously and require no treatment.

Deep lacerations, on the other hand, can cause severe hemorrhage and shock to the extent of endangering the life of the patient. This is particularly so when the laceration extends into the lower uterine segment where the large uterine vessels may be involved. The lacerations may be unilateral or bilateral. The most common sites are at the sides of the cervix, at 3 or 9 o'clock.

Etiology

Etiology of deep lacerations includes precipitate labor, rigid or scarred cervix, the forceful delivery of the child through an undilated cervix, breech extraction, and large baby.

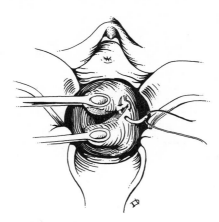

Fig. 9.   Laceration of cervix on the left side. Uppermost suture is placed just above the apex of the tear. The laceration is being closed with interrupted sutures. Figure of 8 sutures may be used.

Diagnosis

Diagnosis is by careful inspection. Some obstetricians inspect the cervix after every delivery. It must be done after all difficult confinements and whenever there is continuous bleeding, especially if it is bright red. Ring forceps are used to grasp the lips of the cervix so that the whole circumference can be examined.

Repair

Repair of tears of the cervix is important. The cervix is exposed with a vaginal speculum or with retractors. An assistant is invaluable. Ring forceps are placed on each side of the laceration. Interrupted or figure of 8 sutures are placed, starting at the apex, and are tied just tightly enough to control the bleeding and to approximate the tissues. Care must be taken not to include the ring of the forceps in the stitch. It is important that the first stitch be placed a little above the apex to catch any vessel which may have retracted. If the tear is high there is danger of injury to the ureter. When the tear has extended into the lower uterine segment or into the broad ligament, repair from below may be impossible, and laparotomy is necessary.

Careful repair of the torn cervix is important, not only to control bleeding but as a prophylaxis against scarring, erosions, and chronic ascending infections. Lacerations over a centimeter in length warrant treatment.

DÜHRSSEN'S CERVICAL INCISIONS

Incisions of the cervix are used to facilitate immediate delivery when the cervix is fully effaced but not completely dilated.   This procedure is used rarely today, the incidence being under 1 percent and being needed more often in primigravidas.

Indications

This operation may be employed in the presence of fetal distress or arrest of progress where it is considered that vaginal delivery would be relatively easy if the cervix were fully dilated.   The obstetrician must beware of diagnosing cervical dystocia when fetopelvic disproportion is the real problem.

Prerequisites

1. There must be no cephalopelvic disproportion.
2. The cervix must be completely effaced.
3. The cervix must be at least half dilated.
4. The station of the fetal skull is at +1 or +2.
5. The patient must have been in good labor for 6 to 8 hours with ruptured membranes.

Technic

The cervix is grasped with ring forceps, and the incisions are made between them at 2, 6, and 10 o'clock.   These are extended to the junction of the cervix and vaginal wall.   When the three incisions have been made, the diameter of the cervix is equivalent to full dilatation.   Because the bladder is pulled upward as effacement takes place, its dissection from the anterior vaginal wall is not required.

Appropriate measures for delivery of the child are then carried out.   The incisions are repaired with continuous, interrupted, or figure of 8 sutures. While there is rarely much bleeding, preparations to treat hemorrhage should be at hand.   Most cervices heal well, and future pregnancies deliver normally.

ANNULAR DETACHMENT OF THE CERVIX

The anterior lip of the cervix may be compressed between the fetal head and the pubic symphysis.   If this situation continues for a long time, edema, local anemia, anoxia, and even necrosis may develop.   Rarely, an entire ring of cervix undergoes anoxic necrosis, and a section of the vaginal part of the cervix comes away.   This is known as annular detachment of the cervix.   Because the prolonged pressure has caused the blood vessels to thrombose, excessive bleeding from the cervix is unusual.

Etiology

1. Seventy-five percent of cases occur in primigravidas.
2. Prolonged labor is almost always the rule.

Fig. 10. Dührssen's cervical incisions at 2, 6, and 10 o'clock.

3. There is often a history of early rupture of the membranes.
4. The fetal head is low in the pelvis.
5. The cervix is well effaced and often quite thin. It is the external os that
    does not dilate. Several observers have reported the cervix as feeling
    rigid to palpation during the first stage of labor.
7. The uterine contractions are strong and efficient.

Mechanism

    The myometrial contractions press the presenting part against the thinned
out rigid external os, and, in addition, the retracting upper segment of the
uterus pulls the cervix upward. This double action leads to poor circulation in
the cervix, anoxia, and necrosis. A tear starts at the cervicovaginal junction,
a line of cleavage develops and continues until the separation is complete. The
characteristic doughnut shaped ring of tissue becomes detached when the cervix
is about 3 to 5 cm dilated. Gross histologic examinations have revealed these
cervices to be no different from the normal term organ.

The Clinical Picture

    The clinical picture is one of good labor obstructed by an unyielding exter-
nal os. In almost every case the fetus was delivered without difficulty once the
cervical obstruction was overcome. Annular detachment is the result of true
cervical dystocia.

Treatment

    Because the vessels are thrombosed, serious bleeding from the stump is
rare. No active treatment is needed. Maternal death has occurred either from

sepsis or from uterine bleeding associated with prolonged labor and postpartum uterine atony. Any hemorrhage which does take place from the cervix must be controlled by figure of 8 sutures.

Prevention

Prevention is by recognizing the situation before the actual detachment takes place. When the cervix is effaced and thin cervical incisions are indicated, delivery usually follows. If the situation is not right for cervical incisions, cesarean section must be done.

Prognosis

Many women avoid future pregnancy. Stenosis and hematometra have been recorded. Several cases have been delivered vaginally with no difficulty. One elective cesarean section and one abortion from an incompetent os have been reported.

RUPTURE OF THE UTERUS

Rupture of the uterus is a dangerous complication of pregnancy. It is responsible for 5 percent of maternal deaths in the United States and Canada, and is an even greater hazard in the underdeveloped countries.

Incidence

The reported incidence varies from 1:93 confinements to 1:8,741, depending on the source of the material. The average incidence is around 1:2,000. Recent publications suggest that the number of uterine ruptures is increasing and blame this fact on 1, the more frequent use of cesarean section; 2, the careless administration of oxytocic drugs; 3, inadequate professional care during labor; and 4, lackadaisical and poor management of labor and delivery.

Types of Rupture

The rupture is complete when all layers of the uterus are involved, and there is direct communication between the uterine and abdominal cavities. This is the more common variety. The incomplete type involves the myometrium, but the peritoneum covering the uterus is intact.

Site of Rupture

Tears which take place during pregnancy are more often in the upper segment of the uterus, at the site of previous operation or injury. During labor the rupture is usually in the lower segment. The longer the labor, the more thinned out the lower segment, and the greater the danger of rupture. The tear may extend into the uterine vessels and cause profuse hemorrhage. Tears in the anterior or posterior walls of the uterus usually extend transversely or obliquely. In the region of the broad ligament the laceration runs longitudinally up the sides of the uterus.

Time of Rupture

It may occur 1, during pregnancy; 2, during normal labor; 3, during difficult labor; and 4, following labor. Most ruptures take place at or near term.
Those happening before the onset of labor are usually dehiscences of cesarean
section scars.

Classification

Spontaneous Rupture of the Normal Uterus: These accidents occur during
labor, are more common in the lower segment of the uterus, and are the result
of mismanagement and neglect. Etiologic factors include:

1. Multiparity
2. Disproportion
3. Abnormal presentation (brow, breech, transverse lie)
4. The improper use of oxytocin

Traumatic Rupture: This is caused by ill-advised and poorly executed operative vaginal deliveries. The incidence is decreasing. Etiologic factors include:

1. Version and extraction
2. Difficult forceps operations
3. Forceful breech extraction
4. Craniotomy
5. Excessive fundal pressure
6. Manual dilatation of the cervix

Postcesarean Rupture: This is the most common variety seen today. It
may occur before or during labor. Classical scars rupture more often than
lower segment incisions. While hysterograms done 3 months after operation
may give an indication as to whether good healing has taken place, there is no
accurate way of predicting the behavior of a uterine scar. All cesarean section
scars present a hazard. Hence, many follow the rule of once a cesarean, always a cesarean.

Rupture Following Trauma Other than Cesarean: The danger is that often
the damage is not recognized, and the accident comes as a surprise. Included
in this group are:

1. Previous myomectomy
2. Too vigorous curettage
3. Perforation during curettage
4. Cervical laceration
5. Manual removal of an adherent placenta
6. Placenta percreta
7. Endometritis and myometritis
8. Hydatidiform mole
9. Cornual resection for ectopic pregnancy
10. Hysterotomy

Silent Bloodless Dehiscence of a Previous Cesarean Scar: This is a complication of lower segment cesarean sections.   Part or all of the incision may be involved.   Usually the peritoneum over the scar is intact.   Many of these windows are areas not of current rupture but of failure of healing of the original incision.   This complication is in no way as serious as true uterine rupture. Features of this complication include:

1. It is usually diagnosed during repeat cesarean section, being unsuspected before operation.
2. No hemorrhage at site of dehiscence
3. No shock
4. Hysterectomy is not necessary
5. No fetal death
6. No maternal mortality

The Clinical Picture

The clinical picture of uterine rupture is variable in that it depends on many factors:

1. The time of occurrence (pregnancy, early or late labor)
2. The cause of the rupture
3. The degree of the rupture (complete or incomplete)
4. The position of the rupture
5. The extent of the rupture
6. The amount of intraperitoneal spill
7. The size of the blood vessels involved and the amount of bleeding
8. The complete or partial extrusion of the fetus and placenta from the uterus
9. The degree of retraction of the myometrium
10. The general condition of the patient

On a clinical basis rupture of the uterus may be divided into four groups:

1. Silent or quiet rupture.   The accident occurs without (initially) the usual signs and symptoms.   Diagnosis is difficult and is often delayed.   Nothing dramatic happens, but the observant attendant notices a rising pulse rate, pallor, and perhaps slight vaginal bleeding.   The patient complains of some pain.   The contractions may go on, but the cervix fails to dilate.   This type is usually associated with the scar of a previous cesarean section.
2. Usual variety.   The picture develops over a period of a few hours.   The signs and symptoms include abdominal pain, vomiting, faintness, vaginal bleeding, rapid pulse rate, pallor, tenderness on palpation, and absence of the fetal heart.   These features may have arisen during pregnancy or labor.   If the diagnosis is not made, hypotension and shock supervene.
3. Violent rupture.   It is apparent almost immediately that a serious accident has taken place.   Usually a hard uterine contraction is followed by the sensation of something having given way and a sharp pain in the lower abdomen. Often the contractions cease, there is a change in the character of the pain, and the patient becomes anxious.   The fetus can be palpated easily and feels close to the examining fingers.   The presenting part is no longer at the pelvic brim and can be moved freely.   Sometimes the uterus and fetus can be

palpated in different parts of the abdomen. Fetal movements cease, and the fetal heart is not heard. The symptoms and signs of shock appear soon, and complete collapse may occur.

4. Rupture with delayed diagnosis. Here the condition is not diagnosed until the patient is in a process of gradual deterioration, unexplained anemia leads to careful investigation, a palpable hematoma develops in the broad ligament, signs of peritoneal irritation appear, or the patient goes into shock (either gradually or suddenly as when a hematoma in the broad ligament ruptures). Sometimes the diagnosis is made only at autopsy.

Diagnosis

The diagnosis is made easily when the classical picture is present, or when the rupture is catastrophic. In atypical cases the diagnosis may be difficult. A high index of suspicion is important. If routine exploration of the uterus is not carried out after every birth, then at least following all difficult deliveries, whenever there is unexplained shock or postpartum bleeding, the interior of the cavity should be explored manually and the lower segment searched for tears.

Palpatory findings, as described in the previous section, may be pathognomonic. The fetal heart beat is absent in most cases. An x-ray of the abdomen may demonstrate the fetus lying in the peritoneal cavity surrounded by the intestines, with the shadow of the uterus to one side.

Treatment

Treatment must be prompt and in keeping with the patient's condition. Laparotomy is performed, and the bleeding is controlled as quickly as possible. Aortic compression (by the hand or by using a special instrument) is useful in reducing the bleeding until the situation can be evaluated. Most patients are critically ill and are unable to stand prolonged surgery.

In most cases total hysterectomy is the procedure of choice. If the patient is in poor condition rapid subtotal hysterectomy may be performed. If, however, the tear has extended into the cervix, the bleeding will not be controlled by subtotal hysterectomy. In such cases, the cervix must be sutured carefully to tie off all bleeding points.

In young women, and in those who desire more children, treatment may be limited to repair of the tear. This should be done only when the uterine musculature can be so reconstituted as to assure a reasonable degree of success and safety for a future pregnancy.

As supportive treatment, blood must be replaced quickly in the amount lost.

Maternal Mortality

The reported maternal death rate ranges from 3 to 40 percent. Spontaneous rupture of the uterus is responsible for the largest number of deaths, followed by the traumatic variety. The amount of hemorrhage is greatest in these types. The lowest death rate is associated with postcesarean ruptures, probably because these patients are observed so carefully during labor.

The main causes of death are shock and blood loss (usually over 1,000 cc). Sepsis and paralytic ileus are contributory factors.

The prognosis for the mother depends on:

1. Prompt diagnosis and treatment. The interval between rupture and surgery is important.
2. The amount of hemorrhage and the availability of blood
3. Whether or not infection sets in
4. The type and site of the rupture

The mortality rate is lower today because of:

1. Early diagnosis
2. Immediate laparotomy
3. Blood transfusion
4. Antibiotics
5. Reduction or elimination of traumatic vaginal operative deliveries
6. Better management of prolonged or obstructed labor

Fetal Mortality

This is high, ranging from 30 to 85 percent. Most fetuses die from separation of the placenta. There is a reduction of blood supply available to the fetus after the uterus has ruptured. Probably the prolonged labor before the rupture plays a part in causing fetal hypoxia. Many of these babies are premature. The highest mortality is associated with fundal rupture where the fetus has been extruded into the abdominal cavity.

INVERSION OF THE UTERUS

Uterine inversion is a turning inside out of the uterus. The incidence is around 1:20,000 confinements. The condition is associated almost entirely with pregnancy. Of the nonpuerperal variety, the most common cause is a fibroid tumor, generally submucous or the pedunculated variety.

Etiology

Some inversions are spontaneous, tend to recur at later deliveries, and are believed to be related to an abnormality of the myometrium. Many are caused by improper obstetric manipulations.

The underlying factors include:

1. Sudden emptying of the distended uterus
2. Thinning of the wall with gradual development of a tumor (fetus or neo-plasm)
3. Dilatation of the cervix
4. Fundal implantation of the placenta

Precipitating factors include:

1. Excessive suprapubic pressure
2. Traction on the umbilical cord or membranes
3. Adherent placenta
4. Mismanagement of the third stage, such as pressure on the uterine fundus when the myometrium is relaxed

Classification

Stage: Classification on the basis of stage is as follows:

1. Acute, occurring immediately after the birth of the baby or placenta
2. Subacute, beginning when contraction of the cervix becomes established
3. Chronic, present for more than 4 weeks

Degree: Classification on the basis of degree is into three types:

1. Incomplete, where the fundus is not beyond the internal os of the cervix
2. Complete, where the fundus protrudes through the external os of the cervix
3. Prolapse, in which the fundus protrudes through the vulva

Pathology

The following stages have been described:

1. Acute inversion
2. Contraction of the cervical ring and lower segment of the uterus around the encircled portion of the uterus
3. Edema
4. Reduction of blood supply
5. Gangrene and necrosis
6. Sloughing

Clinical Picture

Sometimes the symptoms are minor so that the diagnosis is not made, or the condition is recognized but treatment is not carried out at the time. These are the chronic inversions. Those that cause shock and require immediate therapy are the acute ones.

When the inversion is complete the diagnosis is easy. Partial inversions may fool the observer. Classically, shock is greater than expected for the amount of bleeding. The extreme shock is probably caused by tension on the nerves of the broad ligament, which are drawn through the cervical ring, and by the irritation of the peritoneum. In any situation where shock is out of proportion to hemorrhage the accoucheur should think of uterine inversion.

The placenta may have separated or may remain attached. The hemorrhage may be excessive or it may be minimal.

Diagnosis is made by the palpation of the inverted fundus in the vagina and by its absence above the pubis. In every case of unexplained shock or postpartum bleeding vaginal examination and manual exploration of the uterine cavity must be carried out.

Fig. 11. Manual replacement of inverted uterus.

Treatment

Treatment of acute inversion consists of replacement of the uterus and replacement of blood. Blood transfusion should be started as soon as possible.
The patient is anesthetized, and if the placenta is still attached it is removed.
The fingers are inserted through the cervical ring, and replacement is started
by pressure on the site of the inversion. The fundus is gradually pushed through
the ring until a normal shape of the uterus is attained. The hand is kept in the
uterus to prevent recurrence until the uterus is satisfactorily contracted. The
cavity is packed tightly and oxytocics are given.

When immediate replacement is not feasible the patient is treated for shock,
laparotomy is performed, and the accident is corrected surgically.

RETAINED PLACENTA

Retention of the placenta in utero falls into four groups:

1. Separated but retained: Here there is failure of the forces which normally
    expel the placenta.
2. Separated but incarcerated: An hour glas constriction of the uterus, or
    spasm of the cervix, traps the placenta in the upper segment.

3. Adherent but separable placenta: In this situation the placenta fails to separate from the uterine wall. The causes include failure of the normal contraction and retraction of the third stage, an anatomic defect in the uterus, or an abnormality of the decidua which prevents the formation of the normal decidual plane of cleavage.
4. Adherent and inseparable placenta: Here are the varying degrees of placenta accreta. The normal decidua is absent, and the chorionic villi are attached directly to and through the myometrium.

Technic

Manual removal of the retained placenta is not considered to be as dangerous as it once was. Many of the bad results of this procedure were the result of too long a delay in treatment until hemorrhage had put the patient in a precarious state. Where bleeding is present the placenta must be removed immediately. If there is no associated hemorrhage, and the patient is in good condition, a delay of 30 minutes is permissible.

If the patient has been bleeding actively, an intravenous infusion is set up, and blood is made available. Anesthesia is necessary. The procedure is carried out under aseptic conditions.

The uterus is steadied by one hand's holding the fundus through the maternal abdomen. The other hand is inserted into the vagina and through the cervix into the uterine cavity. The placenta is reached by following the umbilical cord. If the placenta has separated it is grasped and removed. The uterus is then explored to be sure that nothing has been left.

If the placenta is still adherent to the uterine wall it must be separated. First some part of the margin of attachment is identified and the fingers inserted between the placenta and the wall of the uterus. The back of the hand is kept in contact with the uterine wall. The fingers are forced gently between the placenta and uterus, and as progress is made they are spread apart. In this way the line of cleavage is extended, the placenta is separated from the uterine wall, and it is then extracted. Oxytocics are given to ensure good uterine contraction and retraction.

PLACENTA ACCRETA

Placenta accreta is an abnormal attachmemt of the placenta to the uterine wall—the result of a defect, deficiency, or absence of the decidua basalis. The villi adhere to, or penetrate into or even through the myometrium.

Incidence

There is a wide discrepancy in the reported frequency. It varies from 1:2,000 to 1:70,000.

Etiology

Anything which results in a defective endometrium plays a part. Included are:

1. Previous curettage
2. Submucous myoma
3. Endometritis
4. Uterine scars
5. Intrauterine radiation
6. Adenomyosis

Pathology

Normally the decidua basalis lies between the myometrium and the placenta. The plane of cleavage for placental separation is in the spongy layer of the decidua basalis. In placenta accreta the decidua basalis is partially or completely absent, so that the placenta is attached directly to the myometrium. The villi may remain superficial to the uterine muscle or may penetrate into it deeply. This condition is caused by a defect in the decidua rather than by any abnormal invasive properties of the trophoblast.

In the superficial area of the myometrium a large number of venous channels develop just beneath the placenta. Rupture of these sinuses by the forceful extraction of the placenta is the source of the profuse hemorrhage which occurs.

Classification

1. By extent
   a. Complete: The whole placenta is adherent to the myometrium.
   b. Partial: One or more cotyledons are adherent
2. By depth
   a. Accreta: The placenta is adherent to the myometrium. There is no line of cleavage.
   b. Increta: The villi penetrate into the uterine muscle.
   c. Percreta: The villi penetrate the thickness of the uterine wall and sometimes perforate the serosa. Rupture of the uterus may occur.

Clinical Picture

There are no characteristic clinical manifestations other than the failure of the uterus to expel the placenta. The amount of bleeding depends on the degree of attachment. In complete placenta accreta, there is no separation of the placenta from the uterine wall and no bleeding. In the partial variety, part of the placenta may be detached spontaneously or by the obstetrician's fingers. The adherent portion prevents the uterus from retracting properly, and the resultant hemorrhage may be catastrophic.

The diagnosis is made by direct intrauterine palpation. No line of cleavage is found, and the examining fingers simply slide over to the fetal surface of the placenta.

The differential diagnosis includes:

1. Incomplete abortion
2. Retained incarcerated placenta
3. Adherent placenta, where there is a line of cleavage

4. Retained placental fragments
5. Subinvolution of the placenta site
6. Choriocarcinoma

Management of Placenta Accreta

The safest treatment is hysterectomy. Since this puts an end to childbearing, a conservative method of therapy has evolved, based on the availability of blood and antibiotics. When placenta accreta is suspected, the following plan of management is useful.

Establishment of Diagnosis: The following steps are taken:

1. An intravenous infusion is started with a wide bore needle.
2. Blood is cross-matched.
3. Expert anesthesia should be available.
4. The operating room must be ready for an emergency.
5. Intrauterine exploration is performed to see whether placenta accreta is present, and if so, whether it is complete or partial.
6. In making the diagnosis an attempt is made to remove the placenta. In most instances placenta accreta will not be present. Overzealous attempts to extract the placenta must be avoided since the uterus can be ruptured.

Indications for Hysterectomy: Indications are:

1. When further pregnancy is not desired
2. Uncontrollable hemorrhage
3. Failure of conservative management
4. Intrauterine suppuration
5. Placenta previa accreta

Conservative Management: Conservative management includes:

1. Total placenta accreta
   a. There will be no bleeding unless attempts are made to remove the placenta.
   b. The cord is cut short and the blood drained from the placenta.
   c. The placenta is left in the uterus.
   d. Broad spectum antibiotics are given.
   e. The placenta will become organized and partially absorbed, and the superficial portion will slough off.
   f. In some cases suppuration takes place and generalized infection may set in.
2. Partial or focal placenta accreta
   a. Manually remove all separated placenta. The part of the placenta which is abnormally attached is left.
   b. An intravenous oxytocin infusion is maintained for 48 hours.
   c. Careful, constant observation of the patient
   d. Broad spectrum antibiotics are given.
   e. If there is no bleeding after 48 hours, the first stage of conservative management has been successful.

Placenta Previa Accreta

Because the decidua of the lower segment is less abundant than that in the fundus, a placenta implanted near the cervix may be abnormally adherent.
The treatment is total hysterectomy.

Maternal Mortality

Before 1937 the mortality rate for all cases was reported as being 37 percent. Where manual removal was the treatment the figure was 65 percent. The mortality has decreased steadily because of: 1, a greater awareness of the problem; 2, the availability of blood; 3, the effectiveness of antibiotics in combatting infection; and 4, the relative safety of timely hysterectomy.

AMNIOTIC FLUID EMBOLISM

This is a syndrome in which, following the infusion of a large amount of amniotic fluid into the maternal circulation, there is the sudden development of acute respiratory distress and shock. Twenty-five percent of women die within 1 hour.
The condition is rare. Probably many cases are unrecognized, the diagnosis being obstetric shock, postpartum hemorrhage, or acute pulmonary edema.

The Clinical Picture

In the typical case an elderly multipara gives birth to a large baby after a stormy and prolonged labor and, suddenly and without apparent reason, develops acute respiratory distress and shock; death follows shortly. The cardinal signs are respiratory embarrassment, cyanosis, cardiovascular collapse, and coma. Convulsions and vomiting are common. Pulmonary edema with pink, frothy sputum occurs quickly. In the few patients who survive the initial insult, afibrinogenemia with bleeding from the placental site is a frequent complication.
Considered in the differential diagnosis are:

1. Thrombotic pulmonary embolism
2. Air embolism
3. Fat embolism
4. Aspiration of vomitus
5. Eclampsia
6. Anesthetic drug reaction
7. Cerebrovascular accident
8. Congestive heart failure
9. Hemorrhagic shock

Predisposing factors include:

1. Tumultuous labor
2. Oxytocin induction or stimulation of labor
3. Oversized fetus
4. Intrauterine death
5. Meconium in the amniotic fluid
6. Multiparity
7. Advanced age of the mother

The one common feature seems to be tumultuous labor or exceptionally strong uterine contractions.

Clinicopathologic Findings

Mode of Infusion

The two major sites of entry into the maternal circulation are the endocervical veins (which may be torn even in normal labor) and the uteroplacental area. Rupture of the uterus increases the chance of amniotic fluid infusion.

Lungs

The significant findings are:

1. Edema
2. Alveolar hemorrhage
3. Emboli composed of the particulate material of amniotic fluid (squames, amorphous debris, mucin, vernix, and lanugo)
4. The pulmonary vessels are dilated at the area of embolization.

Heart

The right side is often dilated. Blood aspirated from the right side will reveal amniotic fluid elements.

Cause of Death

There are two principal theories: 1, there is an overwhelming mechanical blockade of the pulmonary vessels by emboli and 2, death results from an anaphylactoid reaction to the particulate matter in the amniotic fluid, especially meconium.

Etiology of Main Effects

The three major aspects of the syndrome are produced probably by a combination of mechanical and spastic processes.

1. The sudden reduction of the amount of blood returning to the left heart, and the decreased left ventricular output, lead to peripheral vascular collapse.
2. The acute pulmonary hypertension, cor pulmonale, and failure of the right heart produce pulmonary edema.
3. The uneven capillary blood flow with derangement of the ventilation/perfusion ratio leads to anoxemia and tissue hypoxia. This can explain the cyanosis, restlessness, convulsions, and coma.

Coagulation Defects

Many patients who survive the initial episode develop hypofibrinogenemia and hemorrhage. There are three theories as to why the levels of fibrinogen are lowered: 1, a thromboplastic substance, which is present in the amniotic fluid, enters the maternal circulation, produces multiple intravascular fibrin thrombi, and so defibrinates the blood; 2, conditions of stress, shock, and hypoxia increase the fibrinolytic activity. The increased plasma fibrinolysins destroy the fibrin and fibrinogen; 3, a heparin–like compound is present in amniotic fluid, which both blocks the conversion of prothrombin to thrombin and inactivates thrombin.

Management

Prophylaxis

The only precaution that can be taken is to avoid or decrease tumultuous contractions.

Therapy

In severe cases nothing does any good. The following measures have been used:

1. Oxygen under pressure to combat hypoxia and to reduce pulmonary edema
2. Antispasmodics and vasodilators (papaverine, trinitroglycerine, and aminophylin) to reduce vasospasm
3. Hydrocortisone to help the situation of overwhelming stress
4. Parasympathetic drugs (atropine) for the reflex vasospasm
5. Digitalis when heart failure is present
6. Where there is hemorrhage, fresh blood is given, taking care not to overload the circulation.
7. Fibrinogen is used when this is low.
8. Fibrinolytic inhibitor (epsilon amino caproic acid) when there is an excessive amount of fibrinolysin.
9. Manual exploration of the uterus to rule out uterine rupture and to remove retained placental fragments

The most recommended measures are oxygen, papaverine, atropine, and, when indicated, fibrinogen.

SEPARATION OF THE SYMPHYSIS PUBIS

During pregnancy there is relaxation and weakening of the pelvic joints. This begins in the first half of pregnancy and reaches a maximum in the seventh month. Return to normal begins after delivery and is complete by the sixth month.

Incidence

This varies from 1:250 confinements to 1:30,000. Minor degrees of separation take place, but since the symptoms are minimal the diagnosis is not made, and spontaneous correction follows.

Etiology

Rupture of the pubic symphysis occurs in patients with excessive relaxation of the pelvic joints. Precipitating factors include:

1. Tumultuous labor
2. Difficult forceps extractions
3. Cephalopelvic disproportion
4. Excessive abduction of the thighs at delivery
5. Any condition which might place sudden and excessive pressure on the pubic symphysis
6. Many cases occur following spontaneous delivery.

Pathology

There is an actual tear of the ligaments connecting the pubic bones. The rupture is usually incomplete, and a fibrocartilagenous bridge remains. Hemorrhage and edema are present. Arthritis or osteomyelitis are possible complications.

Clinical Picture and Diagnosis

The onset of symptoms is usually sudden but may not be noted until the patient tries to walk. At the time of rupture the patient may experience a bursting feeling or a cracking noise may be heard.

Motion of the symphysis (as by moving the legs) causes great pain. If the patient can walk, she does so with a waddling gait.

There is marked tenderness of the pubic symphysis. Edema and ecchymosis are present frequently. A gaping defect in the joint is often palpable. Walking or pressure causes motion of the loose joint.

Diagnosis is made by the symptoms and signs. X-ray helps, but the degree of separation seen on radiologic study may not be proportional to the clinical manifestations. To be considered pathologic the separation seen on x-ray should be greater than 1 cm.

Treatment

Treatment is governed by the severity of the condition. Some patients require prolonged bed rest, with a tight pelvic belt or corset to keep the separated bones as nearly apposed as possible. When the rupture is minor early ambulation is permissible. A support must be worn for 6 weeks. The period of hospitalization varies with the symptoms and the degree of involvement. In the occasional case surgical correction is necessary.

BIBLIOGRAPHY

Episiotomy

Barter, R. H. , Parks, J. , and Tyndal, C. Median episiotomies and complete perineal lacerations. Amer. J. Obstet. Gynec. , 80:654, 1960.
Soule, S. D. , Wasserman, H. C. , Burstein, R. Oral proteolytic enzyme (Chymoral) in episiotomy patients. Amer. J. Obstet. Gynec. , 95:820, 1966.

Hematomas of Vulva and Vagina

Pedowitz, P, Pozner, S. , and Adler, N. H. Puerperal hematomas. Amer. J. Obstet. Gynec. , 81:350, 1961.
Pieri, R. J. Pelvic hematomas associated with pregnancy. Obstet. Gynec. , 12:249, 1958.

Fig. 12. Manual removal of the placenta.

Duhrssen's Incisions

Carrow, L. A. Cervical incisions in present–day obstetrics. Amer. J. Obstet. Gynec., 79:557, 1960.

Rubovits, F. E., and Cooperman, N. R. The role of Duhrssen's incisions in prolonged labor. Amer. J. Obstet. Gynec., 69:1183, 1955.

Annular Detachment of Cervix

Ingraham, C. B., and Taylor, E. S. Spontaneous annular detachment of the cervix during labor. Amer. J. Obstet. Gynec., 53:873, 1947.

Jeffcoate, T. N. A., and Lister, U. M. Annular detachment of the cervix. J. Obstet. Gynaec. Brit. Emp., 59:327, 1952.

Rupture of Uterus

Cavanagh, D., Membery, J. H., McLeod, A. G. W. Rupture of the gravid uterus: An appraisal. Obstet. Gynec., 26:157, 1965.

Feeney, K., and Barry, A. Rupture and perforation of uterus in association with pregnancy, labor, and the puerperium. Brit. Med. J., 14 Jan. 56 Vol. I, P. 65.

Harris, L. J. A new instrument for control of hemorrhage by aortic compression. Canad. Med. Ass. J., 91:128, 1964.

Keifer, W. S. Rupture of the uterus. Amer. J. Obstet. Gynec., 89:335, 1964.

Prabhavathi, R., and Mukherjee, S. N. Rupture of the uterus. J. Obstet. Gynaec. Ind., 13:455, 1963.

Inversion of Uterus

Bunke, J. W. , and Hofmeister, F. J.   Uterine inversion—obstetrical entity or oddidity. Amer. J. Obstet. Gynec. , 91:934, 1965

Shepler, L. G. Acute inversion of the puerperal uterus. Obstet. Gynec. , 23:598, 1964.

Retained and Adherent Placenta

Brody, H. Placenta accreta. Canad. Med. Ass. J. , 89:499, 1963.

Friesen, R. F. Placenta previa accreta. Canad. Med. Ass. J. , 84:1247, 1961.

Parks, J. , Barter, R. H. , and Hill, R. P. Placenta accreta. Obstet. Gynec., 2:391, 1953.

Thomas, W. O. Manual removal of the placenta. Amer. J. Obstet. Gynec. , 86:600, 1963.

Rupture of Symphysis Pubis

McElin, T. W. , and Scott, R. Rupture of the symphysis pubis during spontaneous labor. Obstet. Gynec. , 25:401, 1965.

Amniotic Fluid Embolism

Russel, W. S. , and Jones, W. N. Amniotic fluid embolism. Obstet. Gynec. , 26:476, 1965.

39 Cesarean Section

Definition: Cesarean section is an operation by which the child is delivered through an incision in the abdominal wall and the uterus.

INDICATIONS FOR CESAREAN SECTION

Indications for cesarean section are absolute or relative. Any condition which makes delivery via the birth canal impossible is an absolute indication for abdominal section. Among these are extreme degrees of pelvic contraction and neoplasms blocking the passage. With a relative indication vaginal birth is possible, but the conditions are such that cesarean section is safer for the mother, the child, or both.

Pelvic Contraction and Mechanical Dystocia

1. Fetopelvic disproportion: Fetopelvic disproportion includes the contracted pelvis, the overgrown fetus, or a relative disparity between the size of the baby and that of the pelvis. Contributing to the problem of disproportion is the shape of the pelvis, the presentation of the fetus and its ability to mold and engage, the dilatability of the cervix, and the effectiveness of the uterine contractions.
2. Neoplasms: Neoplasms which block the pelvis make normal delivery impossible. Invasive cancer of the cervix diagnosed in the third trimester of pregnancy is treated by cesarean section, followed by radiation therapy, radical surgery, or both. The exact procedure varies in different clinics.
3. Uterine dysfunctions: Uterine dysfunction includes incoordinate uterine action, inertia, constriction rings, and inability of the cervix to dilate. Labor is prolonged and progress may cease altogether. These conditions are often associated with disproportion and malpresentations.

4. Malposition and malpresentation: Malposition and malpresentation may make cesarean section necessary where a baby in normal position could be born per vaginam. Sometimes a breech does not descend well, and fetal injury or death results by vaginal extraction. The management of a breech, especially in a primigravida, is a challenge to the skill and judgment of the obstetrician. When the fetus is large and the pelvic architecture faulty, or when labor and progress are unsatisfactory, abdominal delivery is best. Impacted transverse lies are, in most cases, treated better by cesarean section than by version and extraction.

5. Soft tissue dystocia: Soft tissue dystocia may prevent or make difficult normal birth. This includes such conditions as scars in the genital tract, cervical rigidity from injury or surgery, and atresia or stenosis of the vagina. Forceful vaginal delivery results in large lacerations and hemorrhage.

Previous Uterine Surgery

1. Previous cesarean section: There are two schools of thought on the question of repeated cesarean sections. One view is that once a cesarean procedure has been performed, all subsequent pregnancies must be terminated by cesarean section. It is felt that the danger of uterine rupture through the site of the previous incision is too great. The other school holds that, provided the first section was done for reasons other than disproportion and provided that the pelvis is adequate, the fetus is not excessively large, the presentation and position are normal, and the cervix is favorable, a trial of labor should be allowed, with probable vaginal delivery. The patient must be under constant observation, cross-matched blood must be at hand, and the operating room must be ready for immediate surgery should the uterus rupture or threaten to do so. The danger of uterine rupture is less if the previous incision was in the lower segment.

2. Extensive myomectomy: Myomectomy in the past is an indication for cesarean section only if the operation was extensive, the myometrium disorganized, and the incision extended into the endometrial cavity. The previous removal of pedunculated or subserous fibromyomata does not call for cesarean section.

3. Hysterotomy

4. Cervical suture or repair of an incompetent os

Hemorrhage

1. Placenta previa: Cesarean section for central and lateral placenta previa
   has reduced fetal and maternal mortality. The final decision is made by
   vaginal examination in the operating room using a double set-up. Blood is
   cross-matched and available. The operating team stands by in readiness.
   If central or partial placenta previa is found on vaginal examination, cesarean section is performed immediately.
2. Abruptio placentae: Abruptio placentae which occurs before or during early
   labor may be treated by rupture of the membranes and oxytocin drip.
   Where the hemorrhage is severe, the cervix is hard and closed, or uteroplacental apoplexy is suspected, cesarean section may be necessary to save
   the baby, to control hemorrhage, to prevent afibrinogenemia, and to observe the condition of the uterus and its ability to contract and control the
   bleeding. In some cases hysterectomy is necessary.

Toxemia of Pregnancy

1. Preeclampsia and eclampsia
2. Essential hypertension
3. Chronic nephritis

Toxemia of pregnancy may require termination of the pregnancy before
term. In most cases induction of labor is the method of choice. When the cervix is not ripe and induction would be difficult, cesarean section is preferable.

Fetal Reasons

1. Fetal distress: Fetal distress as indicated by severe bradycardia and irregularity of the fetal heart tones sometimes necessitates rapid cesarean
   section to save the infant.
2. Previous fetal death or damage: Especially in older women who have given
   birth to more than one dead or damaged baby, cesarean section may be
   elected.
3. Prolapse of the umbilical cord: Prolapse of the umbilical cord in the presence of an undilated cervix is managed best by cesarean section, provided
   that the baby is in good condition.

4. Maternal diabetes: The fetus of the diabetic mother is inclined to be larger than normal, and this can lead to difficult labor and delivery. Although these infants are large they behave like prematures, and do not withstand well the rigors of a long labor. Death during labor and in the postnatal period is common. In addition a number of babies die in utero before term has been reached. Because of these dangers to the fetus and because a high proportion of pregnant diabetics develop toxemia, the pregnancy should be terminated by the thirty-seventh week of gestation. When conditions are favorable and a rapid and easy labor is anticipated, induction of labor can be carried out. However in primigravidas, and in multiparas with a long, closed cervix or a bad obstetric history, cesarean section is the method of choice.

5. Rhesus incompatibility: When a fetus is becoming progressively damaged by the antibodies of a sensitized Rh-negative mother and when induction and delivery per vaginam would be difficult, the pregnancy may be terminated by cesarean section in selected cases for fetal salvage.

6. Postmortem cesarean: Rarely a live baby can be obtained if rapid cesarean section is performed immediately after the death of the pregnant woman.

Miscellaneous

1. Elderly primigravidity: Elderly primigravidity is difficult to define. While the age varies from 35 to 40 years, other factors are equally important. These include the presence or absence of a good lower uterine segment, the elasticity or rigidity of the cervix and the soft tissues of the birth canal, the ease of becoming pregnant, the number of abortions, the fetal presentation, and the coordination of the uterine powers. When all these points are favorable vaginal delivery should be considered. When the adverse factors are present cesarean section may be the wiser and safer procedure.

2. Previous vaginal repair: Fear that vaginal delivery will cause a recurrence of cystocele, rectocele, and uterine prolapse may lead to an elective cesarean section.

3. Congenital uterine anomaly: Not only does an abnormal uterus often function badly, but in the case of anomalies such as a bicornuate uterus, one horn may block the passage of the baby from the other. In such cases cesarean section must be performed.

4. Bad obstetric history: When a pervious delivery has been difficult and traumatic with extensive injury to the cervix, vagina, and perineum, or when the baby has been injured, cesarean section may be selected for subsequent births.

5. Postterm pregnancy: Postterm pregnancy associated with aging of the placenta may result in a scrawny and weak baby who does not do well in the postnatal period. When there is good evidence of postmaturity, labor should be induced. If this is not feasible the rare case is treated by cesarean section.

6. Lack of progress: Lack of progress and prolonged labor is a valid reason for cesarean. After 24 hours the fetal and maternal morbidity and mortality rise.

7. Failed forceps: Failed forceps is an indication for cesarean section. It is wiser to turn to abdominal delivery than to drag a baby through the pelvis by force.

CONTRAINDICATIONS TO CESAREAN SECTION

Cesarean section should not be performed when the following conditions exist.

1. When the fetus is dead, or in such bad condition that it is unlikely to survive: There is no point in submitting the patient to a needless serious operation.

2. When the maternal birth canal is grossly infected, and the facilities for extraperitoneal cesarean are not available

3. When the operator is inexperienced, when conditions are unfavorable, or when proper assistance is not available

TYPES OF CESAREAN SECTION

Lower Segment: Transverse Incision

In our opinion this is the procedure of choice. The abdomen is opened and the uterus exposed. The vesicouterine fold of peritoneum (bladder flap) which lies near the junction of the upper and lower uterine segments is identified and incised transversely; it is dissected off the lower segment and, with the bladder, is pushed downward and retracted out of the way. A small transverse incision is made in the lower segment of the uterus and is extended laterally with the fingers, stopping short of the area of the uterine vessels. The fetal head, which in most cases lies under the incision, is extracted or expressed, followed by the rest of the body and then the placenta and membranes. The transverse incision is closed with a single or double layer of continuous catgut. The bladder flap is then sewn back to the wall of the uterus so that the entire incision is covered and closed off from the general peritoneal cavity. The abdomen is closed in layers.

Advantages of the Transverse Incision: Included are:

1. The incision is made in the thin lower segment.
2. The muscle is split laterally instead of being cut; this leads to less bleeding.
3. Incision into the placenta is rare.
4. The head is usually under the incision and is extracted easily.
5. The thin muscle layer of the lower segment is easier to reapproximate than the thick upper segment.
6. The entire incision is covered by the bladder flap, and this reduces spill into the general peritoneal cavity.
7. There is less danger of rupture of the uterus in subsequent pregnancies.

Disadvantages of the Transverse Incision: Disadvantages are:

1. If the incision extends too far laterally, as may occur if the baby is very big, the uterine vessels can be torn, causing profuse hemorrhage.
2. The procedure is not advisable where there is an abnormality in the lower segment, such as fibroids or extensive varicosities.
3. Previous surgery or dense adhesions which prevent easy access to the lower segment make the operation onerous.
4. When the lower segment is not well formed, the transverse operation is difficult to perform.

Lower Segment: Vertical Incision

The exposure is the same as with the transverse incision. The vertical incision is made with the scalpel and is enlarged with blunt scissors to avoid injury to the baby.

Fig. 1. Cesarean section: composite illustration to demonstrate the three most frequently used incisions. The bladder flap is shown dissected off the lower uterine segment and held out of the way by a retractor. The fetal position is R.O.T.

The vertical incision has an advantage in that it can be carried upward when necessary. This may be needed when the baby is large, when the lower segment is poorly formed, when there is a fetal malposition such as transverse lie, or when there is fetal anomaly such as conjoined twins.

The main disadvantages are that, since the muscle is cut, there is more bleeding from the incised edges, and that too often the incision extends inadvertently into the upper segment and the value of a completely retroperitoneal closure is lost.

Classical Cesarean Section

A longitudinal midline incision is made with the scalpel into the anterior wall of the uterus and is enlarged upward and downward with blunt nosed scissors. A large opening is needed since the baby is often delivered as a breech. The fetus and placenta are removed and the uterus is closed in three layers.

Indications for Classical Section: Included are:

1. When the lower segment procedure is not possible
2. When the operator is not trained in the lower segment operation
3. When the operator wishes to repair a defect at the site of a previous classical section
4. In some cases of transverse lie and uterine or fetal anomaly
5. In cases of anterior placenta previa: Because of the danger of cutting into the placenta in cases of anterior placenta previa, some obstetricians feel that in this situation classical cesarean section is preferable.

Disadvantages of Classical Section: Disadvantages are:

1. Thick myometrium is cut, large sinuses are opened, and bleeding is profuse.
2. The baby is often extracted as a breech with greater aspiration of amniotic fluid.
3. Should the placenta be attached to the anterior wall of the uterus the incision will cut into it and may lead to dangerous loss of blood from the fetal circulation.
4. The incision lies uncovered in the general peritoneal cavity and there is greater chance of seepage of infected uterine contents with resultant peritonitis.
5. There is a higher incidence of adhesions of abdominal contents to the line of closure in the uterus.
6. There is a higher incidence of uterine rupture in subsequent pregnancies.

Extraperitoneal Cesarean Section

This operation was devised to obviate the need for hysterectomy in neglected and grossly infected cases by preventing general and often fatal peritonitis. There are several methods such as those of Waters, Latzko, and Norton.

The technic of this procedure is relatively difficult, accidental entry into the peritoneal cavity is frequent, and there is an increased incidence of injury to the bladder. Better prenatal care, reduction in the incidence of neglected cases, and the availability of blood and antibiotics have reduced the need for the extraperitoneal technic. The method should not be abandoned but kept in reserve for the occasional case.

Cesarean Hysterectomy

This is the performance of a cesarean section followed by removal of the uterus. Whenever possible total hysterectomy should be performed. However, since the subtotal operation is easier and can be done more quickly, it is the procedure of choice when there has been profuse hemorrhage and the patient is in shock, or when she is in poor condition for other reasons. In such cases the aim is to finish the operation as rapidly as possible.

Indications for Cesarean Hysterectomy: Included are:

1. Hemorrhage from uterine atony after failure of conservative therapy
2. Uncontrollable hemorrhage in certain cases of placenta previa and abruptio placentae
3. Placenta accreta
4. Gross multiple fibromyomata
5. In certain cases of cancer of the cervix or ovary
6. Rupture of the uterus, not repairable
7. As a certain method of sterilization where continuation of menstruation is undesirable for medical reasons
8. In neglected and infected cases where the risk of generalized peritonitis is not warranted by the advantage of preserving the uterus, e.g., in a woman who has several children and is not anxious to have more.

MORTALITY AND MORBIDITY FOLLOWING CESAREAN SECTION

Maternal Mortality

The gross uncorrected maternal mortality rate in the United States and Canada is approximately 30 deaths per 10,000 cesarean sections. In many clinics it is less than this. There has been a steady decline in the number of deaths associated with cesarean section due in part to:

1. Adequate blood transfusion
2. The use of antimicrobial drugs
3. Improved surgical methods
4. Better anesthetic technics and specially trained anesthesiologists
5. The realization that patients with heart disease do better with vaginal delivery than with cesarean
6. The basic treatment of toxemia of pregnancy by medical rather than by surgical methods

Causes of maternal deaths include:

1. Hemorrhage
2. Infection
3. Anesthesia
4. Pulmonary embolism
5. Renal failure following prolonged hypotension
6. Intestinal obstruction and paralytic ileus
7. Heart failure
8. Toxemia of pregnancy
9. Rupture of uterine scar
10. Miscellaneous causes not related to the operation, e.g., cancer

Maternal Morbidity

Maternal morbidity is defined as a temperature of 100.4° F or over occurring on any 2 of the first 10 days postpartum, exclusive of the first 24 hours.

It is more common after cesarean section than after normal delivery, the incidence being between 15 and 20 percent. Antimicrobials, blood transfusions, better surgical technic, use of the lower segment operation, and improved anesthesia have all contributed to the decrease in postcesarean maternal morbidity.

Causes of morbidity include:

1. Genital tract infection
2. Wound infection
3. Urinary tract infection
4. Pulmonary and upper respiratory infection
5. Thrombophlebitis
6. Intestinal obstruction and ileus

Fetal Mortality

While fetal mortality associated with cesarean section has declined steadily, it is, at about 5.5 percent, double that of vaginal delivery.

Reasons for the higher incidence with cesarean section include:

1. Conditions such as toxemia of pregnancy, erythroblastosis, and placenta previa that require treatment by cesarean section result in premature, small infants.
2. There are sometimes errors in estimation of fetal size and maturity in elective or repeat cesareans when the patient is thought to be at term.
3. While respiratory complications such as atelectasis and hyaline membrane disease and the respiratory distress syndrome are more common in premature infants, the incidence is much higher when the premature baby is born by cesarean.
4. Conditions such as placenta previa, abruptio placentae, diabetes, preeclampsia, eclampsia, essential hypertension, chronic nephritis, and prolapse of the umbilical cord result in babies whose general condition and powers of resistance and recuperation are low. When these conditions need treatment by cesarean section fetal mortality is increased.
5. In general, cesarean section does not give as good a prognosis for the infant as does the normal vaginal delivery.

BIBLIOGRAPHY

Douglas, R. G., and Stromme, W. B. Operative Obstetrics, 2nd ed. New York, Appleton-Century-Crofts, 1965.
Eastman, N. J., and Hellman, L. M. Williams Obstetrics, 13th ed., New York, Appleton-Century-Crofts, 1966.

40   Embryotomy: Destructive Operations on the Fetus

The purpose of destructive operations on the unborn child is to reduce its size (head, shoulder girdle, or body) and so enable the vaginal delivery of a baby which is too large to pass intact through the birth canal. This procedure is tolerable only on a fetus that is dead or that is so deformed that survival is impossible. The risk of abdominal delivery to the mother has decreased to the point where embryotomy on the living normal child is never justified. Indeed the operation is so unpleasant and the dangers to the mother are such that destructive procedures are performed rarely today. After delivery the birth canal must be examined thoroughly to be certain that no injury has been caused by the instruments or the sharp edges of the bones of the skull.

Contraindications to Embryotomy

1. Living normal fetus
2. Markedly contracted pelvis
3. Cervix less than three fourths dilated: Full dilatation is preferable.
4. Neoplasms obstructing the pelvis

Dangers of Embryotomy

1. Lacerations of the vagina, cervix, and uterus, as well as fistulae in the bladder or rectum
2. Uterine rupture, especially through the thinned out lower segment, where labor has been obstructed
3. Hemorrhage from lacerations and uterine atony
4. Infection
5. The risks attendant on prolonged deep anesthesia

Types of Embryotomy

Craniotomy: Craniotomy is the opening of the skull. This can be done by perforating the head with Smellie scissors, evacuating the brain, and delivering the head by applying scalp traction with a tenaculum. Sometimes following craniotomy the head is crushed and extracted by special instruments (cranioclast, basiotribe).

The purpose of the operation is to reduce the bulk of the head. The only indication acceptable today is hydrocephalus. The excess cerebrospinal fluid can be removed, even in a live infant, by inserting a large bore needle (16 to 18) through the scalp.   The size of the head is reduced and its delivery made possible.

The most direct approach to encephalocentesis is via the vagina.   The needle is inserted into the cranial cavity through a fontanelle or suture, avoiding the sagittal sinus.   If necessary, the needle can be pushed through one of the cranial bones.   When the presentation is breech, drainage can be achieved by spondylectomy, or, if the head is accessible, by direct entry into the ventricles beneath the occipital plate, or behind an ear.

When the head cannot be reached through the vagina, an alternative route is transabdominal.   The needle is passed through the abdominal and uterine walls, and through the fetal cranial bones into the interior of the skull.

Spondylectomy: Spondylectomy is the transection of the spine of the delivered thorax.   In a breech presentation this may allow drainage of cerebrospinal fluid.   It is done when the back is anterior and the head and neck are out of reach.   In cases of hydrocephalus when there is communication between the ventricles and the spinal cord, the fluid may be drained from the brain in this way, and so the need for craniotomy is obviated.

Decapitation: The head is severed from the body.   This may be done for neglected transverse presentations when the child is dead and version and extraction or cesarean section are contraindicated.   It may be done also when twins have become interlocked, chin to chin.   A blunt hook is placed over the neck to steady the fetus, and decapitation is performed with scissors.   The fingers of the other hand are used to protect the mother's soft tissues.   After decapitation the body is extracted by pulling on an arm or a lower limb.   The head is delivered either by forceps or by inserting a finger in the mouth and exerting traction on the jaw.   This must be done slowly.

Cleidotomy: Cleidotomy is indicated when there is shoulder dystocia and a dead fetus.   One or both clavicles are cut with scissors.   The shoulder girdle then collapses, and delivery is accomplished.

Evisceration: Evisceration is the removal of the organs from the abdomen and thorax to reduce the size of the body of the fetus.

Morcellation: On rare occasions it is necessary to cut the fetus into pieces before vaginal delivery can be accomplished.

BIBLIOGRAPHY

Boring, W. D., and Nathanson, B. N.   Transabdominal fetal encephalocentesis for hydrocephalus.   Obstet. Gynec., 26:399, 1965.

Douglas, R. G., and Stromme, W. B.   Operative Obstetrics, 2nd ed.   New York, Appleton-Century-Crofts, 1965.

O'Neill, E.   Destructive obstetric operations.   Obstet. Gynec., 21:725, 1963.

41 Postpartum Hemorrhage

Definition: This term, in its wider meaning, includes all bleeding following the birth of the baby: before, during, and after the delivery of the placenta. By definition loss of over 500 ml of blood in the first 24 hours constitutes postpartum hemorrhage. After 24 hours it is called "late postpartum hemorrhage." The incidence of postpartum hemorrhage is about 10 percent.

At normal delivery an average of 200 ml of blood is lost. Episiotomy raises this figure by 100 ml, and sometimes more. Pregnant women have an increased amount of blood and fluid, and this enables the healthy patient to lose 500 ml without serious effect. To the anemic patient, however, an even smaller amount of bleeding can be dangerous.

CLINICAL FEATURES

The Clinical Picture

The clinical picture is one of continuing bleeding and gradual deterioration. The pulse becomes rapid and weak, the blood pressure falls, the patient turns pale and cold, and there is shortness of breath, air hunger, sweating, and finally coma and death. A treacherous feature of the situation is that because of compensatory vascular mechanisms the pulse and blood pressure may show only moderate change for some time. Then suddenly the compensatory function can no longer be maintained, the pulse rises quickly, the blood pressure drops suddenly, and the patient is in shock. The uterus can fill up with considerable blood, which is lost to the patient even though there may be little external hemorrhage.

Danger of Postpartum Hemorrhage

The danger of postpartum hemorrhage is twofold:

1. The blood loss, if not arrested, will cause the patient's death.
2. The resultant anemia lowers the patient's resistance and predisposes to puerperal infection.

Studies of Maternal Deaths

Studies of maternal deaths show that women have died from continuous bleeding of amounts which at the time were not alarming. It is not the sudden

475

gush that kills, but the steady trickle. In a large series of cases Beacham found that the average interval between delivery and death was 5 hours and 20 minutes. No woman died within 1 hour and 30 minutes of giving birth. This suggests that there is adequate time for effective therapy if the patient has been observed carefully, the diagnosis made early, and proper treatment instituted.

ETIOLOGY

The causes of postpartum hemorrhage fall into four main groups:

Uterine Atony

The control of postpartum bleeding is by contraction and retraction of the myometrial fibers. This causes kinking of the blood vessels and so cuts off the flow to the placental site. Failure of this mechanism, resulting from disordered myometrial function, is called "uterine atony" and is the main cause of postpartum hemorrhage.

While the occasional case of postpartum uterine atony is completely unexpected, in many instances the presence of predisposing factors will alert the observant physician to the possibility of trouble.

1. Uterine dysfunction: Primary uterine atony is an intrinsic dysfunction of the uterus.
2. Mismanagement of the placental stage: The most common error is to try and hurry the third stage. Kneading and squeezing of the uterus interferes with the physiologic mechanism of placental detachment and may cause partial placental separation with resultant bleeding.
3. Anesthesia: Deep and prolonged inhalation anesthesia is a common cause. There is excessive relaxation of the myometrium, failure of contraction and retraction, uterine atony, and postpartum hemorrhage.
4. Ineffective uterine action: Ineffective uterine action in the first two stages of labor is likely to be followed by poor contraction and retraction in the third stage.
5. Overdistension of the uterus: The uterus which has been overdistended by conditions such as large baby, multiple pregnancy, and polyhydramnios, has a tendency to contract poorly.
6. Exhaustion from prolonged labor: Not only is the tired uterus likely to contract weakly after delivery of the baby, but the worn out mother is less able to stand loss of blood.
7. Multiparity: The uterus which has borne many children is prone to inefficient action in all stages of labor.
8. Myomata of the uterus: By interfering with proper contraction and retraction myomata of the uterus predispose to hemorrhage.
9. Operative deliveries: This includes operative procedures such as mid forceps and version and extraction.

Trauma and Lacerations

Considerable bleeding can take place from tears sustained during normal and operative deliveries. The birth canal should be inspected after each delivery so that the sources of bleeding can be controlled.

Sites of hemorrhage include:

1. Episiotomy. Blood loss may reach 200 cc. When arterioles or large varicose veins are cut or torn the amount of blood lost can be considerably
   more. Hence, bleeding vessels should be clamped immediately to con-
   serve blood.
2. Vulva, vagina, and cervix
3. Ruptured uterus
4. Uterine inversion
5. Puerperal hematomas

In addition, other factors operate to cause an excessive loss of blood where
there is trauma to the birth canal. These include:

1. Prolonged interval between performance of the episiotomy and delivery of
   the child
2. Undue delay from birth of the baby to repair of the episiotomy
3. Failure to secure bleeding vessel at the apex of the episiotomy
4. Neglect of inspection of upper vagina and cervix
5. Nonappreciation of the possibility of multiple sites of injury
6. Undue reliance on oxytocic agents accompanied by too long a delay in ex-
   ploring the uterus

Retained Placenta

Retention in the uterus of part or all of the placenta interferes with contraction and retraction, keeps the blood sinuses open, and leads to postpartum hemorrhage. Once part of the placenta has separated from the uterine wall, bleeding will take place from that area. The part of the placenta which is still attached prevents proper retraction, and bleeding goes on until the rest of the
organ has separated and is expelled.

The retention of the whole placenta, part of it, a succenturiate lobe, a single cotyledon, or a fragment of placenta can cause postpartum bleeding. In
some cases there is placenta accreta. There is no correlation between the
amount of placenta retained and the severity of the hemorrhage. The important
consideration is the degree of adherence.

Miscellaneous

1. Blood dyscrasias: Any of the hemorrhagic diseases can affect pregnant
   women and occasionally will be responsible for postpartum hemorrhage.
2. Afibrinogenemia or hypofibrinogenemia: This condition may follow abruptio
   placenta, prolonged retention in utero of a dead fetus, and amniotic fluid
   embolism. One etiologic theory postulates that thromboplastic material
   arising from the degeneration and autolysis of the decidua and placenta may
   enter the maternal circulation and give rise to intravascular coagulation
   and loss of circulating fibrinogen. This condition, a failure of the clotting
   mechanism, causes bleeding which cannot be arrested by the measures
   usually employed to control hemorrhage. Fibrinogen must be replaced.

INVESTIGATION

1. To obtain a reasonable idea of the amount of blood lost, an estimate is
   made and the figure doubled.

2. The uterine fundus is palpated frequently to make certain it is not filling up with blood.
3. The uterine cavity is explored both for placental remnants and for uterine rupture.
4. The vulva, vagina, and cervix are examined carefully for lacerations.
5. The pulse and blood pressure are measured and recorded.
6. A sample of blood is observed for clotting.

TREATMENT

Prophylaxis

1. Every pregnant woman should know her blood group.
2. Antepartum anemia is treated.
3. Certain patients are susceptible to and certain conditions predispose to postpartum hemorrhage. These include:
   a. The woman who has had more than five babies
   b. History of postpartum hemorrhage or manual removal of the placenta
   c. Abruptio placentae
   d. Placenta previa
   e. Multiple pregnancy
   f. Polyhydramnios
   g. Intrauterine death with prolonged retention of the dead fetus
   h. Prolonged labor
   i. Difficult forceps delivery
   j. Version and extraction
   k. Breech extraction
   l. Cesarean section
4. In cases where uterine atony is anticipated an intravenous infusion is set up before the delivery and oxytocin added to ensure good uterine contractions. This is continued for at least 1 hour post partum.
5. Excessive and prolonged inhalatory anesthesia should be avoided.
6. As long as the child is in good condition and there is no need for rapid extraction, the body is delivered slowly. This facilitates placental separation and permits the uterus to retract sufficiently to control bleeding from the placental site.
7. Once the placenta has separated it should be expelled.
8. Squeezing or kneading the uterus before the placenta has separated is traumatic and harmful.
9. One of the ergot preparations or oxytocin is given after delivery of the placenta to ensure good uterine contraction and retraction.
10. Careful postpartum observation of the patient is made, and palpation of the uterine fundus to prevent its filling with blood is done. The patient remains in the delivery room for at least 1 hour post partum.
11. Fibrinogen studies are done in cases of placental abruption and retained dead fetus
12. When hemorrhage is anticipated adequate amounts of blood should be cross-matched and available.

Fig. 1. Bimanual compression of the uterus.

Supportive Measures

1. The key to successful treatment is the transfusion of blood. The amount must be adequate to replace at least the amount lost. Usually a minimum of 1 liter is needed. It is given quickly. When response to blood replacement is not satisfactory the following conditions must be considered:
   a. Continued unappreciated ooze
   b. Bleeding into an atonic uterus
   c. Silent filling of the vagina
   d. Bleeding behind and into a uterine pack
   e. Hematoma formation
   f. Intraperitoneal bleeding as with ruptured uterus
   g. Afibrinogenemia or hypofibrinogenemia
   h. Bacteremic shock
2. Until blood is available plasma expanders are used.
3. If the blood pressure is falling the foot of the table is elevated.
4. Oxygen is given by face mask.
5. Warmth is provided by blankets.
6. Morphine is given by hypodermic injection.
7. If afibrinogenemia is present, fibrinogen is administered by vein. Two to six grams are injected. Because of the danger of serum hepatitis following the use of fibrinogen, the patient is given gamma globulin.

Placental Bleeding

In the presence of excessive bleeding associated with the third stage no time should be wasted. Manual removal of the placenta is carried out immediately and oxytocics given. The uterus should not be manhandled in efforts to squeeze out the placenta.

Uterine Atony

1. The uterine fundus is massaged through the abdomen.
2. Ergometrine 0.125 or 0.25 mg is given intravenously and/or 0.5 mg intramuscularly.
3. Oxytocin can be given intramuscularly, but the best method is by an intravenous drip with 5 or 10 units of oxytocin in a liter of 5 percent glucose in water. This is run at a speed sufficient to keep the uterus contracted.
4. Manual exploration of the uterus is carried out, and fragments of placenta and membrane and blood clots are removed.
5. The cervix, vagina, and vulva are examined for lacerations.
6. Bimanual compression of the uterus is a valuable method of controlling uterine atonic bleeding. One hand is placed in the vagina against the anterior wall of the uterus. Pressure is exerted against the posterior aspect of the uterus by the other hand through the abdomen. With a rotatory motion the uterus is compressed and massaged between the two hands. This provides twice the amount of uterine stimulation that can be achieved by abdominal massage alone. In addition compression of the venous sinuses can be effected and the flow of blood reduced. As part of this procedure the atonic uterus is elevated, anteverted, and anteflexed.
7. Packing the uterine cavity is a controversial subject. Most authorities condemn its use in that the procedure is unphysiologic. Up to this point attempts had been made to empty the uterus; now it is to be filled. It is not likely that a uterus which will not respond to powerful oxytocic drugs will be stimulated to contract by the gauze pack. It is impossible to pack an atonic uterus so tightly that the blood sinuses will be closed off. The uterus will simply balloon and fill up with more blood. Thus the packing not only does no good but is dangerous in that it leads to a false sense of security by obscuring the flow of blood. Ten yards of three inch packing gauze will absorb 1,000 ml of blood. Furthermore, packing favors infection.
8. In thin women compression of the aorta against the spine may slow down the bleeding.
9. Hysterectomy. If the bleeding continues, the abdomen must be opened and hysterectomy performed. Deaths following and during hysterectomy have been reported, and these have resulted from delaying the operation until the patient was nearly moribund. Performed in time, hysterectomy is effective and lifesaving.
10. Uterine artery ligation. Since most of the uterine blood supply passes through the uterine arteries, their ligation may control postpartum hemorrhage without sacrificing the uterus. The abdomen is opened and the area of the uterine vessels identified. The uterine wall and broad ligament are grasped and a large needle with #1 chromic catgut is passed anteroposteriorly through the myometrium of the lower uterine segment adjacent to the vessels. It is brought out through the avascular area of the broad ligament. The uterine artery distal to the exit of the cervical branch is tied off with a single ligation. The vessels are not divided. The uterus becomes blanched with a pink hue, and bleeding subsides. In some cases the uterus will contract firmly, in others it becomes less soft. If this procedure does not stop the bleeding, hysterectomy is performed.

11. Internal iliac artery ligation. This may be performed in any situation in which pelvic bleeding is uncontrollable. Collateral circulation is so extensive that the pelvic arterial system is never deprived of blood, and there is no necrosis of any of the pelvic tissue. Entry into the abdomen is made by a midline or transverse incision. First the common iliac artery and its bifurcation into the external and internal iliac arteries is palpated and visualized through the posterior peritoneum. The ureter crosses anterior to the bifurcation of the common iliac artery, and it must be identified to prevent its being damaged. The posterior peritoneum is tented and incised in a longitudinal direction beginning at the level of the origin of the internal iliac artery, and extending caudad for 4 to 6 cm. This incision is lateral to the ureter and medial to the internal iliac artery. The ureter usually remains attached to the medial flap of peritoneum. Both the external and internal iliac arteries must be identified to be certain that the correct vessel is tied. Care is taken to avoid injury to the veins. Two #2-0 silk sutures are placed around the interial iliac artery 1 cm apart and then tied. The procedure is repeated on the other side.

Lacerations

1. Rupture of the uterus necessitates laparotomy with either repair of the tear or hysterectomy.
2. Lacerations of the cervix, vagina, and vulva are repaired and the bleeding controlled with figure of 8 sutures.
3. In some cases the bleeding from the vaginal tears cannot be controlled with sutures. Where there are large varicosities each passage of the needle through the tissue seems to provoke fresh bleeding. In such cases the vagina should be packed firmly with gauze, which is left in for 24 hours.
4. Rarely, bleeding from a small superficial laceration in the lower uterine segment can be controlled by packing.

LATE POSTPARTUM HEMORRHAGE

Late postpartum hemorrhage takes place after the first 24 hours. Most occur within 21 days.

Causes

1. Retained fragments of placenta
2. Subinvolution of the uterus and delayed involution of the placental site
3. Intrauterine infection leading to dissolution of the thromboses of the placental vessels
4. Sloughing of sutures from sepsis causing bleeding from the episiotomy or lacerations
5. Uterine fibromyomata, especially the submucous variety.
6. Chorionepithelioma

Treatment

1. Oxytocics are given to try to control the bleeding.
2. If bleeding continues, curettage is performed. This is done carefully to avoid perforating the uterus. In over half the cases no placental tissue is found, the histologic examination showing organized blood clot, decidual tissue, or fragments of muscle. However, the results of curettage seem to be satisfactory whether or not placenta was retained.
3. Secondary hemorrhage from lacerations is treated by sutures and packing.
4. Antimicrobial agents are prescribed.
5. Blood transfusion is given as needed.

BIBLIOGRAPHY

Dewhurst, C. J. Secondary post–partum hemorrhage. J. Obstet. Gynaec. Brit. Comm., 73:53, 1966.

Gordon, C. A., Rosenthal, A. H., and O'Leary, J. L. Postpartum hemorrhage. Amer. J. Surg., 80:587, 1950.

LeCocq, F. Internal iliac artery ligation. Amer. J. Obstet. Gynec., 95:320, 1966.

Lester, W. M., Bartholomew, R. A., Colvin, E. D., Grimes, W. H., Fish, J. S., and Galloway, W. H. Reconsideration of the uterine pack in post-partum hemorrhage. Amer. J. Obstet. Gynec., 93:321, 1965.

MacKay, E. V. Massive post partum hemorrhage. Aust. N. Z. J. Obstet. Gynaec., 5:203, 1965.

O'Leary, J. L., and O'Leary, J. A. Uterine artery ligation in the control of intractable postpartum hemorrhage. Amer. J. Obstet. Gynec., 94:920, 1966.

Paul, W. M., and Kinch, R. A. H. Postpartum hemorrhage. Canad. Med. Ass. J., 87:751, 1962.

Roth, E., and Glynn, R. Internal iliac artery ligation. Obstet. Gynec., 24:49, 1964.

42   Radiography in Obstetrics

As a diagnostic aid the x-ray has a wide range of uses in obstetrics. Because the exact effects of the rays on the maternal ovaries and on the fetus are not known, radiography should be employed in pregnancy only when there is a clear and definite indication. The first trimester is considered to be the most dangerous time.

USES OF RADIOGRAPHY IN OBSTETRICS

Areas in which radiography is helpful include:

1. In cases where hydatidiform mole or chorionepithelioma is suspected and clinical examinations and hormonal tests are inconclusive, a flat plate of the abdomen can demonstrate the presence or absence of a fetus.
2. An abdominal pregnancy can be shown to lie separate from the uterus.
3. The presence of multiple pregnancy can be proved and the positions of the babies in utero shown.
4. Sometimes fetal maturity can be determined. In normally developing fetuses the epiphysis at the distal (lower) end of the femur is visible on x-ray at 36 weeks gestation. The epiphysis at the proximal (upper) end of the tibia appears at 38 weeks.
5. When manual examination is inconclusive, x-ray can be used where it is necessary to establish the lie, presentation, position, and attitude of the fetus.
6. Engagement and descent of the presenting part can be demonstrated.
7. Intrauterine death may be shown. The muscles become flaccid, the limbs are distorted, and there is loss of flexion. Spaulding's sign, the overlapping of the cranial bones as the fetal skull collapses, may be present as early as 7 hours after death.
8. Fetal abnormalities such as hydrocephaly, anencephaly, and spina bifida may be demonstrated. In hydrops fetalis the fetus sometimes assumes the Buddha position.
9. Placental localization is possible by special soft tissue technics, and diagnosis of placenta previa may be established.
10. Bony injuries to the maternal pelvis can be seen.
11. The halo sign. The fetal skull is covered by the scalp. The layers from the deepest to the most superficial are:
    a. The periosteum is closely adherent to the bony skull.

483

b. The galea (an aponeurotic layer) is attached loosely to the periosteum.
c. The subcutis is attached firmly to the galea. In the last months of pregnancy the subcutis is densely infiltrated by fat cells and is the thickest soft tissue layer of the scalp.
d. Outside of the subcutis is the cutis.

The fat-containing subcutaneous layer has a lower density than the other soft tissues, and appears on the x-ray of the fetus in utero as a dark line.

When there is edema of the scalp the fluid lies mainly between the periosteum and the galea and to a lesser degree between the galea and the subcutis. The edema fluid elevates the fat containing subcutis from the skull. On x-ray the fat layer is seen as a dark line, apart from the skull, and more or less parallel to it. This is the halo sign.

The halo sign is seen in both the dead and the living fetus. It occurs in erythroblastosis, and if the baby is alive, it indicates severe hydrops fetalis.

X-RAY PELVIMETRY

X-ray pelvimetry is the most frequently used method of radiography in obstetrics. It is a valuable aid to mensuration of the pelvis, but only when used in conjunction with clinical examination and judgment.

Information gained includes:

1. The shape and inclination of the pelvis
2. The length of the diameters
3. The relationship and fit of the fetal head to the pelvis

X-ray pelvimetry not only provides greater precision of mensuration but makes possible the measurement of many important diameters which cannot be obtained manually, e.g., the transverse diameter of the inlet and the distance between the ischial spines. Moreover, it affords a better understanding of the configuration of the pelvis. This has enabled the female pelvis to be classified according to shape, permitting a more accurate clinical prognosis of the outcome of labor to be made.

A great problem in pelvimetry is the distortion produced by the divergence of the x-rays. The degree of distortion depends on the distance between the object and the film and the distance from the tube to the film. Many methods, such as Caldwell-Moloy, Colcher-Sussman, and Snow, have been described to attempt to correct for the distortion. In our clinic we use Thom's technic. It is sufficiently accurate in its measurements and has the advantage of showing clearly the shape of the pelvis. No complicated calculations are needed, and the average clinician can understand the results.

Three films are taken of which only the last two are part of the Thoms' isometric technic.

The Abdominal View

An anteroposterior view is taken of the abdomen with the patient positioned on her back. This view gives a good picture of the entire fetus.

Information Gained from the Abdominal View

1. The attitude of the fetus
2. The lie, presentation, and position
3. A rough estimate of the size of the baby
4. The presence of more than one fetus
5. Ossification centers that may estimate fetal maturity
6. Fetal abnormalities or death

The Lateral View

A lateral view of the pelvis with the patient erect is taken. The woman stands so that one side is next to the film and the other is facing the x-ray tube. A metal ruler with notches or perforations 1 cm apart is placed in the gluteal folds between the buttocks. The tube is at a distance of 36 inches. If the patient is positioned properly the acetabula should be superimposed. The image of the scale on the film will show the same amount of distortion as the sagittal diameters of the pelvis, and so a reasonably accurate measurement of the diameters is possible. The desired diameters are measured with calipers. These are then placed in the grid scale and the correct length determined.

Information Gained from the Lateral View

1. The inclination, curve, and length of the sacrum
2. The depth of the pelvis
3. The relationship of the promontory of the sacrum to the inlet
4. The sacrosciatic notch, whether it is wide or narrow
5. Anteroposterior diameters of the inlet, the obstetric conjugate; midpelvis, the plane of least dimensions; and the outlet
6. The posterior sagittal diameter of the midpelvis and the outlet
7. The size and shape of the ischial spines. Are they small or large? Are they prominent and posterior? Do they shorten the posterior sagittal diameter and narrow the sacrosciatic notch?
8. The length and inclination of the symphysis
9. The station of the fetal presenting part
10. In cephalic presentations, the presence of synclitism or asynclitism
11. The attitude of the fetus, flexion or extension
12. The relationship or fit of the head to the pelvis

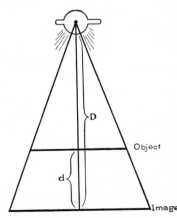

Fig. 1. Principle of divergent distortion. Size of the image depends on object-film distance (d) and tube-film distance (D). (From Eastman and Hellman. Williams Obstetrics, 12th ed., Appleton-Century-Crofts, 1961.)

The Anteroposterior View

The anteroposterior film of the pelvis is taken with the patient on the table using a special backrest which supports her in a semirecumbent position. In order that the plane of the inlet will be parallel to the x-ray table, the patient is positioned so that the perpendicular distance to the table from the juncture of the fourth and fifth lumbar vertebrae and from a point 1 cm below the upper border of the symphysis are equal. The x-ray tube is placed at a height of 36 inches and about 6 cm cephalad to the symphysis. The film is taken and the

Fig. 2. Positioning of patient and markers for the Thoms' antero-posterior pelvic X-Rays. (From Eastman and Hellman. Williams Obstetrics, 12th ed., 1961.)

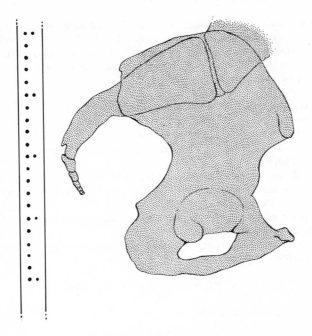

Fig. 3. The relation of the centimeter scale image to the lateral view of the pelvis, Thoms' technic.

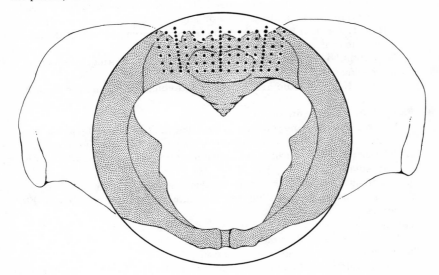

Fig. 4. The relation of the centimeter scale image to the antero-posterior view of the pelvis, Thoms' technic.

patient is removed from the table, but the tube and exposed film are left in place. A lead sheet perforated at intervals of 1 cm is placed in the same plane as the pelvic inlet and a flash film is taken. This superimposes the scale on the picture. The distortion of the pelvis and the grid plate are similar and the diameters can be measured.

Information Gained from the Anteroposterior View

1. The shape of the inlet, the posterior and anterior segments. Is the posterior segment well rounded or heart-shaped? Is the anterior segment round or wedge-shaped?
2. The widest transverse diameter of the inlet
3. The distance between the ischial spines, the transverse diameter of the plane of least dimensions
4. The anterior and posterior sagittal diameters of the inlet
5. The size and shape of the ischial spines
6. The slope of the sidewalls. Are they straight, convergent, or divergent?
7. Classification of the pelvis

INDICATIONS FOR X-RAY PELVIMETRY

1. History of previous pregnancies
   a. Difficult delivery
   b. Fetal damage or death during labor and delivery
   c. Unexplained fetal death
   d. Vaginal delivery being considered after previous cesarean section
2. Manual examination unsatisfactory or suggestive of a small pelvis
   a. Inlet: The sacral promontory can be reached easily; the diagonal conjugate is less than 11.5 cm.
   b. Midpelvis: Large prominent ischial spines, indicating a reduction in the interspinous diameter
   c. Outlet: Narrow pubic arch with the intertuberous diameter less than 8.0 cm
3. Fetopelvic relationships
   a. Failure of engagement of the presenting part in a primigravida near term, especially when the head cannot be pushed into the inlet
   b. Breech presentation in a primigravida or in a multipara who has borne only small babies
   c. Abnormal presentations, such as transverse lie, face, and brow
   d. Impression on examination that this baby is large in relation to this pelvis
4. During labor
   a. When labor is prolonged
   b. When progress is not being made
   c. When molding and caput succedaneum make it difficult to be certain of the station of the bony skull

5. Maternal indications
   a. Elderly primigravida
   b. History of injury to the bony pelvis

BIBLIOGRAPHY

Borell, V., Fernstrom, I., and Ohlson, L. The halo sign in the living and dead fetus. Amer. J. Obstet. Gynec., 87:906, 1963.

Caldwell, W. E., Moloy, H. C., and Swenson, P. C. The use of the roentgen ray in obstetrics: Part I. Roentgen pelvimetry and cephalometry; technic of pelvioroentgenography. Amer. J. Roentgenol., 41:305, 1939; Part II. Anatomical variations in the female pelvis and their classification according to morphology. Amer. J. Roentgenol., 41:505, 1939; Part III. The mechanism of labor. Amer. J. Roentgenol., 41:719, 1939.

Clayton, C. G., Farmer, F. T., and Warrick, C. K. Radiation dosage to the foetal and maternal gonads in obstetrics radiography during late pregnancy. Brit. J. Radiol., 30:291, 1959.

Colcher, A. E., and Sussman, W. A practical technique for roentgen pelvimetry with new positioning. Amer. J. Roentgenol., 51:207, 1944.

Snow, W. Roentgenology in Obstetrics. Springfield, Ill., Charles C. Thomas, 1952.

Thoms, H. The Obstetric Pelvis. Baltimore, The Williams & Wilkins Co., 1935.

_____ Foote, W. R., and Friedman, I. The clinical significance of pelvic variations. Amer. J. Obstet. Gynec., 38:634, 1939.

43 Obstetric Analgesia and Anesthesia

In 1847 Sir James Young Simpson introduced anesthesia into obstetric practice. Intermittently inhaled ether and then chloroform were used to relieve the pains of the final stages of labor and delivery. The perfect method of abolishing the pain of childbirth has not been achieved. It is beyond the province of this book to describe the whole gamut of obstetric analgesia and anesthesia. We shall present general principles of efficiency and safety and some modern technics.

Causes of pain during labor are usually related to one of the following:

1. Myometrial anoxia: Contraction of a muscle during a period of relative anoxia causes pain. When uterine relaxation between contractions is insufficient to allow adequate oxygenation, the severity of pain is increased.
2. Stretching of the cervix: Stretching of the cervix causes pain which is felt mainly in the back.
3. Pressure on the nerve ganglia adjacent to the cervix and vagina
4. Traction on the tubes, ovaries, and peritoneum
5. Traction on and stretching of the supporting ligaments
6. Pressure on the urethra, bladder, and rectum
7. Distension of the muscles of the pelvic floor and perineum

Objectives and methods include:

1. Objectives for the mother
   a. Relief of pain
   b. Freedom from fear
   c. Some degree of amnesia
   d. Safe and relatively painless delivery
2. Objectives for the infant
   a. To improve the progress of labor
   b. To make the delivery less traumatic
3. Objectives for the obstetrician
   a. More deliberate management of the labor
   b. Reduction of pressure from patient and relatives to do something prematurely
   c. Optimum conditions at delivery
4. Methods of achieving objectives
   a. Prenatal training for childbirth which dissipates fear and tension
   b. Sedation by the use of drugs such as barbiturates and tranquilizers
   c. Analgesia by narcotics such as morphine and Demerol

490

      d. Amnesia, provided specifically by scopolamine (hyoscine), but also, to
         a lesser degree, by the sedatives and analgesics
      e. Anesthesia (absence of all sensation) by a wide variety of agents: inhal-
         ant, local, intravenous, and conduction technics
5. Relief of pain during the stages of labor
    a. In the first stage the aim is for sedation, amnesia, and analgesia.
    b. In the second stage the same objectives are sought, with the addition of
       anesthesia when necessary.
    c. The same factors are considered in the third stage.

Criteria for the ideal method must ensure that:

1. The health of the mother will not be endangered.
2. No harm should come to the fetus: Drugs given to the mother cross the
   placenta and reach the infant. Varying degrees of respiratory depression
   result and the baby may be apneic at birth. Some babies are lethargic after birth and require stimulation in the nursery. The long-term effects of
   narcosis on the infant's brain must be considered as well.
3. The agent will have the ability of abolishing or diminishing pain and the
   memory of suffering.
4. The efficiency of the uterine contractions is not decreased: This could
   cause prolonged labor in the first and second stages and atonic postpartum
   hemorrhage in the third.
5. The ability of the patient to cooperate intelligently with the medical and
   nursing staff will be maintained.
6. There should be no need for operative interference solely because of the
   anesthesia.
7. The method will be reasonably simple to use.

    There is no system of analgesia and anesthesia available which fulfils all
these criteria. Compromises are made, but safety must never take second
place to efficiency.

General data on the uses of analgesia and anesthesia:

1. There is wide variation in the degree of analgesia and anesthesia, ranging
   from the minimal dosage designed to take the edge off the pain to the complete abolition of sensation.
2. The smallest effective amount is best.

Fig. 1. Paracervical Block.

3. Unless there is a contraindication, the request of the patient for relief should not be refused.
4. Given too soon or in excessive dosage analgesic preparations interfere with uterine contractions and delay labor. Prescribed at the proper time, pain is relieved, and labor may be speeded up by the relaxation of tension.
5. The widespread use of episiotomy has increased the need for anesthesia.
6. Certain anesthetics, such as spinals, epidurals, or general anesthesia, given too soon, have increased the incidence of forceps extractions.
7. Premature infants are exceedingly susceptible to narcotics of any kind, and best results are attained when the mother is given no narcotics and no general anesthesia.
8. The quality and quantity of nursing supervision determine to an extent the drugs which can or cannot be used safely. Since some agents cause excitement, patients receiving them must be under constant observation.
9. The availability of the obstetrician is important in deciding what drugs can be given. Remote control is never as successful as personal management.
10. The availability of a trained anesthetist is essential if complicated technics are to be employed.

TRAINING FOR CHILDBIRTH

The purpose of training for childbirth is to prepare a woman for labor and delivery so that she approaches the end of her pregnancy with knowledge, understanding, and confidence rather than with apprehension and fear. She should be assured that relief will be provided should pain be excessive and that the modern obstetric armamentarium is available to ensure the safety of herself and her unborn child.

Grantly Dick-Read and Herbert Thoms held that fear stimulates the sympathetic nervous system and causes the circular muscles of the cervix to contract. Thus the longitudinal muscles of the uterus and lower segment have to act against increased resistance, causing tension and pain. This in turn aggravates fear, a vicious cycle is established, and a minor degree of pain is magnified by fear so that it becomes agonizing.

Aims of Prenatal Training

1. To counteract the apprehension of young women caused by the exaggerated tales of horror told by multiparas
2. To give the patient an opportunity to gain confidence, the facts of childbirth are explained, and the methods available to relieve pain are described.
3. Exercises are taught which strengthen certain muscles and relax others.
4. The patient is trained in breech control.
5. The patient is never told that the labor and delivery will be painless. On the contrary, it is emphasized that analgesia and anesthesia are available should they be needed or desired.
6. It is important that the patient is not placed in competition with other women or with an ideal analgesia-free labor and delivery. Too many women who do need assistance are left with a feeling of failure and remain emotionally disturbed.

7. While patients should be encouraged to take part in the training classes, reluctant women must never be forced into participating.
8. Constant emphasis is placed on the fact that most labors are normal.
9. The program has two parts. The education and exercises are beneficial to all. Whether or not an individual is desirous of or able to carry on without any drugs can be decided only during labor.

Whenever possible the patient should be in a private labor room, with an attendant at all times. This may be her husband, some other relative, a friend, a nurse, or her doctor. Peace and quiet in the labor suite are essential. Nothing which might worry the patient should be said in her hearing. Women in labor read erroneous and worrisome significance into innocent remarks. Unruly and noisy patients should be kept out of earshot, since nothing frightens a woman in labor as much as hearing another's screams.

Achievements of Trained Childbirth

1. Women approach labor with confidence.
2. Labors are shorter and less traumatic.
3. Less medication is needed because fewer women complain of unbearable discomfort.
4. There is reduction in the need for operative interference.
5. Blood loss is minimal.
6. Fetal anoxia is unusual.
7. The patient is left with a deep sense of pride and happiness.

On the one hand, there are women who, without having ever attended a training class, are able to go through pregnancy, labor, and delivery with ease and calm. On the other hand, many women will have difficulties no matter how much training they receive.

RELIEF OF PAIN IN THE FIRST STAGE OF LABOR

It is not possible to guarantee complete analgesia and amnesia for the entire labor, and this promise should never be made to the patient. Excessively deep analgesia not only carries risks to mother and child but can complicate the progress and management of labor. However, pain can be relieved safely to a degree that the patient's strength is conserved, she can maintain control, and the apprehension of her family is allayed.

Each patient is handled individually. The types and amount of therapy depends on the patient's personality as well as on the efficiency of the labor. In many cases labor is so short that a single administration of an analgesic is enough to carry the patient to the point of delivery. In difficult labors where multiple doses are required, the program of analgesia and amnesia must be planned carefully. Multiparas generally need less support than primigravidas. The more perfect the result required, the more completely is the personal supervision of the obstetrician necessary.

In the first stage of labor the main objectives are the production of analgesia (relief of pain) and amnesia (loss of memory). Since it is not safe to give doses of narcotics large enough to produce both analgesia and amnesia, scopolamine has been added to enhance the amnesia. Unfortunately drugs which encourage amnesia sometimes lead to excitement and even delirium.

The Narcotics

Morphine

Morphine has been used in obstetrics for many years. The dose is 10 mg (grain 1/6). Because of the danger of fetal narcosis it is prescribed less frequently today during labor. It is useful in the relief of postpartum pain.

Effects on the Mother: The effects on the mother include:

1. The threshold for pain is elevated.
2. Fear and anxiety are replaced by feelings of indifference.
3. Lethargy and sleep are induced.

Effects on the Fetus: Effect on the fetus depends on the time relationship of administration to delivery. The action on the fetus of 10 mg given intramuscularly to the mother reaches a peak in one and a half hours. Administration within three hours of birth is dangerous. The risk of fetal narcosis is increased by general anesthesia and traumatic delivery. Morphine is especially bad for premature infants.

Effect on Labor: The effect on labor varies greatly. Sometimes it weakens or stops uterine contractions. In other cases it improves labor, especially in the colicky uterus where, after a rest, the pattern of the contractions becomes more efficient and coordinate.

Demerol (pethidine, meperidine)

Demerol is a synthetic preparation with a mild atropine-like action. It is an excellent analgesic for labor. The patient is able to rest between her contractions, and can cooperate. The dose is 100 mg given every 3 to 4 hours. Few patients receive more than 200 mg. The analgesic effect is almost equivalent to 10 mg of morphine, but the duration is a little shorter.

Effects on the Mother: Included are:

1. The analgesic effect is good.
2. Transient euphoria and restlessness may occur.
3. Lethargy, mental impairment, and sleep are less than with morphine.
4. The efficiency is increased when combined with scopolamine.

Effects on the Fetus: The effect on the fetus is related to the dosage. Respiratory depression is less than with morphine, but it can be serious. The number of depressed infants is highest when the drug is administered to the mother intramuscularly 2 or 3 hours before delivery. When this narcotic is administered 1 hour or less before birth the incidence of respiratory depression is not significant.

Effect on Labor: Effect on labor is not marked. The action on the uterine contractions is less than with morphine. Often the good relaxation achieved with Demerol seems to speed up cervical dilatation.

Amnesia

Scopolamine (hyoscine)

Scopolamine hydrobromide is an amnesic, the effect of which is achieved without loss of consciousness. It is administered with an analgesic. The dose varies from grain 1/250 to 1/100 (0.25 to 0.6 mg).

Effects on the Mother: The patient is affected:

1. Scopolamine does not affect the pain threshold. Pain is felt, but the memory of it is fragmentary or absent. With large doses amnesia is complete.
2. The patient becomes drowsy and may lose touch with her surroundings. A varying degree of restlessness and even delirium can occur. Because of this fact, constant supervision and sometimes actual physical restraint is necessary.
3. Scopolamine has an action similar to atropine and causes dryness of the mouth and throat.
4. There are no aftereffects.
5. There is great individual variation in response to the drug.

Effects on the Fetus: Although scopolamine passes across the placenta, no ill effects on the fetus have been noted.

Effect on Labor: There is no prolongation of labor or increase in operative deliveries.

The Barbiturates

The barbituric acid derivatives have been used in obstetrics since 1924. They are employed mainly for their hypnotic property and to a lesser degree to produce amnesia. While they can be used for purposes of analgesia, the large doses required to do so produce respiratory depression in both mother and child. Pentobarbital and secobarbital are popular today.

Effects on the Mother: Effects are several:

1. Barbiturates are hypnotics. In small doses (200 mg) they induce lethargy and sleep. The drug can be given orally as soon as good labor is established and takes effect in 20 to 30 minutes.
2. Fear and apprehension are replaced by an attitude of indifference and freedom from anxiety.
3. Sometimes a mood of elation develops and there is release of inhibitions. Some patients become overactive to the point of extreme excitement.
4. There is little effect on the pain threshold as long as the patient remains conscious.

Effects on the Fetus: Included are:

1. The drug passes across the placenta, and a few grains can cause prolonged respiratory depression in the baby.
2. The action on the fetus outlasts that on the mother. Some babies exhibit lethargy and sleepiness long after birth.
3. There is an especially great danger in premature babies.

Effect on Labor: Excessive amounts of barbiturates can prolong labor. The impairment of uterine activity is related closely to the dosage. The cooperation of the patient may be lost.

The Tranquilizers

The ataractics or tranquilizers are depressants of the central nervous system, but they differ from the hypnotics in acting primarily at the subcortic level, affecting the structures concerned with emotion. The most effective drugs are the phenothiazine derivatives, including promazine (Sparine), chlorpromazine (Thorazine), and promethazine (Phenergan). In the usual doses these drugs have tranquilizing and analgesic effects, but in large doses they are hypnotic.

When used with barbiturates or hypnotics the ataractic drugs have an additive or even a potentiating effect. The amount of a sedative or narcotic needed to produce a desired effect is reduced when a phenothiazine derivative is given with it.

The chief objections to the use of these drugs are the side effects, especially hypotension which does not respond well to vasopressors. In some cases delay in the onset of respiration and crying has been reported in the newborn. These drugs should not be employed when the baby is premature.

Paracervical Block

Paracervical block is an effective, easily performed method of achieving relief of pain in the first stage of labor.

In the first stage the sensation of pain (caused by uterine contractions and cervical dilatation) passes by sensory and sympathetic pathways to the area of the uterosacral ligaments, through the pelvic and hypogastric plexuses, to the lower rami of the eleventh and twelfth thoracic vertebras. For this type of pain paracervical block works well.

In the second stage of labor, pain (produced by distension of the vagina and vulva) is transmitted via the sensory fibers of the pudendal nerves to the second, third, and fourth sacral vertebras. Paracervical block is ineffective in this area, and other types of anesthesia are needed.

Technic: The injection is made transvaginally into the posterolateral fornices, thus blocking the sensory pathways at the junction of the uterosacral ligaments with the cervix. The procedure can be carried out in the patient's bed, but it is done more accurately on the delivery table. The block is instituted in the active phase of labor, with the cervix at least 3 to 4 cm dilated.

The equipment consists of a 20 gauge needle, 13 to 18 cm long, with a sheath or needle guide of such length that about 1.5 cm of the tip of the needle protrudes when it is inserted up to its hub.

The needle sheath is guided by the fingers into the vagina and placed in the fornix just lateral to the cervix, at a tangent to the presenting part. The needle (with attached syringe) is introduced through the guide until the point rests against the mucosa. With quick slight pressure the needle is pushed through the mucosa to a depth of 6 to 12 mm. Aspiration is performed to guard against direct intravascular injection. If no blood comes back, the desired amount of anesthetic solution is injected. Mepivacaine hydrochloride 1 percent (Carbocaine) seems to be more effective and lasts longer than most other agents. After one or two contractions have occurred and the fetal heart has been checked, the procedure is repeated on the other side.

The sites of injection vary. Some workers inject the solution at 3 and 9 o'clock. Others give several injections at 3, 4, 8, and 9 o'clock. In any case, 10 cc is given on each side in single or multiple doses.

Effectiveness: Most patients experience complete or partial relief from pain almost immediately. They remain alert and cooperative. The block gives relief for about 1 hour. In many cases a single block remains effective until the cervix is fully dilated. In others a second block is necessary.

For the actual delivery other forms of anesthesia are required. Pudendal block or direct infiltration of the perineum are effective and safe.

Effect on Labor: Opinions vary concerning the effect of paracervical block on labor. Some state that labor is shortened, some say it is inhibited, while others feel that the effect varies from one patient to the next and is not predictable.

Maternal Complications: Minor problems do occur. These include:

1. Transient paresthesis of one or both legs, thought to be the result of inadvertent sciatic nerve block.
2. Rapid absorption or direct intravascular injection causes shaking movements or convulsions.
3. Hypotension down to 80 systolic has taken place.
4. Hematoma at the site of injection may occur.

Fetal Complications: Occasionally fetal bradycardia under 100 per minute has followed the block immediately. These episodes are transient, and the fetal pulse returns to normal within 5 to 15 minutes of giving oxygen to the mother.

A serious possibility, which has been reported with caudal anesthesia, is the accidental direct injection of the fetus with the anesthetic.

Contraindications: These include:

1. Fetal distress
2. Vaginal bleeding at the time or previous to the onset of labor
3. Maternal infection
4. History of sensitivity to local anesthetics

Lumbar Epidural Block

This technic is described later in this chapter.

RELIEF OF PAIN DURING THE SECOND STAGE OF LABOR

The essential requirements for a method of easing pain during this stage are:

1. Short induction
2. Rapid elimination and return to consciousness
3. Safety for mother and child
4. No diminution of uterine activity
5. When possible, the administration should be simple.

Methods in common use include the inhalant gases, perineal infiltration, pudendal block, saddle block, and epidural anesthesia. Methods used for analgesia during the first stage, such as continuous epidural anesthesia, may be enough to carry the patient through the second stage, but in most cases supplementary anesthesia is needed.

In the late first and second stages of labor the patient can be given the inhalant gases to promote analgesia. The gas is given only during the contraction in small concentration, and the patient remains conscious. As the head is being born the plane of anesthesia must be deepened to eliminate the severe pain as the presenting part passes through the introitus.

Inhalant Anesthesia

Nitrous Oxide and Oxygen

Pleasant to take and noninflammable nitrous oxide gas is efficient in supplying analgesia in the last part of the first stage and light analgesia and anesthesia in the second and third stages. Deep anesthesia requires the addition of one of the anesthetic vapors, nitrous oxide being used for the induction.

Effects on the Mother: There are a number of effects:

1. Nitrous oxide is soluble in the tissues and diffuses rapidly so that both induction and recovery are rapid.
2. It is nontoxic and the patient feels well after the administration is discontinued. The gas can be given for long periods.
3. Used as an analgesic, by giving it to the patient with each pain, relief is achieved quickly. The patient is told to take three breaths and to hold the third as she bears down.
4. The depth of the anesthesia can be altered quickly.
5. As the head is being born one of the rapidly acting vapors (Trilene, cyclopropane, Fluothane) must be added to deepen the anesthesia.
6. With safe mixtures of nitrous oxide and oxygen the degree of relaxation is not enough to perform difficult maneuvers such as forceps extractions or versions.
7. Unless anoxia is produced there is no untoward effect on the circulatory, respiratory, or nervous systems.
8. The disadvantage is that a mixture of 80 percent of nitrous oxide and 20 percent of oxygen is needed to produce first plane anesthesia. Deepening the anesthesia by reducing the percentage of oxygen carries the risk of anoxia and is dangerous.

Ether

Given by the simple open drop method ethyl ether has a wide margin of safety for the mother. It does not produce analgesia without anesthesia and cannot be given intermittently with the contractions as can nitrous oxide.

Effects on the Mother: These are both good and bad:

1. It does not damage the liver.
2. In levels used for obstetrics the respiratory or circulatory systems are not depressed.
3. Once induction has been accomplished by nitrous oxide, a small concentration of ether is enough to maintain the anesthesia.
4. Ether is irritating to the respiratory passages and causes much secretion. This makes the prolonged induction unpleasant to the patient.
5. The delayed recovery period is associated with nausea and vomiting.

Effects on the Baby: Ether crosses the placental barrier. Its elimination from mother and child are slow, and if deep and prolonged anesthesia is required, the baby will be depressed.

Effect on Labor: Enough relaxation of the myometrium is attainable to permit intrauterine manipulations. This relaxation can persist into the third stage with resultant hemorrhage from an atonic uterus. When enough ether is given for complete anesthesia the strength of the uterine contractions is reduced.

Cyclopropane

Cyclopropane is a useful and potent anesthetic.

Advantages: Advantages are:

1. It is given with a high concentration of oxygen and this lessens the danger of respiratory depression. Mixtures of 10 percent cyclopropane and 90 percent oxygen are enough to induce first plane anesthesia, while 13 percent to 25 percent cyclopropane provides moderate muscle relaxation.
2. It takes 12 to 15 minutes for the fetal concentration to reach the same level as in the mother. If the baby is born within 8 minutes of the onset of anesthesia, it will not be profoundly depressed.
3. It acts rapidly—two to three breaths achieve analgesia, while four to five breaths permit episiotomy.
4. All levels of anesthesia can be attained.
5. It is eliminated rapidly, so recovery is complete soon after the anesthetic is discontinued.
6. It is pleasant to take.

Disadvantages: Included are:

1. It is extremely flammable and even explosive.
2. It should be used only by expert anesthetists.
3. Cardiac arrhythmias, fibrillation, and, rarely, cardiac arrest have occurred more often than with other anesthetic agents. The danger is increased if pituitary extracts and adrenaline have been used.
4. There is increased bleeding from incised wounds, but excessive uterine hemorrhage is related to the depth of the anesthesia.

Trichloroethylene: Trilene

Trilene is an efficient, safe, and pleasant analgesic and anesthetic. Recovery is not prolonged and there is little vomiting. It causes rapid breathing. Trilene is a liquid and requires vaporization by a gas such as air, oxygen, or nitrous oxide.

A popular method is to employ an inhaler which uses air as the vaporizing agent. The apparatus is adjusted to give a fixed concentration of the anesthetic and can be self-administered by the patient to provide analgesia during the late first and second stages. To produce anesthesia the patient is induced with nirous oxide and oxygen, and then the Trilene is added in the amount needed to maintain the desired level.

Effects on the baby are comparable to other inhalants. Trilene given intermittently for analgesia has a tendency to build up a high level in the mother, and, if continued too long, fetal asphyxia may result.

Halothane: Fluothane

Fluothane is a liquid the anesthetic potency of which is twice that of chloroform and four times that of ether. It acts so rapidly that an excessive depth of anesthesia can be produced before the inexperienced person realizes it. Since the margin of safety is small, observation must be constant, and only trained anesthetists should use this drug.

This is a pleasant anesthetic for the patient. Induction and recovery are so short that coughing or vomiting are seen rarely. It is not inflammable and not explosive.

Fluothane has an effect on the myometrium comparable to that of chloroform. Complete uterine relaxation is attainable quickly. Fluothane may have a place when intrauterine manipulations are to be performed, or in emergencies, such as prolapse of the cord, where rapid anesthesia and relaxation of muscle is essential. However, because of its effect on the myometrium, an increased incidence of atonic postpartum hemorrhage has been reported.

Aspiration of Vomitus during Inhalant Anesthesia

The aspiration of vomit and the resultant pulmonary infection is a great danger. Because of delayed emptying during labor there is often undigested food, fluid, and gas in the stomach at delivery. Regurgitation and vomiting may take place. While the patient is recovering from the anesthetic the cough reflex is poor, and aspiration is especially dangerous at this time.

Women in labor should be given no solid food and a limited amount of clear fluids. If hydration is a problem glucose solution should be infused by vein.

When vomiting does occur the patient must be placed in Trendelenburg position to promote postural drainage, and the airway must be cleaned with an efficient suction machine. If the patient has eaten a large meal within 6 hours of delivery inhalation anesthesia is unwise.

Conduction Anesthesia

General Advantages: There are a number of these:

1. The baby's vital functions are not affected, it is not narcotized, and the respiratory center is not depressed. It is a good method for premature infants.
2. There is no nausea or vomiting, and the patient may take fluids by mouth before, during, and after the delivery.
3. The cough reflex is not depressed and there is no danger of aspiration of vomitus.
4. The mother is awake during the delivery.
5. There is no interference with uterine contractions, and therefore postpartum bleeding is minimal.
6. Since the baby is not affected there is no need to hurry, and the operation can be performed gently and carefully.
7. Postpartum nursing care is easy.
8. There is little or no effect on other parts of the body, and the vital centers are not depressed. Under proper control the complications are minimal.

General Disadvantages: Disadvantages are:

1. Not every patient is suitable.
2. The technic does not work in every case. Practice is needed to acquire proficiency.
3. In rare instances the needle breaks.
4. Care must be taken not to inject into a blood vessel. Intravenous injection may cause convulsions, cardiac arrest, or even death.
5. The rare person is allergic to the anesthetic agent, and every patient should be asked about a history of drug sensitivity.
6. Carelessness in technic may lead to sepsis.

Local Anesthesia

The two methods of local anesthesia are: 1, direct infiltration of the perineal tissues and 2, pudendal nerve block. Local anesthesia is one of the best for obstetrics, but nervous, high strung women and impatient doctors are not associated with a high rate of success.

Special Advantages: Advantages of this type of anesthesia are several:

1. The technic is simple. The obstetrician should administer the drug himself.
2. There are no ill effects on the vital organs, respiratory function is not depressed, and fatalities (with the exception of the rare drug allergy) are almost unknown. It is useful for women with heart disease, tuberculosis, and similar diseases.
3. No special aftercare is needed.
4. The tissues must be handled gently. This reduces trauma.

Disadvantages: However, there are also disadvantages:

1. A blood vessel may be torn during the procedure and lead to formation of a hematoma.
2. Only perineal pain is relieved. The discomfort from the uterine contractions continues.

Direct Infiltration Anesthesia

The main purpose of perineal infiltration is to permit the incision and repair of episiotomy and the suturing of lacerations.

Technic: The procedure is as follows:

1. Because of its rapid and profound action we prefer 1 percent Xylocaine (lignocaine hydrochloride). Procaine or Metycaine can also be used.
2. For the average case 30 to 50 ml of solution are sufficient.

3. Either of two approaches may be used:
    a. The needle is inserted at the posterior fourchette and the injections made laterad.
    b. The needle is inserted at a point halfway between the anus and the ischial tuberosity and the injections made toward the midline.
4. With a small 25 gauge needle a wheal is made by injecting a small amount of the solution into the skin at the point where the needle is to be inserted.
5. The needle is then changed to a number 20 which is inserted through the wheal. Multiple injections are made into the subcutaneous tissue, the muscles, and the fascia.
6. The area to be anesthetized is triangular in shape, the angles being the clitoris, the perianal region, and the point halfway between the anus and the tuberosity.
7. During the procedure the plunger of the syringe must be pulled back repeatedly to be sure that the needle is not in a blood vessel.
8. Adequate anesthesia is achieved in about 5 minutes.

Advantages: The operator will find these factors favorable:

1. The technic is simple; no special anatomic knowledge is necessary
2. The rate of success is almost 100 percent.
3. The injection can be made any time, even when the head is on the perineum.

Disadvantages: Complete perineal anesthesia is not achieved. Only the infiltrated areas are affected.

Pudendal Nerve Block

The pudendal nerve is the main supply of the perineum. It arises from the anterior branches of the second, third, and fourth sacral nerves. These join into a single trunk 0.5 cm to 1 cm proximal to the ischial spine. The nerve passes through the greater sciatic foramen, somewhat diagonally across the posterior surface of the sacrospinous ligament, medial to the pudendal vessels, to enter the lesser sciatic foramen. As the nerve passes medial and posterior to the inferior tip of the spine, it enters the pudendal canal, and proceeds to the lower edge of the urogenital diaphragm. The nerve is blocked most easily where it lies close to the tip of the ischial spine.

The pudendal nerve divides into three main branches: 1, the inferior hemorrhoidal nerve; 2, the dorsal nerve of the clitoris; and 3, the perineal nerve.

1. The inferior hemorrhoidal nerve supplies the lower rectum, the external sphincter ani, and the skin anterior and lateral to the anus. In 50 percent of cases this nerve arises as a separate branch from the fourth sacral nerve, and is not part of the pudendal trunk. In these cases it lies close to pudendal nerve medial to the ischial spine.
2. The dorsal nerve of the clitoris supplies that organ and the area around it.
3. The perineal nerve is the largest branch. It supplies the superficial structures of the vulva and the skin, fascia, and deep muscles of the perineum.

While the ilioinguinal and posterior femoral cutaneous nerves play a small part in innervating the perineum, complete obstetric anesthesia of this area can be obtained (including relaxation of the pelvic floor) by blocking the main trunk of the pudendal nerve.

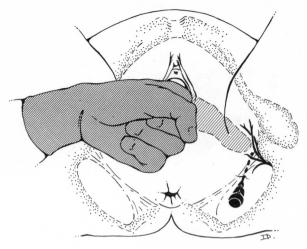

Fig. 2.   Pudendal nerve block: percutaneous transperineal approach.

The time of administration of pudendal anesthesia is important to its success.   Once the head or breech is distending the perineum, it is too late.   In primigravidas the injection is made when the cervix is fully dilated and the presenting part is at station +2.   In multiparas the anesthetic is given when the cervix has reached 7 or 8 cm.   Pudendal anesthesia is sufficient for spontaneous delivery or low forceps extraction, for breech deliveries, and for episiotomy and repair of lacerations.   Many obstetricians combine pudendal block with local infiltration, described above.

Percutaneous Transperineal Approach: The anesthetic agent (1 percent or 2 percent Xylocaine, procaine, or Metycaine) is injected around the pudendal nerve through a 5 inch 20 gauge needle.   After a wheal has been raised the needle is inserted through the skin midway between the anus and the ischial tuberosity.   With a finger in the vagina as a guide (some prefer to put the finger in the rectum), the needle is directed through the ischial fossa toward the posterior surface of the ischial spine.   As the needle nears the spine the vaginal finger directs it posteriorly toward the inferior tip of the spine and into the pudendal canal.   When the needle is in the canal, free from muscle and ligament, it can be moved back and forth without resistance.   If it is not in the correct place it must be withdrawn 3 or 4 cm and reinserted.   One method of ensuring correct location of the tip of the needle is to aspirate the pudendal vessels.   Once this is accomplished the needle is withdrawn from the blood vessel and reinserted medially, where the pudendal nerve lies.

Ten milliliters of the anesthetic solution are deposited.   Three milliliters are injected beneath the inferior tip of the spine.   The needle is then introduced a little deeper, and another 3 ml are placed into the canal just under the superior tip of the spine.   The needle is then inserted a little beyond the spine into the greater sciatic notch, where 4 ml are injected.   This last injection will catch the inferior hemorrhoidal nerve in the case where it arises as a separate branch from the fourth sacral nerve.   Effective anesthesia is achieved in about 15 minutes.

Fig. 3.   Pudendal nerve block: transvaginal route.

Transvaginal Technic: The vaginal route is simple, effective, and safe. The ischial spine is palpable easily through the vagina, and the point where the sacrospinous ligament is attached to it serves as the landmark to locate the pudendal nerve.

A 10 or 20 ml syringe with a 5 inch 20 gauge needle is used. The left pudendal nerve is anesthetized first. The ischial spine is located with the vaginal fingers (left hand). The syringe is held in the right hand. The needle is placed in the groove formed by the apposition of the first and second fingers of the left hand, or the tip of the needle may be pressed against the ball of the index finger. Protected by the fingers the needle is placed into the vagina to the tip of the ischial spine. The syringe is held above the left hand so that the needle can be directed laterally and downward to enter the vaginal mucosa over the sacrospinous ligament and posterior and medial to the tip of the ischial spine. The needle is inserted into the sacrospinous ligament and 3 ml are injected. The needle is pushed deeper, and as it enters the loose tissue behind the ligament, resistance ceases and the fluid flows in easily. Aspiration is attempted to guard against the needle's being in a blood vessel, and then 7 to 8 ml are injected behind the ligament. The needle is withdrawn and the procedure repeated on the right side.

Epidural and Spinal Anesthesia

Innervation and Causes of Pain: Successful anesthesia depends on an understanding of the anatomy involved:

1. Uterus: The sensory nerves are sympathetic and pass via the uterine, pelvic, hypogastric, and aortic plexuses into the dorsal roots of the eleventh and twelfth thoracic segments and into the spinal cord. The motor nerves are also sympathetic. They start in the tenth to twelfth thoracic segments and pass through the aortic, hypogastric, pelvic, and uterine plexuses, to terminate in the uterus.

2. Vulva, vagina, and perineum: The main sensations of pain are carried by the pudendal nerve into the second, third, and fourth sacral segments. A

ity in the epidural space around the sacral roots. Then the patient lies down
with the head slightly elevated. It takes 15 to 20 minutes for good perineal anesthesia to be accomplished. At this time preparations are made for the delivery. During the delivery the mother is given oxygen by mask.

Advantages of Epidural Anesthesia: Advantages of this technic are:

1. Almost the entire labor can be made painfree. In a difficult case epidural
   analgesia brings about a marked change for the better in the patient's general condition and morale. In addition the relatives are placated.
2. The effect can be maintained as long as necessary.
3. The level of anesthesia is controllable by posture.
4. The mother is alert and cooperative. She retains the ability to bear down.
   Delivery may be spontaneous, but even if forceps are used, the patient can
   help by pushing down while the operator is exerting traction.
5. Epidurals are of value in trials of labor. Should cesarean section be necessary the same anesthetic is used.
6. There are no postspinal headaches.

Disadvantages of Epidural Anesthesia: There are several:

1. A specially trained anesthetist is needed.
2. Maternal hypotension is the most frequent complication. Many patients
   show immediate improvement with left lateral posturing. Oxygen administration helps. In some cases vasopressor drugs must be used.
3. Intravascular injection causes twitching, convulsions, or loss of consciousness.
4. The dura may be punctured. Because of the large size of the Tuohy needle
   severe headache results.
5. Fetal bradycardia is a frequent accompaniment of maternal hypotension.
6. Occasionally the uterine contractions become weaker and less frequent.
   An oxytocin infusion will improve the labor and bring about good progress.

Spinal Anesthesia: Saddle Block

Saddle block is a low spinal anesthetic confined to the perineal area. In
practice the region of anesthesia is a little more widespread than the saddle
area, but this does not interfere with the aims of the technic. With the addition
of glucose to the anesthetic agent the solution is made hyperbaric. The subarachnoid injection is made with the patient in a sitting position, so that the
heavy solution gravitates downward. The length of time that the patient sits up
determines the level of anesthesia. Five minutes is sufficient. In this way
complete anesthesia of the perineal region is attained, the perineal muscles
are relaxed, and there is partial loss of sensation of the abdomen and thighs.
The sympathetic fibers which carry the feeling of pain from the uterus are
blocked, and the pains of labor are relieved or abolished. The injection must
not be made during a contraction because the agent would be forced to too high
a level. Nupercaine and pontocaine are popular anesthetic agents.

While uterine contractions do not cease and there is no increase in uterine
atony and postpartum hemorrhage, effective progress of labor halts, so this
anesthetic is used terminally. The patient is not able to deliver the baby her-

self, and extraction with forceps is necessary. Hence the anesthetic can be given only when labor has reached the point where easy low forceps can be performed. The cervix must be fully dilated.

Terminal spinal is an excellent anesthetic for difficult deliveries since it provides good anesthesia and excellent relaxation.

ANESTHESIA FOR CESAREAN SECTION

There is no single "best" anesthesia for cesarean section. Every method has its good and bad features. The choice of the technic to be employed is based on the indication for the operation, the presence of general maternal problems (e.g., heart disease, pulmonary complications), the condition of the fetus, and the availability of trained personnel.

The three main types of anesthesia used today are: 1) local; 2) spinal or epidural; 3) general.

Local Anesthesia

Several agents are available, among them are Procaine (Novocaine) as a 0.5% solution, Lidocaine (Xylocaine), and Mepivacaine (Carbocaine). Addition of adrenaline to make a dilution of 1:200,000 delays absorption and prolongs the effect of the anesthetic. About 300 ml of the solution are used.

Technic: Atropine 0.4 mg is given as premedication 30 minutes before surgery. In nervous patients this may be combined with 50 mg of Demerol.

A skin wheal is made just below the umbilicus with a 25 gauge needle. A 20 gauge needle, 4 inches long, is used to inject the solution intradermally and subcutaneously down to the pubic symphysis for a distance of about 3 cm on each side of the midline. After a few minutes have passed the skin and subcutaneous tissue are incised. The tissue must be handled gently and a minimum amount of traction exerted.

The anterior sheath of the rectus muscle is infiltrated in the same way, in the midline and out to the sides to block the nerves at the lateral margins of the recti. A large amount of solution is placed in the suprapubic region, since this is the area of highest sensitivity. The fascia is then incised.

The peritoneum is then anesthetized and opened to expose the uterus. About 50 to 60 cc of anesthetic is injected under the bladder flap and spread with the fingers under the bladder and to the sides. The bladder peritoneum is cut and pushed caudad.

The uterus is then opened, the baby extracted, the placenta removed, and the incision closed. The nervous patient may be put to sleep with Pentothal just prior to incision of the uterus.

Advantages: Included are:

1. Except for the rare instance of sensitivity to the anesthetic agent or intravascular injection, this method is completely safe for the mother.
2. There is no ill effect on the fetus (no respiratory depression).

Disadvantages: Disadvantages of this technic are:

1. The patient must be prepared to accept this type of anesthesia. It is not suitable for the nervous or hyperexcitable woman.
2. The method is time-consuming and is not good for cases in which rapid operating is necessary.
3. The surgeon must be gentle, patient, and willing to accept slow operating.

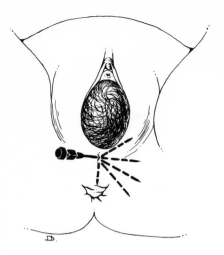

Fig. 4. Local anesthesia: direct infiltration.

2. The vasopressor agent employed to maintain the maternal blood pressure may cause a diminution of uteroplacental blood flow, leading to a decrease in the fetal oxygen saturation.
3. Because of the hypotension this anesthesia is not suitable for cases where hemorrhage is present.

General Anesthesia

Technic: The following steps should be taken:

1. Atropine 0.4 mg is given intramuscularly 30 to 60 minutes prior to surgery.
2. An intravenous infusion of 5 percent glucose in water is set up.
3. Anesthesia is instituted with 250 mg of Pentothal (2.5 percent solution).
4. Succinylcholine, 100 mg is given intravenously to promote muscle relaxation.
5. An endotracheal tube is inserted.
6. The anesthesia is maintained by intermittent positive pressure with nitrous oxide and oxygen.
7. Muscle relaxation is achieved by a succinylcholine drip.
8. Two or three minutes prior to the delivery of the baby the amount of nitrous oxide is reduced, and oxygen and succinylcholine are continued.
9. No more Pentothal is given until the umbilical cord is clamped, at which time it can be injected to deepen the level of anesthesia if this is desired.
10. Timing is important, and, to avoid respiratory depression in the infant, at least 10 minutes should elapse between the injection of the Pentothal and the uterine incision.

Advantages: There are several important advantages to consider:

1. It is highly acceptable to the patient.
2. There is no hypotension.
3. It is effective in cases of hemorrhage or fetal distress where speed is important.
4. Fetal depression or asphyxia are rare.

Disadvantages: The bad features of general anesthesia are:

1. The timing must be accurate or fetal depression may occur.
2. An experienced anesthesiologist is essential to success.

Lumbar Epidural and Spinal Anesthesia

Technic: This has been described in a previous section.

Advantages: There are two major advantages:

1. The use of drugs which depress the infant can be avoided.
2. In those cases where a trial of labor is being carried on under epidural analgesia, the same anesthetic can be continued for the cesarean section.

Disadvantages: Included are:

1. Maternal hypotension is frequent and may be accompanied by fetal bradycardia.

THE PREMATURE INFANT

Premature babies have a low resistance to sedatives, analgesics, and general anesthetics. Small amounts of these agents (whose effects on full term babies may be minor) will depress the respiratory center of the small fetus to the extent of causing severe apnea and asphyxia. Delay in the onset of breathing can result in anoxic brain damage.

We avoid prescribing sedatives and analgesics during labor and where possible do not employ general anesthesia for the delivery. If the patient is able to carry on, we deliver the baby under local infiltration or perineal block. In cases where the pains of labor are severe and the patient needs help, a continuous lumbar epidural block is instituted. This relieves or abolishes the pain of labor, and is an excellent anesthetic for the actual delivery. As the baby is being born the mother is given oxygen by mask. In this way the respiratory center of the fetus is protected during both the labor and the delivery.

CONCLUSION

There are many satisfactory agents and technics available to relieve the suffering of childbirth and to enable operative procedures to be performed when necessary. Our personal preference is for the following:

1. Primigravidas are encouraged to attend prenatal training classes.
2. For nervous patients 200 mg of secobarbital are given orally when labor is well established.
3. When the cervix is 3 cm dilated and the patient is in need of analgesia, we prescribe 100 mg of Demerol with or without the addition of grain 1/200 of scopolamine. This may be repeated in 3 to 4 hours, but in most patients where good progress is being made, one dose is enough.
4. In patients who do not wish a general anesthetic we use local infiltration of the perineum.
5. For patients whose labor is difficult, prolonged, or excessively painful we encourage an epidural when the cervix is 5 to 6 cm dilated in primigravidas and 3 to 4 cm dilated in multiparas. The baby is not narcotized and the same anesthetic will carry over for the delivery.

6. For relief of pain in the latter part of the second stage when the patient is bearing down with the contractions, she is given a Trilene inhaler or nitrous oxide and oxygen to breathe with each contraction.
7. Patients who wish to be put to sleep during the delivery are given nitrous oxide, Trilene, or Fluothane.
8. For operative deliveries we prefer epidural anesthesia, with one of the inhalants as second choice. A narcotized baby is less resistant to the trauma of a difficult birth.

BIBLIOGRAPHY

Bromage, P. R. Continuous lumbar epidural analgesia for obstetrics. Can. Med. Ass. J., 85:1136, 1961.

Brown, E. O., Engel, T., and Douglas, R. G. Paracervical block analgesia in labor. Obstet. Gynec., 26:195, 1965.

Cowles, G. T. Experiences with lumbar epidural block. Obstet. Gynec., 26:734, 1965.

Crawford, J. S. Obstetric analgesia and anaesthesia—the current scene. Postgrad. Med. J., 42:351, 1966.

Hartridge, V. B. Anesthesia for obstetrics. Surg. Clin. N. Amer., 45:961, 1965.

_____ and Wilson, R. B. Balanced anesthesia for cesarean section. Amer. J. Obstet. Gynec., 85:619, 1963.

Kandel, P. F., Spoerel, W. E., and Kinch, R. A. H. Continuous epidural analgesia for labour and delivery. Canad. Med. Ass. J., 95:947, 1966.

Klink, E. W. Perineal nerve block. Obstet. Gynec., 1:137, 1953.

Kobak, A. J., Evans, E. F., and Johnson, G. R. Transvaginal nerve block. Amer. J. Obstet. Gynec., 71:981, 1956.

Masters, W. H., and Ross, R. W. Conduction anesthesia: Protection afforded premature infants. J. A. M. A., 141:909, 1949.

Ranney, B. Paracervical block for first-stage pain in primigravidas. Obstet. Gynec., 27:757, 1966.

Sheridan, C. A., and Robson, J. G. Fluothane in obstetrical anesthesia. Canad. Anaes. Soc. J., 4:365, 1959.

Shnider, S. M., and Moya, F. Effects of meperidine on the newborn infant. Amer. J. Obstet. Gynec., 89:1009, 1964.

Tafeen, C. H., Freedman, H. L., and Harris, H. A system of continuous paracervical block anesthesia. Amer. J. Obstet. Gynec., 94:854, 1966.

Wilds, P. R. Transvaginal pudendal nerve block. Obstet. Gynec., 8:385, 1956.

44 The Newborn

ASPHYXIA NEONATORUM

The normal healthy infant should breathe within one half minute to one minute of birth. Asphyxia of the newborn (mild or severe) is a syndrome in which apnea is the principal clinical manifestation. In severe cases the infant is flaccid, there is bradycardia, the color is blue to white, and the response to stimulation is poor or nonexistent. Frequently the baby is covered with meconium, a sign of intrauterine distress. The infant is hypoxic, and if the state of lack of oxygen is prolonged, permanent brain damage will occur.

There are two large groups:

1. Central nervous system failure resulting from:
   a. Narcosis by maternal sedatives, analgesics, and anesthesia
   b. Prenatal or paranatal anoxia
   c. Intracranial trauma or hemorrhage
   d. Congenital anomalies

In this group either the children are born with apnea, or the breathing ceases after a few ineffectual gasps.

2. Peripheral respiratory difficulty:
   a. Respiratory distress syndrome
   b. Aspiration of meconium and amniotic fluid
   c. Pneumonia
   d. Congenital anomalies

In this category the breathing begins fairly promptly, but is or soon becomes labored and inadequate. The central nervous system seems to function, but the grunting, retraction, and cyanosis point to disturbances in the peripheral respiratory apparatus. This is the more common of the two groups.

Hyaline Membrane Disease: Hyaline membrane disease is found in the lungs of infants, especially prematures, who have died in the early neonatal period. The air passages are lined with a homogeneous eosinophilic material which prevents adequate transfer of oxygen. The exact mechanism of formation of the membrane is not known.

Respiratory Distress Syndrome: The respiratory distress syndrome is often associated with hyaline membrane disease. The great majority of fatal cases are in premature infants, and the condition is more common after cesarean section than following normal vaginal delivery. Many infants are born in reasonably good condition, but within a few hours they develop dyspnea, cyanosis, retraction, and apnea. Death may result. In severe cases a state of acidosis is added to the hypoxia, and this chemical imbalance must be corrected if the baby is to survive.

Etiology of Asphyxia Neonatorum

During Pregnancy

1. Maternal
   a. Anemia
   b. Hemorrhage and shock
   c. Cardiorespiratory disease
   d. Toxemia of pregnancy
   e. Age of mother over 40 years
   f. Grand multiparity
2. Placenta
   a. Placental diseases (syphilis, infarction)
   b. Hemorrhage (placenta previa, abruptio placentae)
3. Umbilical cord
   a. Prolapse
   b. Knots and entanglements
   c. Compression
4. Fetal
   a. Congenital anomalies
   b. Prematurity
   c. Premature rupture of the membranes leading to infection, especially pneumonia
   d. Prolonged gestation

At Labor and Delivery

1. Anoxia from uterine contractions that are too strong and last too long
2. Narcosis from excessive analgesia and anesthesia
3. Maternal hypotension from spinal anesthesia
4. Obstruction of the airway by aspiration of blood, mucus, and vaginal debris
5. Prolonged labor
6. Difficult delivery (with or without forceps) causing cerebral hemorrhage or damage to the central nervous system

Diagnosis

Antepartum

Signs which indicate intrauterine fetal distress and hypoxia include:

1. Bradycardia under 100 beats per minute between uterine contractions
2. Gross irregularity of the fetal heart

3. Tachycardia, over 160. This is not of great significance by itself; however, when it alternates with periods of bradycardia it is an ominous sign.
4. The passage of meconium in a cephalic presentation. This indicates relaxation of the sphincter ani, a result of insufficient oxygenation.

Postpartum

Apgar has elaborated a method of grading newborn infants: 0, 1, or 2 points are awarded for each of 5 signs, depending on their presence or absence. The grading is done at 1 minute after birth and may be repeated at 5 minutes. A score of 10 indicates that the infant is in the best condition. At 5 to 9 there is minimal to mild asphyxia calling for supportive treatment. A score of 4 or less is diagnostic of severe asphyxia, and prompt and active therapy is necessary.

Sign	0 points	1 point	2 points
Heart rate	absent	under 100	over 100
Respiratory effort	absent	slow, irregular	good, crying
Muscle tone	limp	flexion of extremities	active motion
Reflex irritability: response to catheter in nostril	no response	grimace	cough or sneeze
Color	blue-white	body pink, extremities blue	completely pink

Treatment

1. Gentleness in handling the infant is of paramount importance. It is in a state of shock or close to shock.
2. The correct temperature and humidity must be maintained. This is achieved best in an incubator. The baby should be kept warm, but excessive heat is contraindicated.
3. A clear airway to the lungs must be established.
   a. Except in cases where cerebral hemorrhage is suspected the baby should be postured, head down, at an angle of about 30 degrees with the horizontal.
   b. Mucus and debris are sucked out of the nose and throat by means of a soft rubber catheter.
   c. When simple methods are not successful, direct endotracheal intubation is performed. This must be done carefully to avoid damage to the larynx and trachea. The tube is available for both aspiration of secretion and administration of oxygen.
4. The most important principle of therapy is to supply oxygen to the fetal lungs and to maintain pulmonary ventilation until the respiratory center can take over this function. Oxygen is the essential therapeutic agent, the phys-

iologic stimulant to the anoxic respiratory center. It can be administered in the incubator, by positive pressure mask or by mouth to mouth breathing where better methods are unavailable.

5. When the infant has been narcotized by the administration of analgesics to the mother, Nalline (N-allyl-nomorphine) can be given to counteract certain drugs. Effective in combatting respiratory depression caused by morphine, codeine, Demerol, Pantapon, Dilauded, Nisentil, and heroin, Nalline is of no value against the barbiturates, the anesthetic gases, or other causes of respiratory failure. It may act as a respiratory depressant when given to nonnarcotized infants. Repeated administration is of no value and may be harmful. It can be given to the narcotized mother intravenously (5 to 10 mg) 15 minutes before delivery. The most effective route is by injection into the umbilical vein of the infant in the dose of 0.2 to 0.4 mg diluted in 2 ml of saline. Another drug used for the same purpose is Lorfan Tartrate (0.05 to 0.1 mg) to the baby. Drugs, such as alpha-lobeline, Coramine, caffeine, and Metrazol are of no value as respiratory stimulants, may cause convulsions, and are no longer used.

6. Especially in babies born by cesarean section the stomach should be aspirated to remove the large amounts of fluid.

7. Antibiotics are given to combat possible pneumonia.

8. The baby should be kept in an incubator under close observation until its condition is good. In this way the body temperature, humidity, and oxygen concentration can be maintained at proper levels.

Prevention

1. Trauma must be kept to the minimum. Prolonged labor and difficult vaginal operations should be avoided whenever possible.

2. Oxygen is given to the mother for at least 5 minutes before and during difficult deliveries.

3. Excessive narcosis and deep prolonged inhalation anesthesia should not be used. Local or conduction anesthesia is preferable. If inhalation anesthesia must be used, that one is chosen which will give the mother and infant the highest oxygen saturation with the least physiologic alterations. Conduction anesthesia sometimes causes hypotension in the mother. This must be treated with hypertensive drugs or the baby will be affected by the decreased oxygen availability.

4. Careful observation so that fetal distress (fetal bradycardia, irregular fetal heart rate, passage of meconium in a vertex presentation) can be diagnosed and prompt treatment carried out both during the labor and after birth.

FETAL INJURY

Intracranial Hemorrhage

The brain is enclosed in a tough membrane, the dura mater. The falx cerebri and the tentorium cerebelli are extensions of the dura inside the skull and act as scaffolding to give support to the brain. The falx occupies a vertical plane between the two cerebral hemispheres. The tentorium lies in a horizontal plane separating the cerebral hemispheres above from the cerebellum below. Venous sinuses are enclosed in the margins of the falx and tentorium.

Excessive compression of the fetal head, either by natural forces or by instruments, can cause hemorrhage or brain damage. Death, mental retardation, epilepsy, or cerebral palsy may follow. Compression of the fetal skull acts in several ways:

1. The pressure is transmitted to the interior of the calvarium and overcomes the intravascular pressure. This leads to arrest of the cerebral circulation, followed by anoxia and then degeneration of the brain cells and the blood vessels. The latter become more permeable, and bleeding into the brain takes place.
2. The falx and the tentorium may be torn. If the laceration extends into the venous sinuses, extensive hemorrhage will occur.
3. A fractured skull bone may lacerate the underlying brain.

Thus, hemorrhage in the fetal brain is the result of mechanical trauma and/or anoxia. It is more common in premature infants. The improvement in general obstetric care and the elimination of heroic vaginal operations have contributed to the reduction in the incidence and severity of cerebral hemorrhage.

Subdural Hematoma

This type of hemorrhage is the result of difficult labor and delivery. There is a collection of blood between the dura mater and the pia arachnoid. Usually the venous sinuses are torn, often at the junction of the falx and tentorium. Sometimes the great vein of Galen is lacerated.

Subdural hemorrhage is especially liable to occur with:

1. Prolonged labor
2. Precipitate labor
3. Cephalopelvic disproportion
4. Mid or high forceps
5. Breech extraction
6. Elderly primigravida

The symptoms and signs may not appear for 24 to 36 hours. They include:

1. High pitched cry
2. Bulging fontanelle
3. Irritability or convulsions
4. The circumference of the head may enlarge.
5. Death may result from pressure on vital centers.
6. The diagnosis is confirmed by subdural tap.

Subarachnoid and Intraventricular Hemorrhage.

This type of bleeding is seen almost entirely in premature infants and is often the result of anoxia rather than trauma.

Intracerebral Hemorrhage and Edema

Bleeding into the brain tissue may be gross, or it may be petechial and associated with edema. External compression causes venous engorgement with subsequent bleeding from capillaries and small veins. The falx and tentorium may be torn. This type of bleeding is seen after difficult births.

Treatment of Intracranial Hemorrhage

1. Traumatic deliveries should be avoided and cesarean section performed where there is disproportion.
2. The baby is kept in an incubator.
3. The temperature is controlled.
4. Extra oxygen is given as needed.
5. The secretions are removed from the throat.
6. The baby is handled as little as possible.
7. Vitamin K is administered when indicated.
8. Convulsions are controlled by sedatives.
9. The head should not be lowered, since this may increase the bleeding.
10. If there is suspicion of a subdural collection of blood, lumbar puncture is done to relieve pressure as well as for diagnosis.
11. Prophylactic antibiotics are given.

Cerebral Palsy

The incidence of cerebral palsy is from 4 to 7 per 1,000 births. It is the greatest neurologic crippler of children today. While the reduction of traumatic vaginal deliveries has lowered the incidence of cranial damage, the occurrence of cerebral palsy has not decreased.

Although Little (who gave his name to the disease) believed that asphyxia was the prime etiologic factor, many observers considered that trauma at birth was the main cause. However, most children traumatized at birth do not develop cerebral palsy. Today it is felt that anoxia is, by far, the leading agent in the production of permanent cerebral damage, and that prematurity is the greatest contributing factor. Since every premature infant does not develop cerebral palsy, it may be that the same factors caused both conditions.

A recent concept is that of an unfavorable intrauterine environment producing hypoxia or anoxia. If this anoxia is compounded by other factors, the requirements for permanent brain damage may be met.

Conditions associated with cerebral palsy include:

1. Maternal age
2. Relative sterility
3. Bleeding during pregnancy
4. Multiple pregnancy
5. Prolonged second stage of labor
6. Fetal distress, as it points to anoxia
7. Abnormal delivery—higher incidence with breech presentation
8. Frequency of poor condition at birth, probably a reflection of previously occurring damage which also caused the palsy

9. Prematurity
10. The role, in modern obstetrics, played by traumatic delivery in the etiology of cerebral palsy is probably under 10 percent.

Cephalhematoma

This is a subperiosteal hemorrhage occurring most often over one of the parietal bones. It results from trauma to the periosteum during labor or delivery. The incidence is between 2 and 3 percent. It is more common after midforceps operations, especially where there is drag on the scalp by rotation of the head. There is no evidence that the brain is affected. No treatment is required. Spontaneous resolution takes place (see Ch. 6).

Damage to Brachial Plexus

This injury is caused by stretching or tearing of the roots of the brachial plexus. It is associated with breech delivery when there is difficulty with the arms, and with shoulder dystocia in cephalic presentations when there is excessive flexion of the head obliquely toward one shoulder.

Erb's palsy occurs when C-5 and C-6 are involved. The arm hangs limply to the side and is rotated internally. The elbow is extended and the wrist flexed with the palm upward.

Klumpke's paralysis occurs when C-8 and T-1 are damaged. There is weakness and wasting of the muscles supplied by the median and ulnar nerves. Flaccid paralysis of the small muscles of the hand is a part of the syndrome.

Facial Paralysis

This is the result of damage to the seventh nerve. It may be seen after spontaneous delivery, but the majority follow forceps extractions. The tips of the forceps press on the stylomastoid foramen where the nerve leaves the skull. In some cases the nerve is actually damaged. In others the edema causes loss of function. Occasionally facial palsy follows central nervous system injury. The facial muscles, including those of the eyelids, are paralyzed. The characteristic sign is the failure of one side of the mouth to move. Often spontaneous resolution takes place after the edema subsides. In some cases surgery to relieve pressure on the nerve helps. In others the paralysis is permanent with resultant weakness or atrophy of the facial muscles.

Sternomastoid Muscle

This muscle may be damaged during delivery. A hard, painless, nonfluctuant swelling appears in the lower part of the muscle. The underlying pathology is uncertain. Theories include hemorrhage, venous thrombosis, or an exudate from ruptured muscle fibers. Treatment includes local massage and passive stretching of the neck to the opposite side. Occasionally contracture of the muscle takes place resulting in torticollis (wry neck).

Bony Injuries

This group includes fractures of the clavicle, humerus, and femur. These are seen most often following difficult breech deliveries and shoulder dystocia.

CONGENITAL MALFORMATIONS

Of the many anomalies which may occur, only two of those which complicate labor and delivery will be described.

Anencephalus

This is the absence of the vault of the skull with complete or partial absence of the brain. What brain tissue there is is uncovered and unprotected.

The diagnosis is established by x-ray, but the condition may be suspected by the inability of the attendant to feel the head and by hyperactive movement of the fetus after rectal or vaginal examination. The examining finger abuts against the exposed lower brain tissue and stimulates the fetus to move vigorously. Anencephaly is the most common cause of polyhydramnios and should be suspected in all cases of unexplained excessive amniotic fluid.

Most anencephalics deliver without difficulty. Since the head is small it does not dilate the cervix well, and traction on the head with clamps may be necessary to pull the shoulders through. In general it is better to await the spontaneous onset of labor than to attempt induction through an unripe cervix. It is impossible for an anencephalic monster to survive.

Hydrocephalus

This is the accumulation of cerebrospinal fluid in the ventricles of the brain. The amount varies between 500 and 1,500 ml, but much larger amounts have been reported. The obstetric problem is one of gross disproportion between the head and the pelvis. Breech presentation occurs in about 30 percent of cases. In these cases labor proceeds normally in the early part, and it is often not until the aftercoming head cannot be extracted that the attendant suspects hydrocephaly.

Diagnosis is made by abdominal, vaginal, and radiologic examination. When the head is extremely large, one can recognize the abnormality by palpation, and the x-ray confirms the clinical impression. In borderline cases, however, it may be difficult to be certain of the diagnosis, and rash action must not be taken lest a normal child be damaged.

The danger of hydrocephaly to the mother is rupture of the uterus during the obstructed labor. Because of the disproportion the lower segment of the uterus becomes distended and thin, and rupture may take place spontaneously or as a result of obstetric manipulations. After labor is in progress, the cervix is dilated, and the diagnosis is that the baby is dead, the size of the head should be reduced by evacuating the fluid through a large bore needle. This will make the head smaller and delivery will ensue. In breech presentations, when the aftercoming head cannot be extracted, the obstetrician must resist the temptation to pull the head through by force since this will surely rupture the lower uterine segment. The fluid should be drained either by perforating the skull or by transecting the spinal canal in the thoracic region.

PERINATAL MORTALITY

Perinatal mortality has been defined as the number of infants dying before birth, during birth, or in the first 7 days of life and weighing more than 1,000 g at birth. Of the babies that die during the first month, 90 percent do so in the first week.

Death before or during delivery is caused, usually, by anoxia, preceded frequently by a period of hypoxia. In the first week of life most deaths are the result either of damage from intrauterine hypoxia, or of inefficient pulmonary ventilation after birth.

Anoxia

Anoxia is of four kinds:

1. Anoxic anoxia is the low uptake of oxygen as a result of insufficient supply from the mother. Included here are the following:
   a. Low oxygenation of maternal blood (anemia, intoxication)
   b. Reduction of blood flow through the placenta
   c. Insufficiency of the placenta (poorly developed and inadequate number of villi, placental degeneration, abruptio placentae, placenta previa)
   d. Umbilical cord problems (prolapse, entanglements)
2. Anemic anoxia signifies inefficient oxygen transport in the fetus, and includes:
   a. Fetal anemia (erythroblastosis, umbilical cord hemorrhage)
   b. Carbon monoxide poisoning
   c. Congenital malformations
3. Stagnant anoxia is the poor uptake of oxygen in the tissues and includes conditions such as postnatal shock.
4. Histotoxic anoxia is reduced oxygenation in the cells, as under the effect of narcotics and anesthetics.

Etiology

The main causes of perinatal mortality include:

1. Anoxia
2. Congenital malformations
3. Trauma during birth
4. Umbilical cord complications
5. Respiratory distress
6. Infection
7. Erythroblastosis
8. Prematurity is a contributory factor to all causes of perinatal death.

Fetal mortality is increased in the following groups:

1. Maternal
   a. Women over 40 years of age
   b. Primigravidas over 35
   c. Grand multiparas
   d. Women of low economic and social strata
2. Factors at birth:
   a. The larger the fetus, the greater the risk during birth.
   b. The smaller the infant, the higher the danger after delivery.
   c. The mortality is increased with abnormal presentations.
3. Fetal conditions include:
   a. Multiple pregnancy
   b. Male infants
   c. Premature babies
   d. The dysmature infant

Fetal Dysmaturity

This term refers to the syndrome where, presumably because of placental malfunction, either the infant's stage of development does not correspond to the period of gestation, or he shows the regressive changes and signs of intrauterine hypoxia.

The appearance of the child is characteristic:

1. The weight is low in relation to body length.
2. The limbs are long and lean.
3. The baby looks undernourished and has only a small amount of subcutaneous fat.
4. The vernix is scanty or absent and when present is yellow or green.
5. The hair is abundant.
6. The nails are long.
7. The skin hangs in folds. There is a tendency to desquamation, especially on the palms and soles. The skin dries after birth and becomes parchmentlike.
8. The skin, nails, umbilical cord, and amniotic fluid are stained with meconium.
9. In advanced cases the amniotic fluid becomes scanty and thick with meconium. There is a tendency to aspiration of this fluid with subsequent pulmonary complications.

BIBLIOGRAPHY

Ahvenainen, E. K. A study of the causes of perinatal death. Acta. Obstet. Gynec. Scand., 39:438, 1960.

Apgar, V. Evaluation of the newborn infant. J. A. M. A., 168:1985, 1958.

Chefetz, M. D. Etiology of cerebral palsy. Obstet Gynec., 25:635, 1965.

Churchill, J. A., Stevenson, L., and Habhab, G. Cephalhematoma and natal brain injury. Obstet. Gynec., 27:580, 1966.

Cook, C. D., Lucey, J. F., Drorbaugh, J. E. Segal, S., Sutherland, J. M., and Smith, C. A. Apnea and respiratory distress in the newborn infant. New Eng. J. Med., 254:562, 1956.

Ginsburg, S. J., and Gerstley, L. Fetal tachycardia in labor. Amer. J. Obstet. Gynec., 92:1132, 1965.

Gruenwald, P. Asphyxia, trauma, and shock at birth. Arch. Pediat., 67:103, 1950.

Kaern, T. Perinatal mortality. Acta. Obstet. Gynec. Scand., 39:392, 1960.

Lister, U. M., and Buchanan, M. F. G. Foetal distress and neonatal asphyxia. J. Obstet. Gynaec. Brit. Emp., 64:233, 1957.

O'Brien, J. R., Usher, R. H., and Maughan, G. B. Causes of birth asphyxia and trauma. Canad. Med. Ass. J., 94:1077, 1966.

Rubin, A. Birth injuries: Incidence, mechanisms, and end results. Obstet. Gynec., 23:218, 1964.

Todd, R. M. Birth injuries. The Practitioner, 197:297, 1966.

INDEX

Date Due

DE 15 70				